W0050558

Physical Modalities in Dermatologic Therapy

Physical Modalities
in Dermatologic Therapy

Radiotherapy, Electrosurgery,
Phototherapy, Cryosurgery

edited by
Herbert Goldschmidt

with 317 illustrations
including 16 color plates

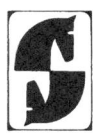

Springer-Verlag New York Heidelberg Berlin

Herbert Goldschmidt, M.D., F.A.C.P.
Clinical Professor of Dermatology
University of Pennsylvania Medical School
3400 Spruce Street
Philadelphia, Pennsylvania 19104

Library of Congress Cataloging in Publication Data

Main entry under title:

Physical modalities in dermatologic therapy.

   Includes bibliographical references and index.
   1. Skin—Diseases—Radiotherapy. 2. Phototherapy.
3. Skin—Surgery. 4. Electrosurgery. 5. Cryosurgery.
I. Goldschmidt, Herbert.
RL113.P45   616.5'06   78-2318
ISBN-13: 978-1-4612-6261-9

All rights reserved.

No part of this book may be translated or reproduced in any form
without written permission from Springer-Verlag.

Copyright © 1978 by Springer-Verlag New York Inc.

Softcover reprint of the hardcover 1st edition 1978

9 8 7 6 5 4 3 2 1

ISBN-13: 978-1-4612-6261-9   e-ISBN-13: 978-1-4612-6259-6

DOI: 10.1007/978-1-4612-6259-6

Preface

A number of vital therapeutic modalities are not covered adequately in current dermatology textbooks. This book is intended to fill that gap. It originated in a series of special lectures on modern applications of physical modalities given at recent annual meetings of the American Academy of Dermatology; the main topics were radiotherapy, electrosurgery, phototherapy, cryosurgery, and related therapeutic modalities.

The authors, recognized authorities in their field, have included much additional information which could not be covered in the original lectures because of time limitations. The indications for modern dermatological x-ray therapy reflect the basic views of the recently published guide lines of the National Academy of Sciences—National Research Council. Both text and illustrations are oriented toward the practical aspects of therapy with physical modalities. A special effort was made to bring the contributions up to date; pertinent references have been added for those who wish to pursue particular topics still further. Where there is an apparent overlap between chapters, it was felt to be advantageous because different authors approached their subject from different perspectives.

I am most grateful to the various authors who generously contributed despite their many other commitments. I wish, also, to thank the staff of Springer-Verlag for their advice and assistance in the preparation of the manuscript.

HERBERT GOLDSCHMIDT
Philadelphia, June 1977

Contents

Contributors

Bart, Robert S., M.D.
Associate Professor of Dermatology
New York University
566 First Avenue
New York, New York 10016

Crumay, Hugh M., M.D.
Associate in Dermatology
University of Pennsylvania School of Medicine
Address:
Crumay Parnes Associates Inc.
104 Erford Road
Camp Hill, Pennsylvania 17011

Daniels, Farrington, Jr., M.D.
Professor of Medicine and Head,
Dermatology Division
The New York Hospital
Cornell Medical Center
1300 York Avenue
New York, New York 10021

Davis, Lawrence W., M.D.
Professor of Radiation Therapy
and Nuclear Medicine
Thomas Jefferson University
925 Chestnut Street
Seventh Floor
Philadelphia, Pennsylvania 19107

Everett, Mark Allen, M.D.
Professor and Head, Dermatology
University of Oklahoma College of Medicine
Oklahoma City, Oklahoma 73190

Fromer, John L., M.D.
Assistant Clinical Dermatologist
Massachusetts General Hospital
Boston, Massachusetts
N. E. Deaconess Hospital
Boston, Massachusetts
Address:
66 Arnold Road
Wellesley Hills, Massachusetts 02181

Gladstein, Arthur H., M.D.
Professor of Clinical Dermatology
New York University
566 First Avenue
New York, New York 10016

Goldman, Leon, M.D.
Department of Dermatology
Director, Laser Laboratory
University of Cincinnati Medical Center
231 Bethesda Avenue
Cincinnati, Ohio 45267

Goldschmidt, Herbert, M.D., F.A.C.P.
Clinical Professor of Dermatology
University of Pennsylvania Medical School
3400 Spruce Street
Philadelphia, Pennsylvania 19104

Gorson, Robert O.
Professor of Medical Physics
Department of Radiology
Stein Research Center
Division of Medical Physics
Jefferson Medical College
of Thomas Jefferson University
Philadelphia, Pennsylvania 19107

Hauss, Helga, Dr. med.
Department of Dermatology
University of Kiel
West Germany
Address:
Moltkestrasse 37
2300 Kiel
West Germany

Hollander, Mark B., M.D.†
Formerly:
Instructor in Dermatology
Johns Hopkins University School of Medicine

Kopf, Alfred, W., M.D.
Professor of Dermatology
New York University
566 First Avenue
New York, New York 10016

Lassen, Margit, Ph.D.
Assistant Professor of Medical Physics
Department of Radiology
Stein Research Center
Thomas Jefferson University
Philadelphia, Pennsylvania, 19107

Lewis, Henry M., M.D.
Clinical Professor of Dermatology
University of Colorado Medical Center
Civilian Consultant in Dermatology
Fitzsimons Army Medical Center
Denver, Colorado 80206

Lukacs, Stefan, Prof. Dr. med.
Department of Dermatology
University of Munich
Frauenlobstrasse 9
8 Munich 15
West Germany

Malkinson, Frederick D., M.D., D.M.D.
Professor and Chairman
of Dermatology Department
Rush-Presbyterian-St. Luke's Medical Center
Chicago, Illinois 60612

Proppe, Albin, Prof. Dr. med.
Professor Emeritus of Dermatology
Department of Dermatology
University of Kiel
West Germany
Address:
Moltkestrasse 37
2300 Kiel
West Germany

Rudolph, Robert, M.D.
Instructor in Dermatology
University of Pennsylvania Medical School
Philadelphia, Pa.
Address:
400 N. Fifth Street
Reading, Pennsylvania 19601

Willis, Isaac, M.D.
Chief of Dermatology
Atlanta Veterans Administration Hospital
Associate Professor of Dermatology
Emory University School of Medicine
1670 Clairmont Road
Decatur, Georgia 30033

Zacarian, Setrag, A., M.D., F.A.C.P.
Associate Clinical Professor of Medicine
(Dermatology)
Albany Medical College of Union University
50 Maple Street
Springfield, Massachusetts 01103

Physical Modalities
in Dermatologic Therapy

1

Physical Aspects of Dermatologic Radiotherapy[4]

Robert O. Gorson and Margit Lassen

X-ray Phenomena

X rays are electromagnetic radiations of high energy. Figure 1-1 shows the relative position of x rays in the electromagnetic spectrum. γ rays also cover the same energy range as do x rays and are indistinguishable from them. γ rays originate from within the atomic nucleus whereas x rays are generated outside the nucleus. As do all other electromagnetic radiations, X and γ rays consist of oscillating electric and magnetic fields characterized by the following parameters.

Velocity	c (2.997925 $\times$ 10^8 m/sec)
Wavelength	λ
Frequency	ν
Period	T
Energy	E

The velocity of all electromagnetic radiation is the same in a vacuum, ie, approximately 3 $\times$ 10^8 m/sec. The wavelength (λ) is the distance between any two corresponding points on two adjacent waves, which is the same as the distance traveled during the time for one cycle. The time for one cycle is the period (T). The frequency (ν) is the number of cycles per second and is expressed in hertz (Hz), which is a special unit of frequency equal to one cycle per second. The period and frequency are inversely related, so that $T = 1/\nu$. By definition of velocity,

$$c = \lambda/T = \lambda\nu \qquad (1)$$

In addition to their wavelike characteristics, electromagnetic radiations exhibit particlelike qualities in their interactions (transfers of energy) with matter. Each x ray is characterized by a definite amount of energy which is directly proportional to its frequency and inversely proportional to its wavelength. These "packets" of energy are called *photons* or *quanta*. The relationship between the energy of a photon and its frequency is

$$E = h\nu \qquad (2)$$

where $h = 6.625 \times 10^{-34}$ joule-seconds (Planck's constant) and E is expressed in joules (J). By combining equations (1) and (2) the following relationship between photon energy and wavelength is obtained:

$$E = hc/\lambda \qquad (3)$$

The joule is a relatively large unit of energy for use in radiation physics. A more convenient unit is the *electron volt* (eV). An electron volt is the amount of energy that an electron acquires when it is accelerated through a difference of potential of one volt. Multiple units are 1000 eV (1 keV) and 1,000,000 eV (1 meV). One eV equals 1.6 $\times$ 10^{-19} J.

When values for the velocity of light and Planck's constant are substituted into equation (3) and when the wavelength is expressed in

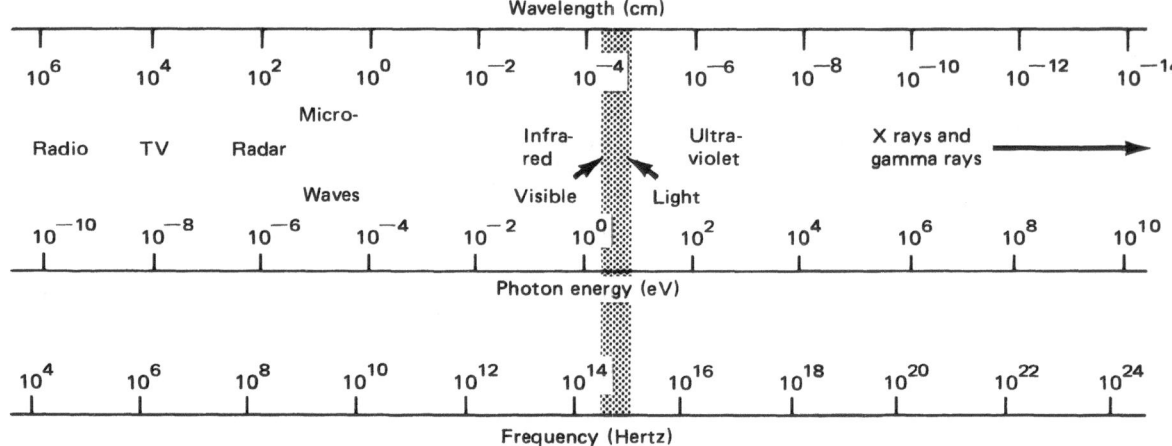

Figure 1-1. Diagram of the electromagnetic spectrum indicating the relative position of different parts of the spectrum in terms of wavelength, photon energy, and frequency.

angstroms (1 Å = 10^{-10} m) and the energy in keV, the following useful relationship can be derived:

$$E = 12.4/\lambda \qquad (4)$$

Table 1-1 lists various photon energies and their corresponding frequencies and wavelengths derived from equations (1) and (4).

Production of X Rays

X rays are produced by two processes involving the deceleration of high-energy electrons in matter. High-energy electrons are readily obtained by accelerating electrons boiled off a heated filament (thermionic emission) through a high electric potential in an evacuated tube (x-ray tube). Figure 1-2 diagrams the principal parts of an x-ray tube. By varying the electric potential between the filament (cathode) and the anode, the kinetic energy of the electrons striking the target in the anode may also be varied. Most of the electrons striking the target

Table 1-1 *Photon Energy, Wavelength, and Frequency*

Energy (keV)	Wavelength (Å)	Frequency (Hz × 10^{18})
0.5	24.8	0.12
1.0	12.4	0.24
6.2	2.0	1.5
12.4	1.0	3.0
24.8	0.5	6.0
49.6	0.25	12

lose their energy by "colliding" with orbital electrons of the atoms of the target material (usually tungsten). Many of the orbital electrons are knocked out of the atoms or into higher energy levels within the atoms. As the target atoms return to the ground state, electromagnetic photons are released. Some of the photons may have sufficient energy to be categorized within the x-ray region of the electromagnetic spectrum. Most of the photons have energies in the ultraviolet, visible light, or infrared regions. In any case, radiation produced by excited atoms returning to the ground state is called *characteristic* radiation because the energies of the released photons correspond to differences in the energy levels of the orbital electrons of the target atoms, and the energy differences depend upon the atomic number of the atoms comprising the target. Characteristic (or fluorescent) radiation consists of a line spectrum of energies corresponding to the energy differences of the electron levels in the excited and ground states.

X rays are also produced when high-energy electrons are decelerated by the nuclei of the target atoms. This radiation is called *bremsstrahlung* or braking radiation. Usually only part of the kinetic energy of a decelerating electron is converted into an x-ray photon; hence, most of the x rays generated have energies less than the kinetic energies of the striking electrons. On rare occasions, all of the energy of an electron is converted into an x ray. Thus, the maximum energy of x rays generated in an x-ray tube, when expressed in electron volts, is numerically equal to the accelerating voltage across the x-ray tube. Figure 1-3 illustrates two kinds of electron interaction. Figure 1-3a (collision loss) shows the ejection of a K electron followed by the emission of a K-characteristic x ray when the vacancy in the K shell is filled. Figure 1-3b (radiation loss) shows the emission of a bremsstrahlung x ray when the striking electron is deflected from its path by the atomic nucleus.

The intensity (I) of x rays of a given energy is the number of x rays with that energy (N) times the energy (E): $I \simeq N \times E$. It can be shown that the relative intensity of the bremsstrahlung of a given energy generated in a thick target is given by the following:

$$I = kZ(E_{max} - E) \qquad (5)$$

where I is the intensity of the photon with energy E, Z is the atomic number of the target atoms, k is a proportionality constant, and E_{max} is the maximum photon energy which may be produced, equal to the energy of the bombarding electrons. The relative intensities of x rays generated by 50- and 100-keV bombarding electrons are shown in Fig. 1-4 by dashed lines. The solid lines show the relative

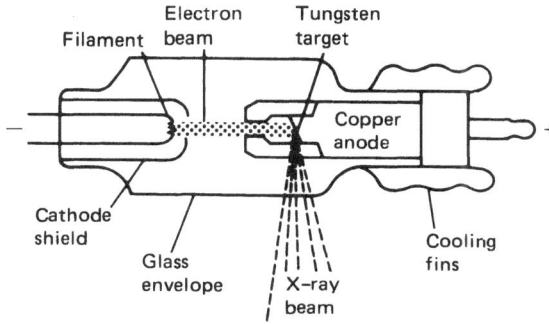

Figure 1-2. The principal parts of an x-ray therapy tube. Electrons emitted by the heated filament are accelerated to the copper anode where they strike the tungsten target from which the resultant x rays are emitted.

intensity distribution of the x rays transmitted through the x-ray tube. The difference between the two curves is the intensity of the x rays absorbed in the target material and the glass envelope of the x-ray tube. Note that all of the x rays below a certain energy level are absorbed within the x-ray tube. If more filtration is added to the x-ray tube, an even greater proportion of lower-energy photons will be removed and the peak of the curve will shift to higher energies and the effective energy of the

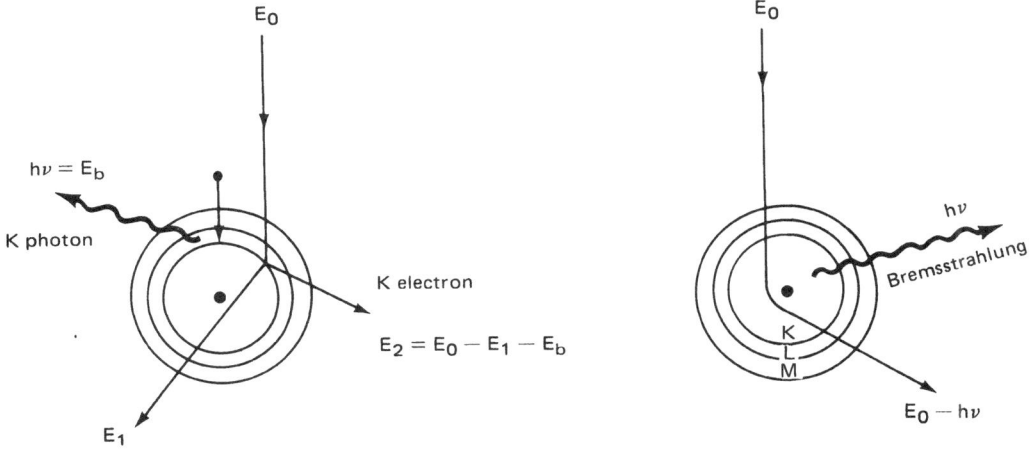

Figure 1-3. Electron interactions. *a*. Collision loss. The incident electron with energy E_0 collides with a K electron, knocking it out of the atom. This is followed by the emission of the K-characteristic x-ray photon when the vacancy in the K shell is filled by another electron. E_b is the binding energy of the K electron; *b*. Radiation loss. The incident electron loses energy as it is decelerated by the atomic nucleus, producing an x-ray photon (bremsstrahlung).

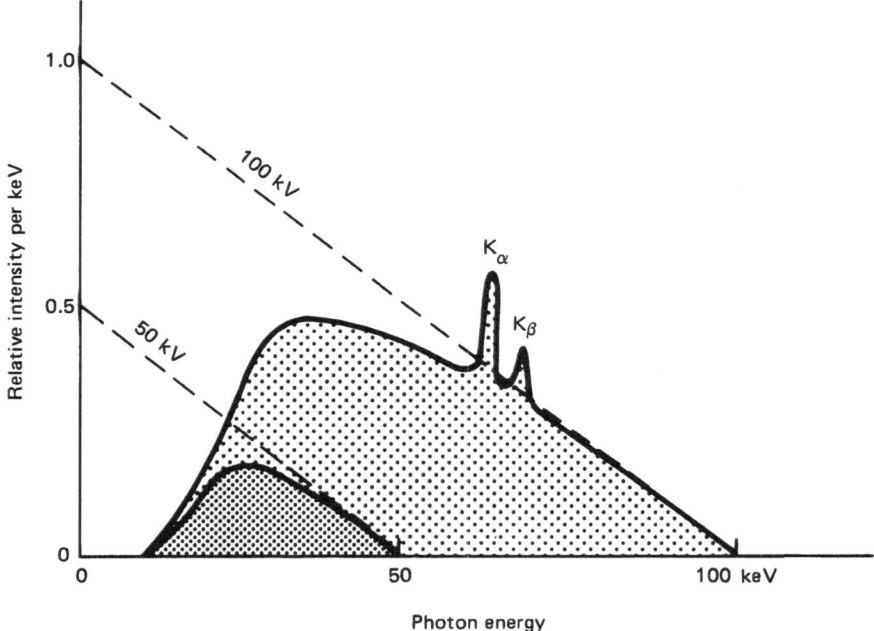

Figure 1-4.   Energy distribution of x rays generated by x-ray tubes operated at 50 and 100 kV. The dashed curves show the theoretical distribution of bremsstrahlung generated within a thick tungsten target. The solid curves show the energy distribution of the x rays that escape from the target and penetrate the x-ray tube. In both cases, the maximum energy of the x rays expressed in electron volts is numerically equal to the voltage across the x-ray tube. Also shown are the K_α- and K_β-characteristic x rays for tungsten which are produced by electrons having energies above approximately 69 keV.

transmitted x-ray beam will increase. Increasing the accelerating voltage of the x-ray tube, and hence the kinetic energy of the bombarding electrons, will produce a similar shift.

Superimposed upon the bremsstrahlung intensity spectrum is the line spectrum of the characteristic x rays. The characteristic x-ray spectrum constitutes a small fraction of the total x-ray intensity and can usually be disregarded. This is particularly the case for x-ray tubes operated at tube potentials below 69 kV since the binding energy of the tungsten K electrons is about 69 keV.

Since most of the electrons striking the target suffer collision losses with orbital electrons and only a small portion undergo bremsstrahlung-producing interactions with atomic nuclei, the efficiency of x-ray production is low. For x-ray tubes operating at potentials below 100 kV, less than 1% of the total energy of the electron beam striking the target appears in the emerging x-ray beam.

X-ray Absorption

In general, when an x-ray beam is directed at a human body, some x rays will be absorbed or scattered and some will pass through as though the body were not present. The probability that a given x-ray photon will be absorbed depends upon the energy of the photon, the atomic number of the constituent atoms of the body, and the density and thickness of the part of the body through which the photon passes. When x rays are used to treat superficial lesions, the energy spectrum of the x-ray beam is adjusted (by selecting an appropriate combination of x-ray tube voltage and filtration) so that most of the energy is absorbed within the tissue volume to be treated. The absorption process involves the interaction of photons with orbital electrons producing ionization and excitation of the affected atoms. There are two such processes which are of importance in the energy range of x rays used in superficial radiation therapy.

These are illustrated in Fig. 1-5. The first process, called the *photoelectric* effect, occurs whenever a photon transfers *all* of its energy to an orbital electron. The photon disappears and the electron is ejected from the atom with a kinetic energy equal to the photon energy less the binding energy of the electron. The second process, called the *Compton* effect, occurs whenever a photon interacting with an orbital electron transfers only part of its energy to the electron. The electron, called a *Compton electron,* leaves the atom with a kinetic energy equal to the transferred energy less the electron-binding energy. The remaining energy appears in the form of another photon of lower energy than that of the original (longer wavelength), emitted in a different direction. The Compton scattered photon will either pass out of the body or will interact with another atom in the body by either the Compton or photoelectric process. In any case, the energies of the photoelectric and Compton electrons are dissipated by subsequent interactions with other electrons (collision losses) producing fur-

ther ionization and excitation or, very infrequently, by bremsstrahlung production (radiation losses). Since it takes approximately 34 eV of energy (on the average) to produce an ion pair, the complete absorption of a 34-keV photon will result in the production of about 1000 ion pairs. Some of the ions recombine; some initiate chemical changes and the production of free radicals leading to further chemical reactions. The energy not used in chemical changes is degraded into heat. The increase in temperature, however, is negligible.

X-ray Quality

X-ray quality is a term loosely used to denote the relative penetrating characteristics of an x-ray beam. If the photons were monoenergetic, as, for example, γ rays emitted by certain radioisotopes, they would all have the same probability of being absorbed per unit thickness of an absorbing material, and each additional unit thickness of the same material would remove

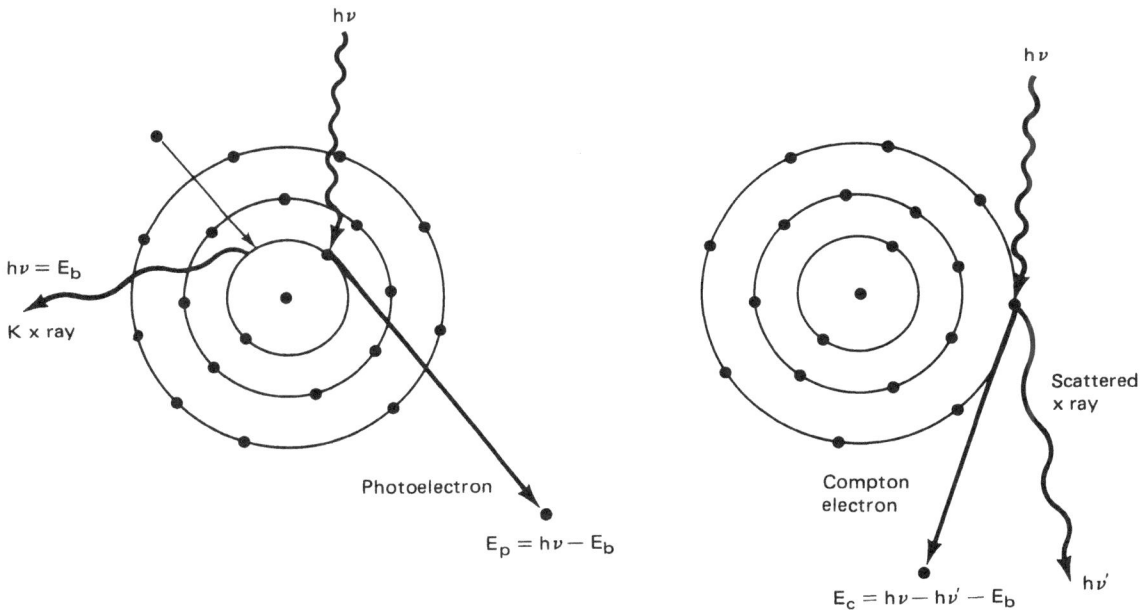

Figure 1-5. X ray interactions with electrons. Left: An x-ray photon transfers all of its energy to a K electron which is ejected from the atom with a kinetic energy equal to the photon energy less the electron-binding energy. A K x ray is emitted when the vacancy in the K shell is filled by another electron. Right: An x-ray photon interacts with one of the outer orbital electrons transferring only part of its energy to the electron. The remaining energy appears in the form of a scattered x-ray photon of longer wavelength.

the same fraction of the incident photons. Suppose 1 mm of aluminum absorbs $2/3$ and transmits $1/3$ of the incident monoenergetic photons comprising a narrow x- or γ-ray beam. Then, 2 mm of aluminum would transmit $1/3 \times 1/3$ or $1/9$ and 3 mm would transmit $(1/3)^3$ or $1/27$ of the incident photons. Hence, the transmission of monoenergetic photons decreases exponentially with increasing thickness of absorbing material and can be expressed as follows:

$$N = N_0 e^{-\mu t} \qquad (6)$$

where N is the number of photons remaining in the transmitted beam after passing through an absorbing material of thickness t, N_0 is the original number of photons in the incident beam (the number of photons removed from the beam by the photoelectric and Compton processes is $N_0 - N$), and μ is the probability

of absorption per unit thickness and is called the attenuation coefficient. The value of μ depends upon the energy of the photons and the atomic number of the absorbing material. Hence, one index of radiation quality is the value of the attenuation coefficient for a given material. Another index is the *half-value layer* (HVL), ie, the thickness of a given material which will attenuate a narrow beam of photons to 50% of its original intensity. Thus, $N/N_0 = 1/2$ when $t = T_{1/2}$ or 1 HVL. When these values are substituted into equation (6) and natural logarithms of both sides are taken, the following relationship is derived:

$$T_{1/2} = \ln 2/\mu = 0.693/\mu \qquad (7)$$

When attenuation data for a monoenergetic photon beam are plotted on semilog paper, the points fall along a straight line, as is expected

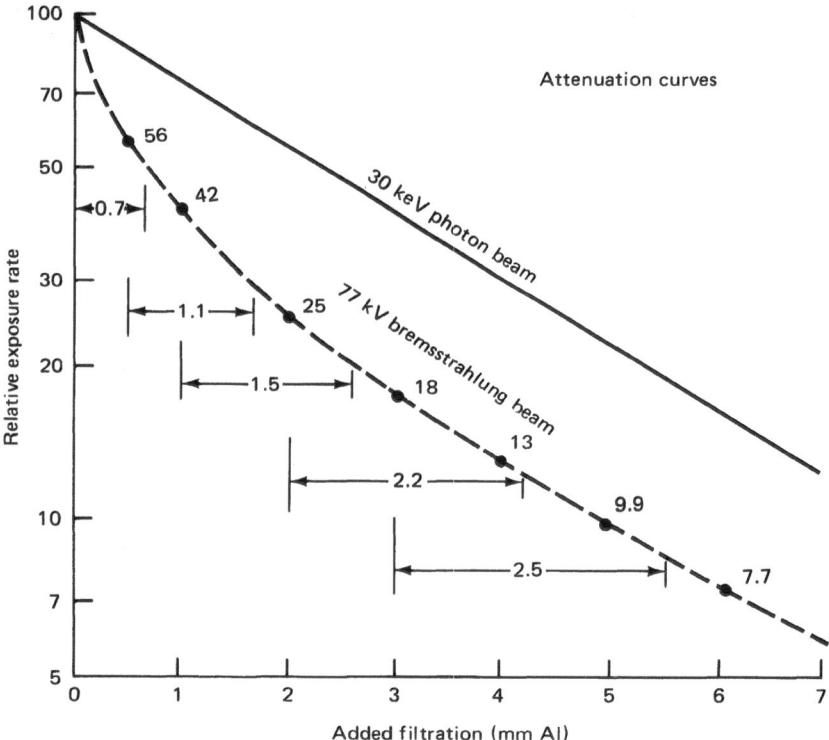

Figure 1-6.   X-ray attenuation curves. The upper curves illustrates the attenuation of a narrow 30-keV monoenergetic x- or γ-ray beam in aluminum. The curve is a straight line on semilog paper showing that the HVL and the energy of the beam remain constant with added filtration. The lower curve illustrates the attenuation of a 77-kV bremsstrahlung beam emitted by an x-ray tube. Since the beam contains a wide spectrum of energy, the attenuation curve is not a straight line and the average energy and the HVL, shown below the curve, increase with increased filtration.

for an exponential function. However, when attenuation data for a heterogeneous photon beam, such as the bremsstrahlung produced by an x-ray tube, are plotted on semilog paper, a curve is obtained which asymptotically approaches a straight line as the absorber thickness increases. Such a beam has a wide spectrum of energies, each of which with its own attentuation coefficient, so that the resulting attenuation curve is the sum of a large number of exponential curves. Figure 1-6 shows attenuation curves for two photon beams: a monoenergetic beam of γ rays and a heterogeneous beam of x rays. For the monoenergetic beam, all the HVLs are equivalent. For the bremsstrahlung beam, the slope of the curve decreases with absorber thickness and the half-value layers increase. For x-ray machines, it is customary to use the *first* HVL as an index of x-ray beam quality. Sometimes, the ratio of the first to the second HVL, called the *homogeneity factor,* is used to denote the degree of energy homogeneity. The homogeneity factor is equal to one for a monoenergetic beam. It is less than one for a bremsstrahlung beam, but it approaches unity as greater thicknesses of absorbing material (filters) are placed in the beam.

Other indices of radiation quality are the *equivalent energy, equivalent kilovoltage,* and *equivalent wavelength.* The equivalent energy of a heterogeneous beam of x rays is defined as the energy of a monoenergetic beam that would have the same HVL as the first HVL of the heterogeneous beam. The effective attenuation coefficient can be derived from the first HVL using equation (7), and the corresponding energy can be obtained from a table of attenuation coefficients. The equivalent kilovoltage is numerically equal to the equivalent energy in keV. The equivalent wavelength can then be calculated from equation (4). The effective energy, half-value layer, and effective attenuation coefficient of an x-ray beam are functions of the magnitude and waveshape of the x-ray tube potential and the total filtration of the x-ray beam. The x-ray tube potential in keV and the added equivalent filtration in mm of aluminum are sometimes specified together as an index of x-ray quality. The index most commonly used, however, is the half-value layer (or thickness) of aluminum (Al) (for x-ray machines operating below 120 kV) or copper (above 120 kV). The

HVL increases with increasing tube potential and increasing added filtration.

Dosimetry

In order to treat tumors with x rays, there must be some method for specifying not only the quality of the beam of radiation used, but also the quantity of radiation absorbed at various points in the tissue volume [2]. It is not practical to measure the amount of radiation absorbed directly. This must be calculated from measurements made on the x-ray beam in air prior to tissue penetration. These measurements are made during the calibration of the x-ray machine. One of the calibration parameters is the *exposure rate* measured under specified conditions of distance, x-ray tube potential, tube current, and collimation (x-ray beam size).

Exposure

One of the oldest concepts in radiation dosimetry was that of *radiation dose* or *dosage,* which later became *exposure dose* and now is called *exposure.* It refers to the amount of ionization produced in a small volume of air around a point of interest under certain defined conditions of measurement. Figure 1-7 illustrates the concept of exposure. As the x-ray beam passes through the incremental air volume surrounding the point of interest, a very small fraction of the photons interact with the air atoms within

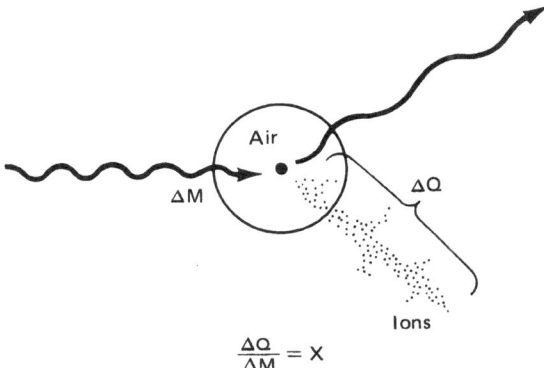

Figure 1-7. The concept of exposure. ΔM is an incremental mass of air surrounding the point of interest. ΔQ is the sum of the electric charges of all the ions, of either sign, produced by primary electrons released by the interaction of x rays within the air mass.

the volume releasing primary (photoelectric and Compton) electrons which produce additional ionization, releasing secondary electrons within and outside the incremental air volume. The total absolute charge produced is the charge of one electron multiplied by the sum of all of the primary electrons released within the air volume plus all of the secondary electrons. The total charge is divided by the mass of the incremental volume. The exposure is the limiting value of this ratio as the volume becomes infinitely small.

In 1971 the International Commission on Radiation Units and Measurements (ICRU) adopted the following formal definition [3]:

The *exposure, X,* is the quotient *dQ/* by *dm,* where *dQ* is the absolute value of the total charge of the ions of one sign produced in air when all of the electrons liberated by photons in a volume element of air having a mass *dm* are completely stopped in air:

$$X = dQ/dm \qquad (8)$$

In the International System (SI) of Units, the unit of exposure is the coulomb per kilogram. Historically, the special unit of exposure has been the roentgen (R).* The roentgen was originally defined as the exposure required to produce one electrostatic unit of charge (of either sign) per cubic centimeter of air at standard temperature and pessure (0°C, 760 mm Hg). The new equivalent definition in terms of SI units is:

$$1 \text{ R} = 2.58 \times 10^{-4} \text{ C/kg} \quad \text{(exactly)}$$

At present, exposure and exposure rate, which describe the ability of an x-ray beam to ionize air, are generally used for x-ray machine calibration purposes as the first step in determining the amount of radiation energy absorbed by the patient. This is done by taking ionization measurements in air at the position where the surface to be treated will be placed subsequently. One can, however, refer to the exposure at some locus within the patient. In such a case, the exposure value would be determined for a small quantity of air inserted at the point of interest in the patient.

It is not easy to measure exposure rates directly, even in free air. In practice, appropriately designed ionization chambers are used which have been compared directly or indirectly with standard ionization chambers at the National Bureau of Standards or with secondary chambers maintained by regional calibration centers approved by the American Association of Physicists in Medicine (AAPM). The chambers must be calibrated for the same quality of x rays as those which will be used for irradiation. The concept of exposure is limited only to ionization in air and only to x and γ-rays.

Absorbed Dose

An easier concept to understand than that of exposure and a more relevant one for biologic purposes is that of *absorbed dose.* This is simply the energy absorbed per unit mass at the point of interest. According to the 1971 formal definition of the ICRU [3],

"The absorbed dose, *D,* is the quotient of *dē* by *dm,* where *dē* is the mean energy imparted by ionizing radiation to the matter in a volume element and *dm* is the mass of the matter in that volume element."

$$D = d\bar{e}/dm \qquad (9)$$

In SI units, the unit for absorbed dose is the joule per kilogram. In 1974 the ICRU recommended and in 1975 the International Committee of Weights and Measures (CIPM) adopted the following new special unit [6]:

the gray, symbol Gy, equal to the joule per kilogram (J/kg). Historically, the special unit of absorbed dose has been the rad.* The rad was defined as the absorbed dose equal to 100 ergs of energy per gram of absorbing material, Since one joule equals 10^7 ergs, and one kilogram equals 10^3 grams,

one gray = 10^7 ergs/10^3 grams
= 10^4 ergs per gram = 100 rads.

The concept of absorbed dose is illustrated in Fig. 1-8. Note that the concept of absorbed dose is not restricted to x and γ rays, but also applies to all other ionizing radiations and to any absorbing medium.

In general, one cannot readily measure absorbed dose directly. However, in the case of x and γ rays, the absorbed dose at any point is proportional to the exposure at that point; if the exposure is known, the absorbed dose can

*1975, the ICRU recommended that the special units the roentgen, the rad, (and the curie) be gradually abandoned over a period of not less than 10 years and be replaced by the SI units the coulomb per kilogram (C/kg), the gray (Gy), (and the becquerel (Bq)), respectively. [6]

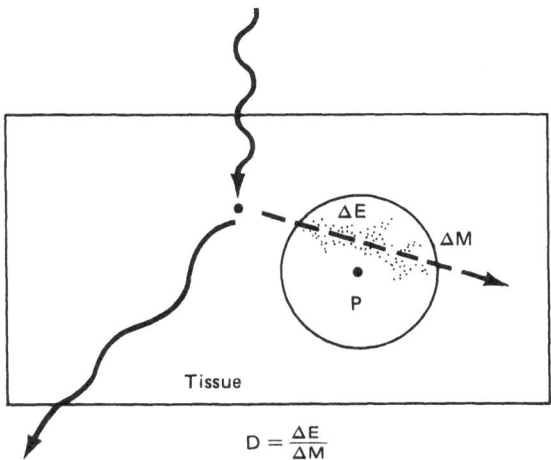

$$D = \frac{\Delta E}{\Delta M}$$

Figure 1-8. The concept of absorbed dose. ΔM is an incremental mass (of tissue) surrounding the point of interest, P. ΔE is the total energy dissipated by the primary (photo- or Compton) electron *within* the incremental mass. The absorbed dose at P is the ratio $\Delta E / \Delta M$ as ΔM surrounding P becomes vanishingly small [3].

be calculated taking into account the differences between the x-ray absorption coefficients of air and the absorbing medium. The first step is to determine the energy equivalence of a roentgen (R) in order to evaluate the absorbed dose in air.

The charge of an electron is equal to 1.6 $\times$ 10^{-19} coulombs. If we divide 2.54×10^{-4} coulombs/kg used in the definition of a roentgen by the electronic charge, we obtain 1.61×10^{15} electrons/kg. Each electron represents one ionization or the release of one ion pair (ie, electron and positive ion). Therefore, an exposure of 1 R produces 1.61×10^{12} ion pairs/g of air. The average amount of energy required to produce an ion pair is 33.7 eV (to convert to ergs, multiply by 1.6×10^{-12} ergs/eV). The result is that an exposure of 1 R produces an absorbed dose of 86.9 ergs/g in air or 0.869 rads. Thus,

$$D_{\text{air}} = 0.869 \, \frac{\text{rads}}{\text{roentgen}} \\ \times X \text{ roentgens} = 0.869 \, X \text{ rads} \quad (10)$$

If after measuring the exposure at some point of interest we wish to determine the absorbed dose in a tiny mass of some other medium at that point, we can do so by taking into account the difference in the mass energy absorption coefficients for the medium and for air.

$$D_{\text{med}} = \left(0.869 \frac{\mu_{\text{med}}}{\mu_{\text{air}}} \right) \times X = f \times X \quad (11)$$

The quantity in parentheses is of such importance in absorbed dose calculations that it is often referred to as the roentgens-to-rad conversion factor or f-factor. The value of the mass energy absorption coefficient (μ) depends upon the energy of the photon beam and the effective atomic number of the absorbing material. It is less than the attenuation coefficient used in equation (6) since it refers only to that part of the energy removed from the beam by the incremental mass which is also absorbed by the mass. The radiation scattered from the beam at the point of interest does not contribute to the absorbed dose at that point.

The f-factor has been calculated for a number of photon energies and HVLs for bone, muscle, and water (soft tissue). These are plotted in Fig. 1-9.

Depth Dose Calculations

Exposure measurements are not normally made in the patient since it is not practical to insert calibrated air ionization chambers at all points of interest. Instead, exposure measurements are made in "phantom patients" composed of tissue equivalent material, or in tanks of water, for a wide range of exposure conditions. Readings below the surface are usually normalized in terms of a percentage of the maximum readings that occur at the surface for x-ray energies used in dermatology. These depth dose data have been collected and published by others [1]. In order to apply this information to dose calculations in radiation therapy, we need to introduce the concepts of *backscatter factor, skin dose,* and *percentage depth dose.*

Backscatter Factor and Skin Dose

Figure 1-10 illustrates the steps necessary to determine the absorbed dose at some point P on the central axis of the x-ray beam located d cm below the skin surface (Fig. 1-10d). S represents the target–skin distance (TSD), ie, the distance from the target in the anode of the x-ray tube to the surface of the patient when in position for treatment. The first step (Fig. 1-10a) is to take ionization readings for a given

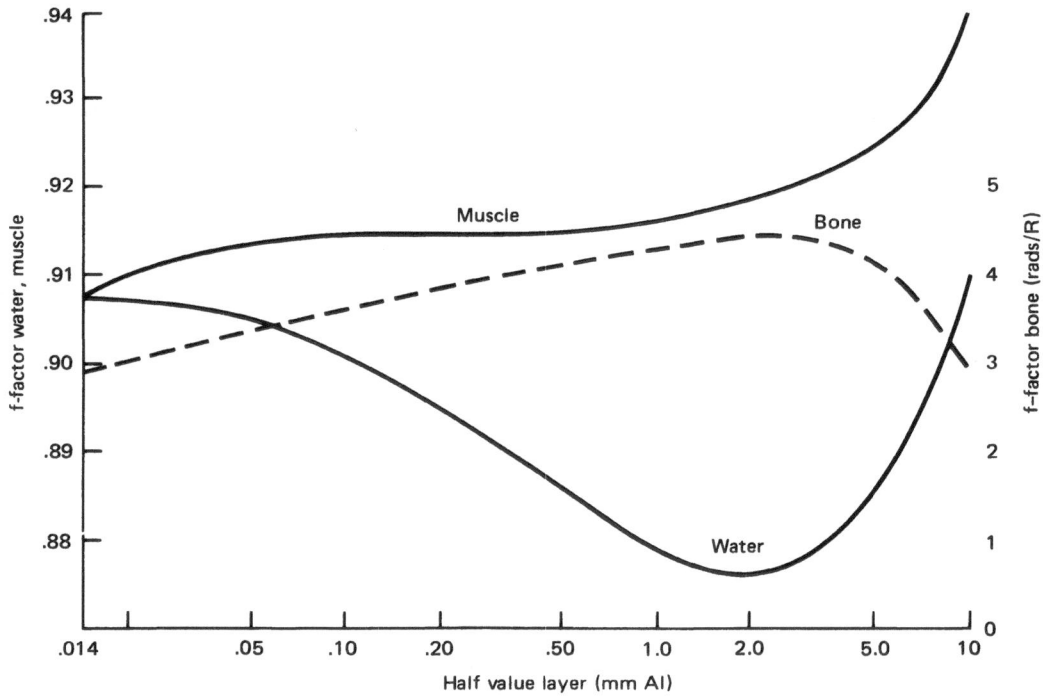

Figure 1-9.   The rads/roentgen *f*-factor is shown as a function of HVLs of aluminum for bone, muscle, and water (soft tissue).

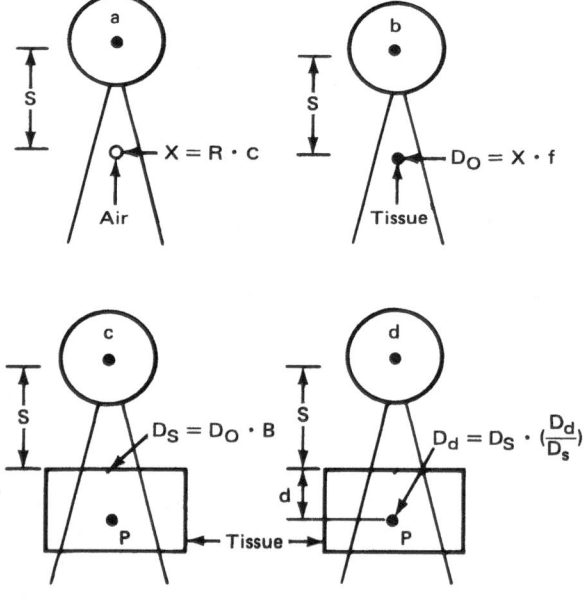

Figure 1-10.   a–d. The steps necessary to determine the absorbed dose at some point *P* on the central axis of the x-ray beam located *d* cm below the skin surface.

exposure time with a calibrated ionization chamber in air, with the TSD, added filtration, kVp, mA, and collimation values that will be used for treatment. The exposure *X*, in roentgens, is obtained by multiplying the average reading *R* by the calibration factor *C,* and making any necessary corrections for air temperature and pressure. These data are obtained at the time the x-ray machine is calibrated and are part of the calibration report. Figure 1-10b shows an imaginary tiny spherical mass of tissue (radius equal to the maximum range of the photoelectric and Compton electrons) located at the position of the ionization chamber. The absorbed dose, D_o, of this incremental mass of tissue suspended in air is $f \times X$ rads, according to equation (11). Figure 1-10c shows the same mass element as part of the skin at the surface of the area to be treated. The absorbed dose, D_s, at the skin *(skin dose)* will be greater than D_o because of the additional contribution from x rays scattered back from tissue below the skin. This scattered radiation is often called *backscatter,* and the ratio D_s/D_o is called the *backscatter factor, B.*

The magnitude of the backscatter depends upon the radiation quality (HVL) and the area and geometric shape of the x-ray beam at the skin. Backscatter factors have been measured for a wide range of HVLs and areas and some of the data of interest for superficial radiation therapy are plotted in Fig. 1-11. Note that the backscatter factor increases with x-ray beam size and increases with HVL over the range shown. It reaches a maximum at about an HVL of 10 mm of aluminum, much beyond the range of interest in dermatology.

Percentage Depth Dose

In Fig. 1-10d, the absorbed dose at P is D_d. The ratio D_d/D_s is known as the *fractional depth dose*. When multiplied by 100, the ratio is called the *percentage depth dose*. The percentage depth dose is a complicated function of the depth d, the HVL, the area A, the shape of the field, and the TSD. Depth dose data have been obtained in water phantoms over a wide range of these parameters. Some data are plotted in Fig. 1-12 for a 30-cm TSD and a 4.4-cm diame-

ter beam size over the HVL range of interest in dermatologic radiation therapy.

The following example will further illustrate the calculation of absorbed dose at a given depth below the skin. Suppose we wish to treat a superficial lesion so that the base of the tumor 5 mm below the skin surface receives 200 rads per treatment and we need to determine the treatment time. We decide to operate the beryllium-window x-ray tube at 29 kV, 25 mA, with a 0.3 mm Al filter and a 30-cm TSD, 4-cm diameter cone. Under these conditions, according to the calibration of the machine, the exposure rate is 115 R/min and the HVL is 0.17 mm Al. According to Fig. 1-9, the roentgen-to-rad conversion factor f is about 0.88 for water (soft tissue) at this HVL. The backscatter factor B is about 1.05 for an x-ray beam size of 12.6 cm², as obtained by interpolation in Fig. 1-11. Hence the absorbed dose rate at the skin is:

$$D_s = 115 \text{ R/min} \times 0.88 \text{ rads/R}$$
$$\times 1.05 = 106.3 \text{ rads/min}$$

By interpolation of the depth dose data in Fig. 1-12, we find that the percentage depth dose at

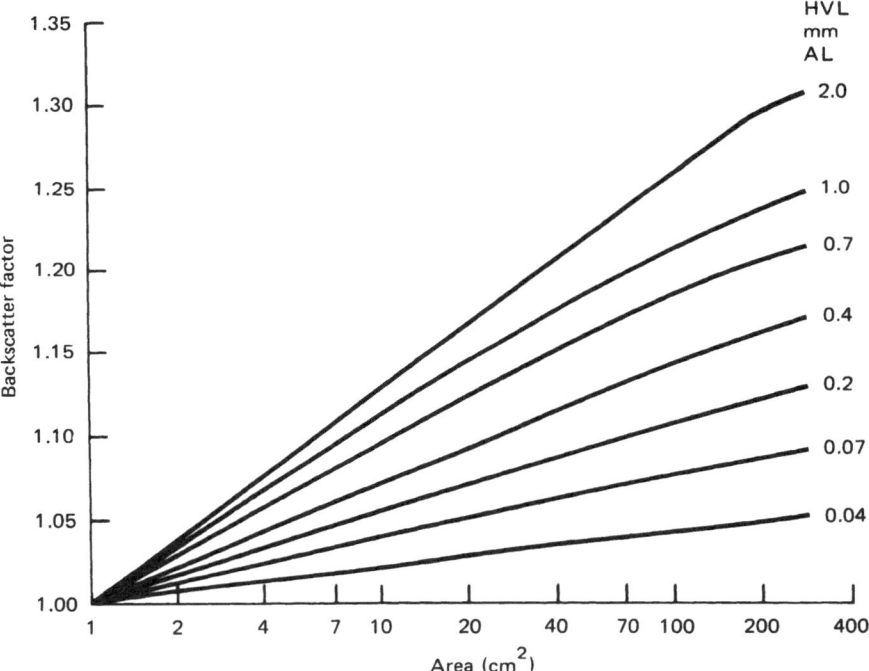

Figure 1-11. The backscatter factor plotted as a function of circular area of x-ray beams for different HVLs of aluminum.

5 mm is approximately 37% for a 4.4-cm diameter field, 30-cm TSD, and a 0.17-mm HVL of aluminum. Therefore, the absorbed dose rate at the base of the lesion is:

$$D_p = 106.3 \text{ rads/min} \times 0.37 = 39.3 \text{ rads/min}$$

The treatment time (*T*) to deliver 200 rads is:

$$T = \frac{200 \text{ rads}}{39.3 \text{ rads/min}}$$
$$= 5.09 \text{ min} = 5 \text{ min} + 5 \text{ sec}$$

Factors Affecting Percentage Depth Dose

Three factors are involved in determining the percentage depth dose at some reference point below the skin on the central axis. These are (1) the geometric divergence of the x-ray beam, (2) the attenuation of the primary beam by the tissue between the surface and the point of reference, and (3) the contribution of radiation scattered from the surrounding tissue to the point of reference. The geometric diver-

gence of the x-ray beam is described by the inverse square law. If there were no tissue attenuation of the primary beam and if there were no scattered radiation, the dose at depth *d* in Fig. 1-10 would be related to the dose at the surface as follows:

$$D_d = D_s \times \left(\frac{S}{S + d}\right)^2$$

For example, if the TSD were 30 cm, the percentage depth dose at a depth of 4 cm due to divergence alone would be the following:

$$\frac{D_d}{D_s} \times 100 = \left(\frac{30}{30 + 4}\right)^2 \times 100 = 78\%$$

Hence, the divergence of the beam from a distance of 30 to 34 cm decreases the x-ray intensity, exposure rate, and absorbed dose rate by 22%. At a distance of 60 cm, the beam intensity would drop to $(30/60)^2$, or 25%. The effect of beam divergence on percentage depth dose is illustrated by curve 1 in Fig. 1-13, which is a plot of the inverse square factor for a TSD of 30 cm. Curve 2 in Fig. 1-13 is a plot of the depth

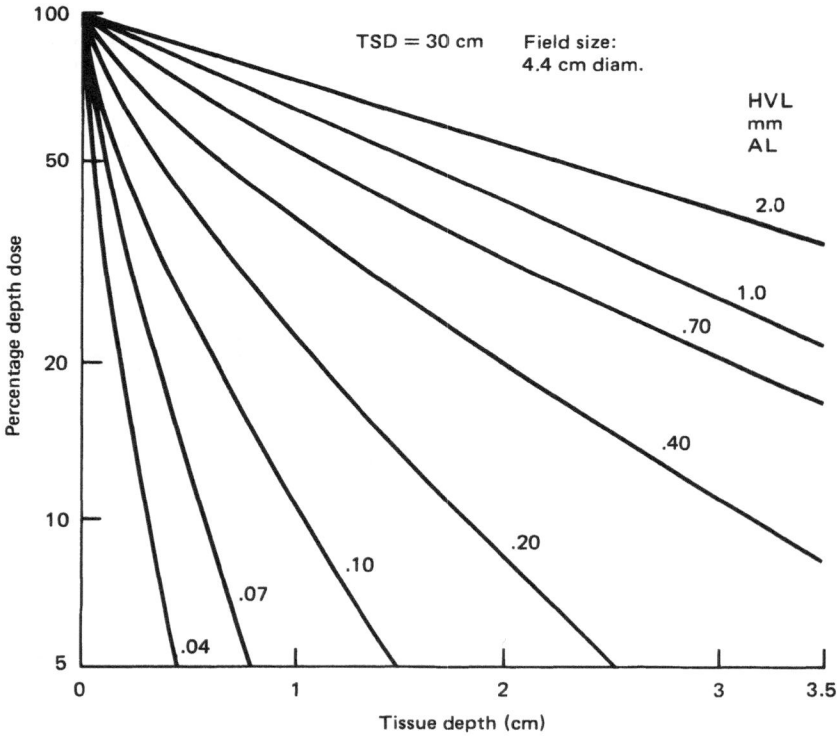

Figure 1-12. Percentage depth dose plotted for various HVLs as a function of tissue depth.

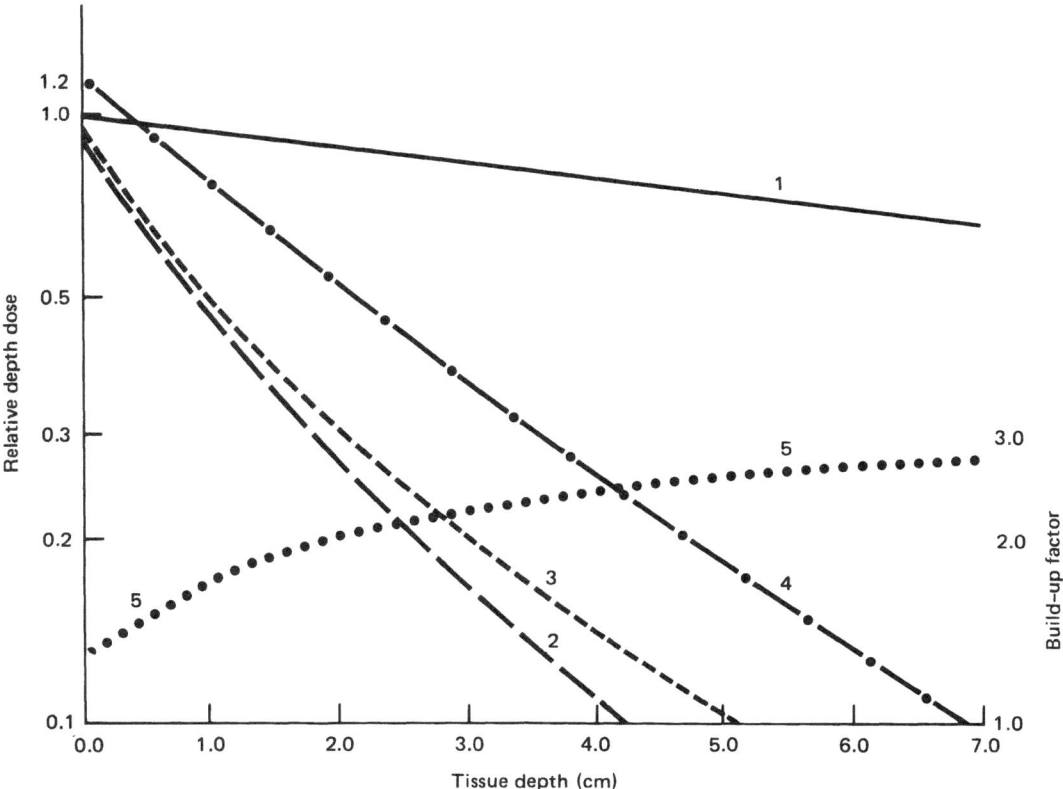

Figure 1-13. The component parts of a depth dose curve. Curve 4 is a depth dose curve for a 1-mm Al HVL x-ray beam, with a 30-cm TSD and a circular area of 100 cm². Curve 1 is the component part due only to the inverse square factor. Curve 2 is a plot of depth dose data for the same x-ray beam as in Curve 4, except that the cross-sectional area has been reduced to essentially zero, thus eliminating scattered radiation. Curve 3 is Curve 2 divided by Curve 1, eliminating the inverse square factor. Hence, it is a plot of the tissue attenuation of the x-ray beam. Curve 5 is the result of dividing Curve 4 by Curves 1 and 3 to eliminate both the tissue attenuation and inverse square factors, leaving only the build-up factor due to scattered radiation.

dose data for a narrow beam of x rays with essentially zero cross-sectional area, 1-mm HVL of aluminum, and 30-cm TSD. Since the beam is so narrow, there is virtually no contribution from scattered radiation at the surface (backscatter) or below the surface (build-up factor). Hence, curve 2 is the result of attenuation of the primary beam by tissue and the inverse square law divergence. If the ordinate values of curve 2 are divided by the corresponding ordinate values of curve 1, the beam divergence is factored out, producing curve 3. Curve 3 shows the contribution of tissue attenuation of the x-ray beam on the depth dose curve, $e^{-\mu d}$, where μ is the effective attenuation coefficient for a 1-mm HVL beam in tissue. Curve 4 is a plot of the depth dose data for

a circular beam of 100-cm² area, with the same HVL and TSD as above. This curve has been normalized to 100% of the skin dose for zero area. Hence, the skin dose for 100-cm² area is 1.2 times the zero-area skin dose because of the backscatter factor. Curve 4 includes the effects of tissue attenuation, inverse square divergence, and scattered radiation (build-up factor). If curve 4 is divided by curves 3 and 1 to factor out tissue attenuation and inverse square factors, only the build-up factor due to scattered radiation is left. The result is plotted in curve 5. The build-up factor increases rapidly with depth, so that at 5 cm the scattered radiation contributes considerably more to the dose than does the energy absorbed from the primary beam.

Isodose Distributions

The central axis depth dose tables or graphs are of limited value for describing the absorbed dose distribution throughout the treatment volume. The dose drops off rapidly toward the edge of the x-ray field. To take this effect into account, one must either treat an area considerably larger than the tumor or refer to two-dimensional depth dose distributions usually presented graphically as families of isodose curves. An isodose curve is the locus of points along which the percentage depth dose is constant. A set of isodose curves for a particular combination of HVL, TSD, and beam size is shown in Fig. 1-14. Isodose curves usually are drawn full scale on transparent sheets, which can be overlayed on an outline of the area to be treated in order to select an x-ray field size which will adequately treat the entire tumor volume. While the central axis depth dose data measured in a tissue equivalent phantom for one x-ray therapy machine is reasonably reliable for use with other x-ray machines operated under the same conditions of HVL, TSD, and x-ray beam size, isodose curves should be gen-erated with the same type of machine as the one to be used.

Half-Value Depth and Fall-Off Ratio

The half-value depth, or $D_{1/2}$, is the tissue depth at which the dose drops to 50% of the surface dose. In like manner, $D_{9/10}$ is the tissue depth at which the dose falls to 10% of the surface dose. The fall-off ratio for a given set of treatment parameters is defined as $D_{9/10}$ divided by $D_{1/2}$. The fall-off ratio is a clinical index of the rate the dose decreases with increasing tissue depth. The $D_{1/2}$ and fall-off ratio depend, of course, on all of the parameters that determine percentage depth dose. Figure 1-15 shows how the $D_{1/2}$ varies with HVL for various field sizes at a TSD of 30 cm. Additional data for a wide range of parameters have been published by Tuddenham [5].

Summary

In radiotherapy, one major objective is to maximize the amount of absorbed dose in the region occupied by the lesion and to minimize the dose to other adjacent tissues. In deep therapy, where the lesion to be treated is some distance below the surface, multiple fields intersecting at some internal point are often used or sometimes the primary beam (or patient) is rotated, with the axis of rotation in the vicinity of the tumor. In superficial therapy, however, the tumor volume is at or near the surface and it generally is not advisable to treat with more than one field. The problem then is to select the treatment parameters (kV potential, added filtration, TSD, and field size) so as to deliver an adequate dose to the base and edges of the lesion while sparing the underlying structures as much as possible. If isodose curves are available, one can readily visualize the expected dose distribution for the given treatment conditions and select the combination of parameters that provides a reasonable compromise. When isodose curves are not available, as is often the case, one must consult central axis percentage depth dose tables or $D_{1/2}$ tables or graphs to estimate the percentage dose reaching the base of the tumor and underlying tissues. One must also keep in mind that the dose rate falls off sharply near the edge of the field. This must be taken into consideration when choosing the size of the primary beam to adequately treat the entire tumor volume.

Table 1-2 summarizes qualitatively the effects of varying the physical parameters used in radiologic treatment of superficial lesions.

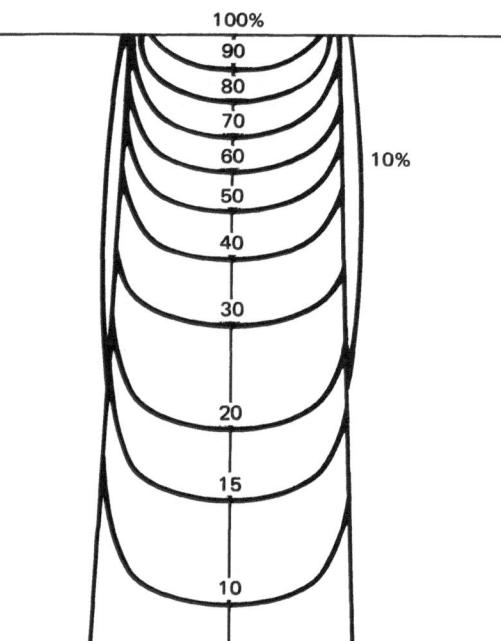

Figure 1-14.   A set of isodose curves indicating dose distribution normalized to 100% of the skin for a given HVL, TSD, and beam size.

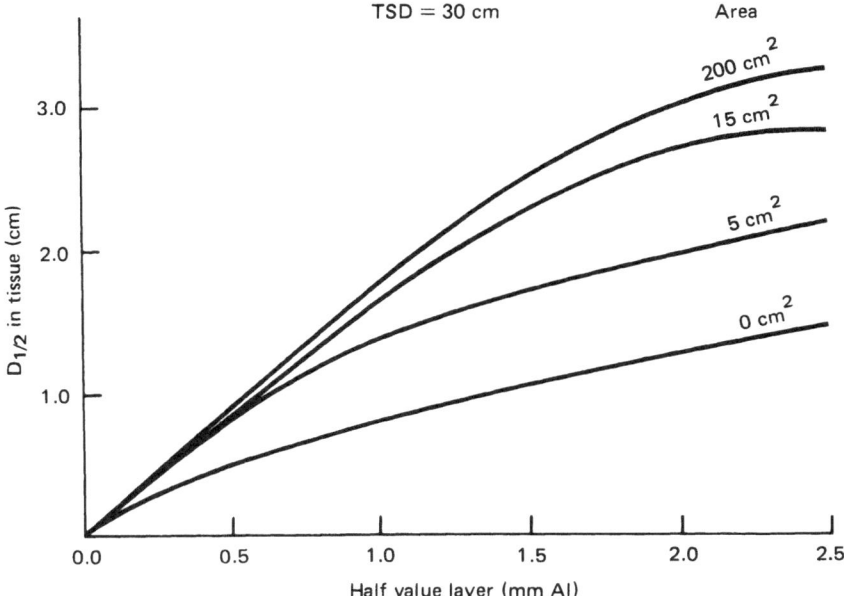

Figure 1-15. $D_{1/2}$ in tissue as a function of HVL and beam size.

Table 1-2 *Qualitative Effect of Increasing Physical Parameters Used in Dermatologic X-ray Therapy*

	Physical Parameters					
Related Parameters	X-RAY TUBE POTENTIAL *(kV)*	X-RAY TUBE CURRENT *(mA)*	ADDED FILTER *(mm Al)*	TARGET-TO-SKIN-DISTANCE *(TSD)*	COLLIMATOR OR CONE SIZE	EXPOSURE TIME *(T)*
Exposure rate (R/min) in air*	↑	↑	↓	↓	—	—
Absorbed dose rate (rads/ min) at the skin†	↑	↑	↓	↓	↑	—
Total skin dose (rads)‡	↑	↑	↓	↓	↑	↑
Effective energy (half-value layer) of the x-ray beam§	↑	—	↑	—	—	—
Maximum photon energy ‖	↑	—	—	—	—	—
Minimum photon wavelength ‖	↓	—	—	—	—	—
Backscatter factor#	↑	—	↑	—	↑	—
Percentage depth dose**	↑	—	↑	↑	↑	—
$D_{1/2}$ value**	↑	—	↑	↑	↑	—
Surface area in the primary beam††	—	—	—	↑	↑	—

↑, increases; ↓, decreases; —, no change.

*The exposure rate increases with increased production of x rays. The number of x rays produced per second depends upon the number of electrons striking the target per second (ie, the tube current). X-ray production also depends upon the energy of the electrons striking the target. The electron energy increases with tube potential (kV). Exposure rate decreases with added filter which absorbs the weaker x rays. Exposure rate also decreases with increasing target-to-skin distance (TSD) because of the inverse square divergence.

†The absorbed dose rate is directly proportional to the exposure rate. At the skin surface, it also increases with the beam size because of increased scatter.

‡The total skin dose depends upon the absorbed dose rate and the exposure time.

§As the tube potential (kV) is increased, the energy of the electrons striking the tube target increases, thus increasing the average energy of the emitted x rays. Increasing the aluminum filtration selectively absorbs the lower energy (weaker) x rays, thus effectively increasing the energy of the transmitted x-ray beam.

‖ The maximum photon energy and minimum photon wavelength depend only upon the energy of the striking electrons, and hence only upon the tube potential.

#The backscatter factor increases with photon energy and reaches a maximum at about an HVL of 10 mm Al (0.6 mm Cu), depending upon field size. Hence, the backscatter radiation increases with tube potential and with added filtration for the ranges of interest in dermatologic radiation therapy. The backscatter factor also increases with field size.

**The percentage depth dose and $D_{1/2}$ value increase with photon energy (hence, with tube potential and added filtration) because of the greater penetrating ability of higher-energy x rays. They also increase with target-to-skin distance (TSD) because of the reduced effectiveness of the inverse square law factor at increasing distances.

††The surface area in the primary beam increases, of course, with field size or cone size and increases with target-to-skin distance (TSD) because of the inverse square divergence of the beam.

References

1. British Institute of Radiology: Central axis depth dose data for use in radiotherapy. Radiol (Suppl) 11, 1972
2. International Commission on Radiation Units and Measurements: ICRU Report No. 17. Radiation Dosimetry: X Rays Generated at Potentials of 5 to 150 kV. Washington, DC, 1970
3. International Commission on Radiation Units and Measurements: ICRU Report No. 19. Radiation Quantities and Units. Washington, DC, 1971
4. Johns HE, Cunningham JR: The Physics of Radiology, 3rd ed. Springfield, Ill, Thomas, 1969
5. Tuddenham WJ: Half-value depth and fall-off ratio as functions of portal area, target-skin-distance and half-value layer. Radiology 69:79, 1957
6. Wyckoff HO (chairman): Statement by the ICRU. Medical Phys 3:52, 1976

2

Radiobiology

Lawrence W. Davis

In this chapter we will review some of the information available concerning the response of cells to radiation and how this information helps to explain the response of normal tissues and tumors to radiation.

Interaction of Radiation with Matter

Radiation damage results from the deposition of energy in matter, and the unit of radiation dose, the rad, is a measure of the amount of energy deposited. With respect to the biologic effects produced, the amount of energy deposited by radiation is relatively small. A small portion of the energy may be transformed into heat, but the greater portion interacts with atoms and molecules along the path of the photon (x or γ ray) or charged particle (proton or electron). Photons may interact directly with molecules by increasing the energy level of the orbiting electrons (excitation) or by displacing an orbital electron (ionization). In a common interaction of photons with atoms (Compton effect), a portion of the photon energy is used to displace an outer electron. In addition to the displaced electron, this results in a scatter photon with slightly less energy than that of the original photon. The scattered photon may then interact with other atoms until all of its energy is dissipated. Photons may also deposit energy by displacing the inner, bound electrons of atoms. These interactions occur along the paths

of the photons and displaced electrons and result in "tracks" of ionization. The frequency of these ionizations along the track is related to the type and energy of the radiation. Some heavy, charged particles, such as α particles, cause a great many ionizations over a very short track, while lighter particles, such as electrons, cause relatively few ionizations over a very long path.

LET and RBE

Linear energy transfer (LET) is a measure of the energy transferred along the track and is measured in keV/micron of path length. LET is related to the mass, charge, and energy of the ionizing particle. Very densely ionizing particles have a high LET while sparsely ionizing radiations have a low LET. If ionizations occur infrequently, the probability of biologic damage occurring is low since it is unlikely that a critical area of the cell will be the site of the ionization; however, if the ionization is very dense along the track, the cells in the track will be damaged, but a great number of the ionizations will not have an effect. The LET for electrons resulting from x rays used in radiotherapy ranges from 0.25 to 3, for neutrons from 3 to 80, and for α particles from 95 to 260 [3,12,15].

The rad is a measure of energy deposited in matter; however, 1 rad from 100 kilovolt potential (kVp) x rays will have a different pattern of ionization than will 1 rad from a neutron or α particle, even though each had deposited 100 ergs/g. Likewise, the biologic effects of these radiations will be different even though 1 rad of each had been delivered. The radiobiologic equivalent (RBE) is a comparison of the dose of one radiation producing a given biologic effect with the dose of a standard radiation necessary to produce the same biologic effect. The standard radiation is usually 250 kVp x rays. A given radiation may have several RBEs depending on the biologic effect being measured, ie, the RBE of neutrons for tumor control may be different than that for skin necrosis or damage to the small intestine.

Interaction of Radiation with Water

Since cells are largely composed of water, the transfer of energy from ionizing radiation to water is important. In some body fluids where the concentration of solute is low, almost all of the energy from radiation is transferred to water. Although many of these reactions are incompletely and imperfectly understood, a number of complex reactions have been identified. Three highly reactive species with extremely short lifetimes (1 to 100 μsec) seem to result from most of these reactions [3]. These are the hydrated electron, the hydrogen radical, and the hydroxyl radical. The hydrated electron and the hydrogen radical act as the primary reducing species in the reactions with water. The hydrogen radical sometimes acts as an oxidizing species, although the major oxidizing species is the hydroxyl radical. These products may then react with the solutes present. The radicals may abstract hydrogen from C— H and —OH bonds, may dissociate organically bound functional groups, or may add to unsaturation centers in the solute.

Site of Radiation Damage

The processes of energy deposition described thus far do not directly result in the death of cells; however, this energy may be transferred to vital cell areas resulting in injury and cell death. This is an "indirect" action of radiation. On the other hand, the ionizing event may occur close to a vital part of the cell resulting in damage and death of the cell—a "direct" action. While such damage may occur to the cell

membrane or the lysosomes resulting in immediate cell lysis, there is evidence to support the view that the most sensitive area for radiation damage within the cell is the DNA [13]. In viruses with single-stranded DNA, there is evidence that radiation damage to the DNA is 100% effective in causing cell death; but in viruses with double-stranded DNA, radiation damage to a single strand is relatively ineffective in inactivating viruses [20,21]. Freifelder [9] has presented evidence that double-strand breaks are necessary for cell inactivation. However, double-strand breaks account for only a portion of lethal events; the remaining number are ascribed to base damage.

Some ionizing events may result in immediate cell lysis, but damage to DNA more often causes reproductive death, ie, cells undergo normal metabolic functions but are unable to undergo cell division. It has also been shown that some cells undergoing reproductive death may undergo division one or more times before cell death occurs; however, the majority of cells damaged by radiation are unable to undergo any cell divisions. As a result of this reproductive death, the effect of a radiation dose is delayed. The length of this delay varies with the irradiated cells and is related to such factors as the phase of the cell cycle at the time of irradiation, the proportion of resting cells in an irradiated population, and the intermitotic time.

Cell Survival Curves

The early work on mammalian cell radiosensitivity was done by Puck and Marcus [17] and followed the development of their technique for culturing mammalian cells. In their experiments, HeLa cells, derived from a human uterine carcinoma, were used. In this technique, a known number of cells are plated onto a suitable medium, and the number of colonies formed are counted to determine the plating efficiency of the method. A known number of cells are then plated and irradiated. The number of colonies resulting are counted to determine the proportion of cells surviving that dose of radiation. This process is repeated with different radiation doses. When the proportion of surviving cells is plotted against the radiation dose, a curve similar to that in Fig. 2-1 is obtained. This curve is similar to that observed

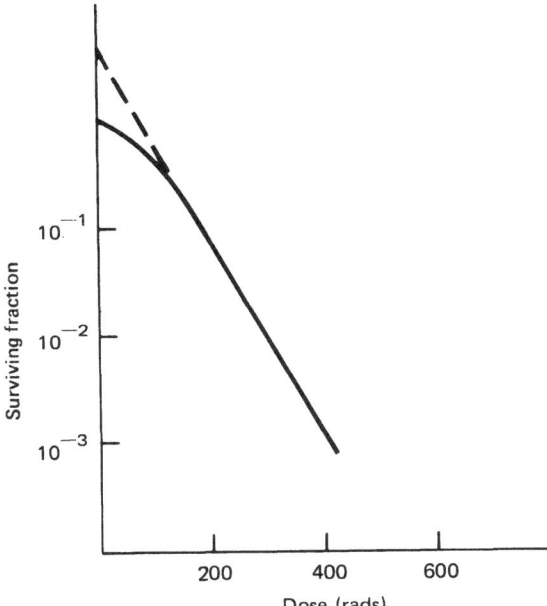

Figure 2-1. Typical cell survival curve for x-irradiated cells.

in many biologic experiments and similar to that for the decay of radioactive materials or the attenuation of a radiation beam by an absorber. When these data are plotted with the log of the survivors on the vertical axis and the radiation dose on the horizontal axis, a straight line results. The exponential portion of the curve is described by the following formula [12]:

$$N = N_o e^{-D/D_o}$$

where N are the survivors remaining after a dose D
N_o is the original number of cells
e is the base of the natural logarithm
D_o is the mean lethal dose

If D is set equal to D_o, the expression becomes:

$$N = 0.37\,N_o$$

Thus, D_o, or the mean lethal dose, is the dose required to reduce the population to 37% of its initial value, ie, the dose which kills 63% of the cells.

The section of these curves of clinical interest is that part with very few survivors, since cure of tumors is dependent on that part of the curve. Unfortunately, this is the most difficult portion of the curve to determine.

Hewitt [11] has fit data to the curve for murine leukemia cells for a surviving fraction of approximately 10^{-7}, and Dewey [5] has fit data on bacteria for a surviving fraction of 10^{-9}.

An example of the effect of the exponential portion of the curve is shown in Table 2-1. In this example, a dose of 300 rads will kill 90% of the irradiated cells. Since the 300 rads kills a constant fraction of the irradiated cells, the absolute number of cells killed is related to the number irradiated. On the basis of the exponential portion of these curves, the following points can be made concerning the response of cells to radiation:

1. A specified dose of radiation kills a constant fraction of irradiated cells.
2. The fraction of cells killed is independent of the number of cells irradiated.
3. The absolute number of cells killed varies with the number of cells irradiated.

On closer examination of the curve in Fig. 2-1, it can be seen that while most of the curve is exponential, the initial portion is not but curves back to the vertical axis. This initial part of the curve is called the "shoulder" region. If the exponential portion of the curve is extrapolated back to the vertical axis, the second descriptor of the curve is obtained—the extrapolation number or N_e. The curve in Fig. 2-1 has an extrapolation number of 4. In current theory, the extrapolation number represents the number of "targets" in the sensitive part of the cell which must be "hit," ie, damaged, to cause cell death. All of these targets must be hit or the cell will recover. The shoulder portion of the curve represents the accumulation of sublethal damage in the cells, and the curve becomes exponential when all but one of the targets in the cells have been hit. This is the "multitarget" theory of cell survival. While other models of cell survival curves exist, the multitarget one seems to fit the existing data best.

Table 2-1 *Exponential Cell Death*

No. Cells Irradiated	No. Cells Killed	No. Cells Remaining
1,000,000	900,000	100,000
100,000	90,000	10,000
10,000	9000	1000
1000	900	100

Three hundred rads will kill 90% of irradiated cells.
Modified after Suit [19].

D_o and N_e have been determined for a large number of animal tumors. In spite of the large variability of tumor response, the values of D_o and N_e are relatively constant. N_e ranges from 1.5 to 10 and D_o from 110 to 240 [16,18,-19]. The larger D_o and N_e values are related to cells which are more radioresistant, since a larger dose of radiation is required to kill a given proportion of cells.

Time Required for Repair of Radiation Injury

Thus far we have considered the effects of a single dose of radiation. Consider next the results of a second dose of radiation following some time interval after the first dose. Elkind and Sutton [6,7] performed an experiment in which cells were irradiated with 505 rads and then incubated at 37 C for 18.1 hours. At that time, the cells were irradiated with 487 rads. They found that instead of a survival equivalent to a single dose of 992 rads, the survival was actually less by an amount equivalent to the shoulder portion of the original cell survival curve. They concluded that repair had occurred within 18.1 hr. To determine how quickly repair occurs, they irradiated cells with a second dose at varying times following the first dose. Figure 2-2 illustrates the results of those experiments. Within 2 hr, the cells had reached their preirradiation sensitivity; however, following this, the cells were more sensitive to radiation and this sensitivity reached a peak approximately 4 hr following the first

dose. Sensitivity then slowly decreased and within 10 hr the cells had reached a plateau of full recovery.

How can this complex pattern of recovery be explained? Several processes must obviously contribute. Within 2 hr following the first dose of radiation, repair of sublethal damage occurred and accounts for the early rapid rise of the curve. Since the radiosensitivity of cells varies with the cell cycle, this first dose kills more cells in the sensitive phases of the cycle than in the resistant portions (Chapter 3). This first dose of radiation also produces a delay in mitosis and a piling up of cells in G_2. At this point, the cells become partially synchronized, and the remaining portion of the curve can be explained by the varying radiosensitivity of the cells as they progress through the cell cycle. The exact curvilinear shape and length of time for this total process to occur will vary with the cell system studied.

From these experiments, several general statements can be made.

1. Repair of sublethal damage occurs quickly and is usually complete within 2 hr of irradiation.
2. For a short time, cells become synchronized following this first dose of radiation.
3. The sensitivity of cells to a second dose of radiation will depend on the phase of the cell cycle at the time the radiation is given.
4. The rate of movement of the cells through the cell cycle will determine the shape of the curve.

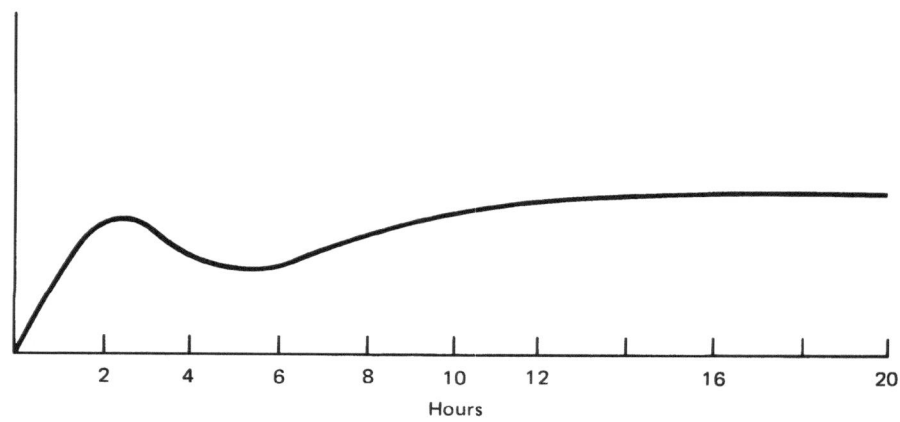

Figure 2-2.   Response to a second dose of x rays given at varying times after the first dose [6].

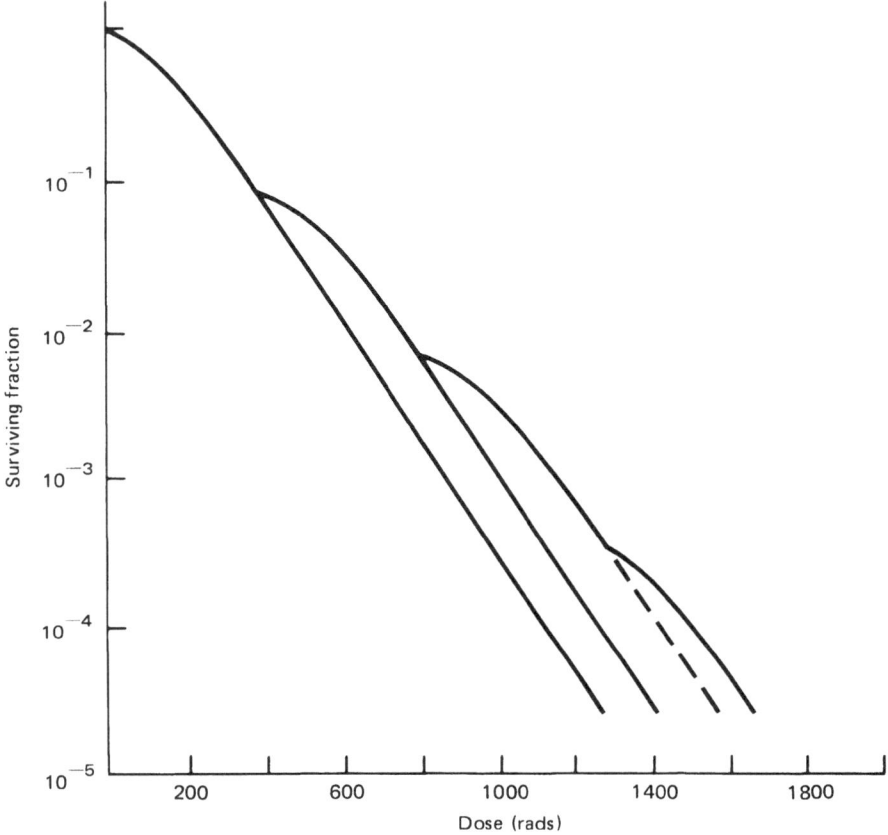

Figure 2-3. Effect of number of fractions on proportion of surviving cells.

Although sublethal damage is quickly repaired by cells, Sinclair [18] has noted that the total repair process is an incomplete one since the irradiated cells have properties which differ from those of nonirradiated cells. He has noted the following differences in irradiated cells.

1. An increased radiosensitivity (smaller D_o)
2. A change in the median cell volume
3. Chromosome abnormalities
4. A lengthened intermitotic time
5. An increased number of deaths of daughter cells

Effect of Multiple Doses on Cell Survival

Since, in clinical radiation therapy, a single dose of radiation is given daily for 5 days each week, we will next consider the effects of this process in terms of cell survival curves. This practice of dividing the total radiation dose into a number of daily doses or fractions is called

fractionation, and the dose is said to be protracted over the total number of days. Figure 2-3 illustrates the effectiveness of one, two, and four fractions of radiation. Since in each case full recovery has occurred between doses, the shoulder portion of each curve has reappeared. Because of the reappearance of the shoulder between fractions, a larger total dose is required to reduce the surviving fraction to a given number; ie, the greater the number of fractions, the larger the total dose required for a given biologic effect.

One of the earliest and best known studies attempting to correlate radiation dose with time is that of Strandquist [12]. Figure 2-4 illustrates Strandquist's data for carcinoma of the skin. In this study, the time–dose relationships of 280 irradiated carcinomas of the skin were plotted on a log–log scale. A line was drawn that separated the incidence of skin necrosis from that of recurrences; ie, doses above the line resulted in a radiation complication, while

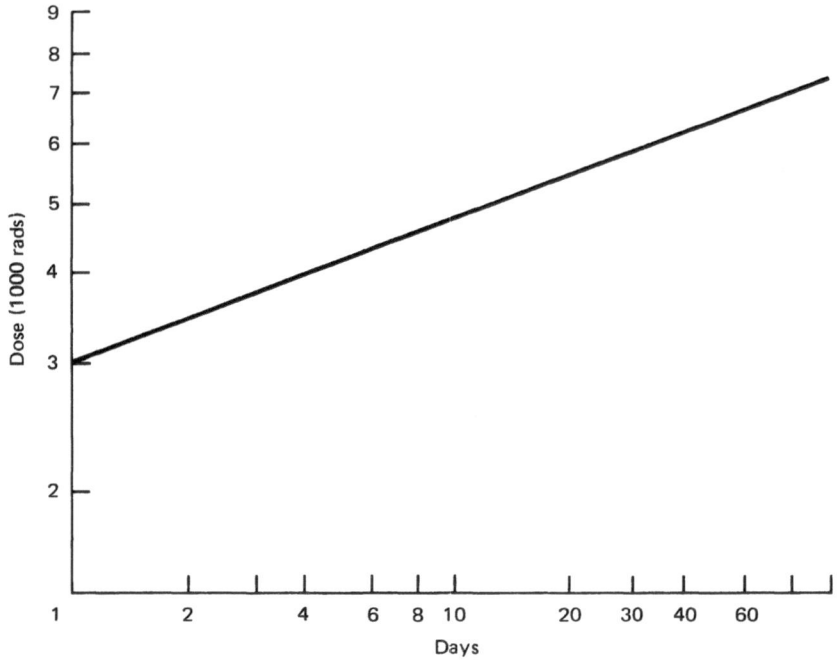

Figure 2-4.   Strandquist curve for carcinoma of the skin. Modified after Johns [12].

those below the line were inadequate for control and resulted in recurrence. The usefulness of this curve can be illustrated if the dose or time factor of a treatment course is being changed. For example, if a skin carcinoma is usually treated with 3000 rads in 4 days but for some reason one wanted to change either the dose or time, the same effect could be obtained with 4000 rads in 11 days or 6000 rads in 45 days.

Strandquist's data imply that a biologic effect is only related to the radiation dose and the time over which it is delivered. This is an oversimplification of the problem since several other factors are important, including the total number of fractions and the volume being irradiated.

Ellis [8] has attempted to correlate the number of fractions with the dose and total time of a treatment series. He introduced the concept of the nominal single dose (NSD), which might be considered as the single dose equivalent of a total dose, protraction, fractionation scheme. This permits the comparison of various treatment schemes or the changing of a given scheme to a different one of equivalent biologic effectiveness. The NSD can be calculated from the formula

$$NSD = Dose \times F^{-0.24} \times T^{-0.11}$$

where Dose is the total dose in rads
    F is the number of fractions
    T is the number of elapsed treatment days

The unit of NSD is the ret and typical clinical treatment techniques deliver doses between 1700 and 1950 rets.

While the NSD is a useful concept, it also does not account for all the factors involved in radiation response. It is probably helpful in changing or comparing doses involving a small range of fractions or total time; however, for large variations in treatment technique such as a change from a 6-week to a 1-week protraction, the results of this calculation should be accepted with caution.

Mixed Cell Populations

Until now we have considered the response of a uniform population of cells. Figure 2-5 shows a survival curve for a population consisting of two types of cells, a more sensitive group with a D_o of 150 rads and a more resistant group with a D_o of 250 rads. The initial response of this mixed population of cells is due to the response of the sensitive cells. However, as the radiation dose increases, the proportion of resistant cells in the population increases due to the death of the sensitive cells. Eventually, the response of the cells follows the survival curve of the resistant cells, since they finally form the bulk of the total cell population. Thus, while the initial response of this mixed population follows the sensitive cell survival curve, the final response is due to the resistant cells, so that the final cell survival is predicted by the resistant cells rather than the sensitive ones. This is important in clinical applications since the overall response of a tumor to radiation is due, not to the radiosensitive cells of the tumor, but to the most radioresistant cells present.

Oxygen Effect

One of the earliest radiation sensitizers studied was molecular oxygen. In almost all mammalian cell systems studied, the effectiveness of radiation is increased by the presence of oxygen. Figure 2-6 shows two survival curves: one with cells irradiated in the presence of oxygen and one irradiated in the absence of oxygen. It can be seen that the D_0 for the cells irradiated in the presence of oxygen is smaller than that for those cells irradiated without oxygen. The change in sensitivity of the cells with and without oxygen can be calculated by comparing the

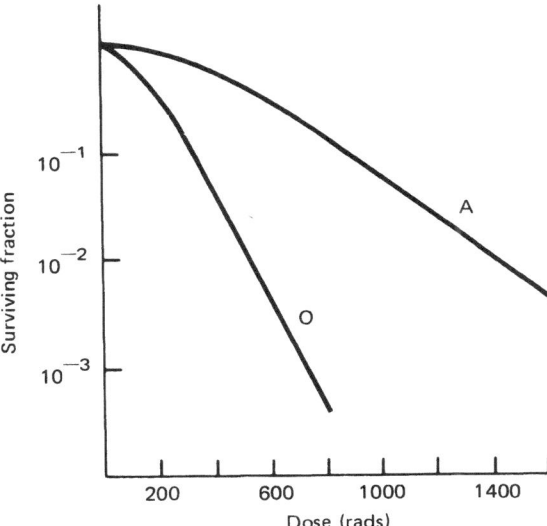

Figure 2-6. Cell survival curves of oxygenated (O) and anoxic (A) cells.

respective D_0s. The ratio of the D_0s is called the oxygen enhancement ratio (OER) and is most often between 2 and 3 for x rays; ie, cells are 2 to 3 times more sensitive to radiation in the presence of oxygen than in the absence of oxygen.

Deschner and Gray [4] studied the relationship between oxygen pressure and radiosensitivity in Ehrlich ascites cells. This relationship is shown in Fig. 2-7. It can be seen that most of the oxygen effect occurs at very low oxygen pressure, and that the radiosensitivity curve rises very quickly and reaches a plateau by a pressure of 30 mmHg. The amount of oxygen in venous blood is in excess of this amount, so that the oxygen effect is not a factor in the response of normal tissue to radiation. However, as will be seen later, this is not the case with tumors.

Cell Survival Curves and High LET Radiation

As was mentioned earlier, LET describes how frequently ionizations occur along the track of ionizing radiation. Since the ionizations from x and γ rays are due to electrons, the ionizations are relatively infrequent; however, some types of radiation, such as protons, α particles, and neutrons, cause more densely ionizing tracks and the biologic effects of these radiations are

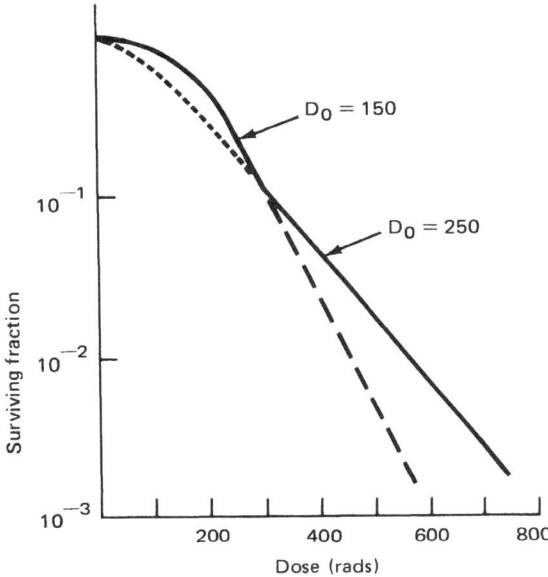

Figure 2-5. Radiation response of mixed cell population.

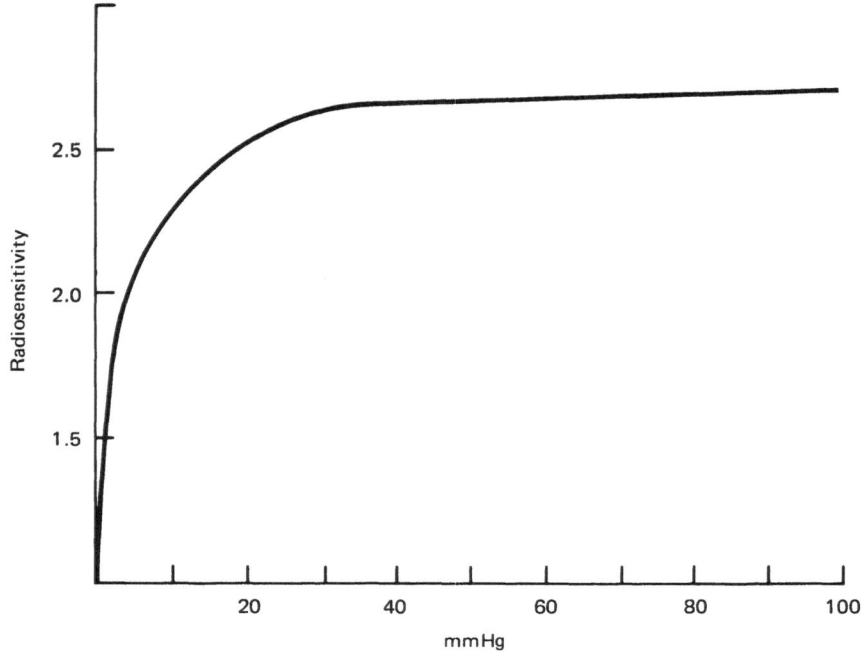

Figure 2-7. Effect of oxygen concentration on radiosensitivity.

different from those of x rays. Figure 2-8 shows two cell survival curves from neutron-irradiated cells—one determined in the presence and one in the absence of oxygen. Several differences can be noted from the cell survival curve shown in Fig. 2-1. First, although the curves in Fig. 2-8 have shoulders, they are much smaller than that with x rays; therefore, the response to this high LET radiation is more exponential. Furthermore, since the shoulder portion represents accumulation of sublethal damage, there is thus less sublethal damage with neutrons and therefore a smaller effect will result from fractionation.

In addition, the difference between the oxygenated and unoxygenated cell survival curves is smaller than with x rays, so that the relative protection conferred by the absence of oxygen is less. With neutrons, the OER is between 1.2 and 2. Because of these differences, neutrons and other high LET radiations are currently being studied for their possible clinical applications.

Clinical Applications of the Oxygen Effect

Although the amount of oxygen in normal tissue is sufficiently adequate to be on the plateau

of the radiosensitivity curve, this does not seem to be the case with tumors. Tumors normally derive their blood supply from the tumor periphery. As the tumor increases in volume, it reaches a size where nutrition from the peripheral blood supply cannot diffuse across the tumor cord. This generally occurs when the tumor diameter is greater than 150 μ. At this point the central cells become anoxic and die, but between the well-oxygenated peripheral cells and the central anoxic cells is a zone of hypoxic cells. The importance of this hypoxic zone was first recognized by Gray [10] and has since been confirmed by others.

In clinical radiotherapy several techniques have been used to overcome the decreased sensitivity of these oxygen-starved cells.

1. Fractionation. Fractionated radiotherapy may partly overcome the problem of hypoxic tumor cells. It may be that as well-oxygenated cells die from a dose of radiation, the existing hypoxic cells become better oxygenated and are no longer protected. On the other hand, it has been suggested that some of the anoxic cells are in a resting state and these cells move into the hypoxic zone. Whether fractionation and protraction

overcome this protective effect of hypoxia remains to be proved; the outcome will probably be shown by clinical trials with high LET radiation.

2. Hyperbaric oxygen. In several studies patients with advanced tumors were treated under several atmospheres of oxygen pressure using a hyperbaric oxygen chamber. Most of these studies have used altered fractionation schemes for the experimental group but not for the controls. While some of the studies suggest an advantage for hyperbaric oxygen therapy, at this time the advantage has not been clearly demonstrated [2,14,22].

3. Anoxia. A few studies have attempted to decrease the sensitivity of the normal tissue by decreasing the blood supply. This overcomes the protective advantage of the hypoxic tumor; however, the tumor sites for these studies have been limited to the extremities and results are too few to demonstrate an advantage for this type of therapy.

4. High LET radiation. Two trials are currently in progress using neutrons. At Hammersmith Hospital in London, where neutron radiotherapy has been under study for

the longest period of time, encouraging results have been reported in treating a selected number of very advanced tumors [1]. As a result of these initial reports, a prospective, randomized study has been started.

Other types of high LET radiation are being studied for their possible use in radiotherapy. At the Los Alamos, New Mexico, laboratory, studies are underway with the use of mesons; however, it will be several years before clinical trials are started.

Conclusions

A number of factors have been presented that influence the biologic response to radiation. These factors include the mass and charge of the ionizing particle, the number of fractions, the total radiation dose, protraction and fractionation, and modifying factors such as oxygen.

The reaction of tissue to radiation may differ from the reaction of cells due to such factors as repair, reoxygenation of hypoxic cells, and repopulation of normal tissue. Although the D_o and N_e of tumor and normal tissue have been found to be similar [23], clinical observation has shown that a differential effect is obtained between tumor and normal tissue by fractionation and protraction of treatment. Furthermore, the radiosensitivity of tumors varies to a greater extent than would be predicted by the variation in D_o and N_e; therefore, a number of other factors must contribute to the observed response of tumor and normal tissue to radiation. More of these factors must be identified for a better understanding of radiation effects on tumor and normal tissue.

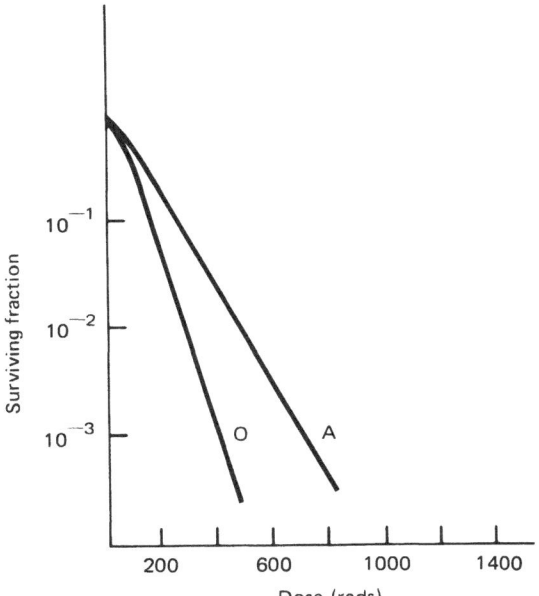

Figure 2-8. Cell survival curves for neutron-irradiated cells in the presence (O) and absence (A) of oxygen.

References

1. Catterall M: Clinical experience with fast neutrons from the Hammersmith cyclotron. Eur J Cancer 7:227, 1971
2. Churchill-Davidson I, Sanger C, Thomlinson RH: High pressure oxygen and radiotherapy. Lancet 1:1091, 1955
3. Dalrymple GV, Gaulden ME, Kollmorgen GM et al: Medical Radiation Biology. Philadelphia, Saunders, 1973
4. Deschner EE, Gray LH: Influence of oxygen tension on x-ray induced chromosomal damage in Ehrlich ascites tumor cells irradiated in vitro and in vivo. Radiat Res 11:115, 1959
5. Dewey DL: The x-ray sensitivity of *Serratia marcescens.* Radiat Res 19:64, 1963

6. Elkind MM, Sutton H: X ray damage and recovery in mammalian cells in culture. Nature 184:1293, 1959

7. Elkind MM, Sutton H: Radiation response of mammalian cells grown in culture. Radiat Res 13:556, 1960

8. Ellis F: Dose, time, and fractionation. A clinical hypothesis. Clin Radiol 20:1, 1969

9. Freifelder D: Lethal changes in bacteriophage DNA produced by x-rays. Radiat Res (Suppl) 6:80, 1966

10. Gray LH, Conger AD, Eibert M, et al: The concentration of oxygen dissolved in tissues at the time of irradiation as a factor in radiotherapy. Br J Radiol 26:638, 1953

11. Hewitt HB: Radiation Effects in Physics, Chemistry, and Biology. Amsterdam, North-Holland, 1963

12. Johns HE, Cunningham JR: The Physics of Radiology. Springfield, Ill, Thomas, 1969

13. Kaplan HS: Enzymatic repair of radiation-induced strand breakage in cellular DNA and its chemical inhibition. Radiology 105:121, 1972

14. Kunkler PB, Henk JM, Shah NK, et al: Radiotherapy and hyperbaric oxygen in malignant tumours of the oral cavity and oropharynx with lymph node metastases. Gann Monograph No. 9. Tokyo, Maruzen, 1970

15. Lawson RC, Watt DE: The LET distribution of the recoil proton dose from DD and DT neutrons. Phys Med Biol 22:217, 1967

16. Lockart RZ, Elkind MM, Moses WB: Radiation response of mammalian cells grown in culture. II. Survival and recovery characteristics of several subcultures of HeLa S 3 cells after x-irradiation. J Natl Cancer Inst 27:1393, 1961

17. Puck TT, Marcus PI: Action of x rays on mammalian cells. J Exp Med 103:653, 1956

18. Sinclair WK: X-ray–induced heritable damage (small colony formation) in cultured mammalian cells. Radiat Res 21:584, 1964

19. Suit HD: Radiation biology. A basis for radiotherapy. In Fletcher GH (ed): Textbook of Radiotherapy. Philadelphia, Lea & Febiger, 1966

20. Tessman I: Mutagenesis in phages ϕ-X174 and T4 and properties of the genetic material. Virology 9:375, 1959

21. Tessman I, Tessman ES, Stent GS: The relative radiosensitivity of bacteriophages S13 and Ts. Virology 4:209, 1957

22. Van den Brenk HAS, Madigan JP, Kerr RC: Experience in Melbourne with the use of hyperbaric oxygen combined with megavoltage radiation in 614 cases of advanced malignant disease. In Vaeth JM (ed): Frontiers of Radiation Therapy and Oncology. New York, Karger, 1968

23. Whitmore GF, Till JE: Quantitation of cellular radiobiological responses. Ann Rev Nucl Med 14:347, 1964

3

Radiation and Cell Kinetics

Frederick D. Malkinson

The dermatologist must treat a large number of benign and malignant diseases characterized by increased rates of epidermal cell proliferation [45]. For some of these disorders radiotherapy, chemotherapy, or combined treatment measures may be either curative or effective in achieving disease control. The usefulness of these regimens, locally applied or systemically administered where indicated, has stimulated great interest in the biology of cellular responses to ionizing radiation and to chemotherapeutic agents as well.

Bergonié and Tribondeau first showed that radiosensitivity of a tissue depends critically on that tissue's rate of cell proliferation [6]. Cells in the division cycle are now known to be more radiosensitive than nondividing cells, as measured by several different parameters of radiation damage. Moreover, among actively dividing cells, radiosensitivity is much greater in some phases of the cell division cycle than in others [65]. These findings suggest, for example, that if even partial synchrony could be produced in abnormally proliferating cell populations, delivery of ionizing radiation in radiosensitive phases of the cycle could intensify treatment effects with relative protection of more slowly dividing normal tissue cells.

This paper briefly considers several interrelationships of ionizing radiation and cell kinetics, and some of their possible implications for radiotherapy.

Cell Division Cycle and Age Responses to Radiation

In any tissue or organ cell population, the critical therapeutic target for ionizing radiation is the stem cell pool, upon which continued cell population growth is dependent. The reproductive cell cycle is defined as the time interval between completion of mitosis in a cell and completion of the following mitosis in a daughter cell. The division cycle has been divided into four major phases [33]: G_1, the time interval between the completion of mitosis and the initiation of chromosomal replication; S, the period of DNA synthesis; G_2, the period separating the end of chromosomal replication from the onset of cellular division (prophase); and M, the period of mitosis. In normal mammalian cells in culture the durations of S, G_2, and M phases are fairly constant: S phase lasts 6 to 8 hr, G_2 phase lasts 3 to 5 hr, and mitosis lasts 1 hr or less. The duration of the G_1 period is highly variable: overall, short or long cell cycle times differ from each other almost entirely in the length of the G_1 phase (which may last hours, days, or weeks).

RNA synthesis occurs throughout the cell cycle, ceasing in mitosis [70]. Protein synthesis occurs during the entire cycle, but is at a minimum during cell division [3]. In our current

This manuscript was completed and submitted for publication in December, 1973.

understanding, G_1 and G_2 phases represent time intervals during which no highly specific or absolutely critical molecular events have yet been identified. Phase differences in biochemical and metabolic events occurring throughout the cell cycle, however, apparently account for significantly different responses to radiation. These differences can be clearly demonstrated in cultured populations of proliferating cells synchronized by a variety of techniques, eg, selective harvesting during mitosis; phase blockade, particularly with DNA inhibitors such as hydroxyurea or methotrexate; and selective killing by tritiated thymidine "suicide" (for a review of synchronization methods used, see [51]).

Experimentally, radiation damage was first measured by the presence or absence of division in cultured cells [58]. Significant phase-dependent differences in postradiation survival were first demonstrated for HeLa cells with the finding that radiosensitivity varied by a factor of 2.5 throughout the phases of the cycle [71]. These studies and other investigations [25,36,68] indicated that G_2- and M-stage cells were the most responsive to radiation, though in many cell lines late G_1 cells also displayed high radiosensitivity (Fig. 3-1). The early G_1 stage was relatively radioresistant in cells where the G_1 phase lasted several hours or longer. Radiosensitivity increased markedly in late G_1 and early S periods, but declined again with a second radioresistant peak occurring in late S phase. It is clear from Fig. 3-1 that cell phase differences in radiation response are greatly magnified by increasing doses of radiation.

Cyclic effects of irradiation in proliferating cell populations in vivo are not as clear-cut as are the findings described for in vitro stud-

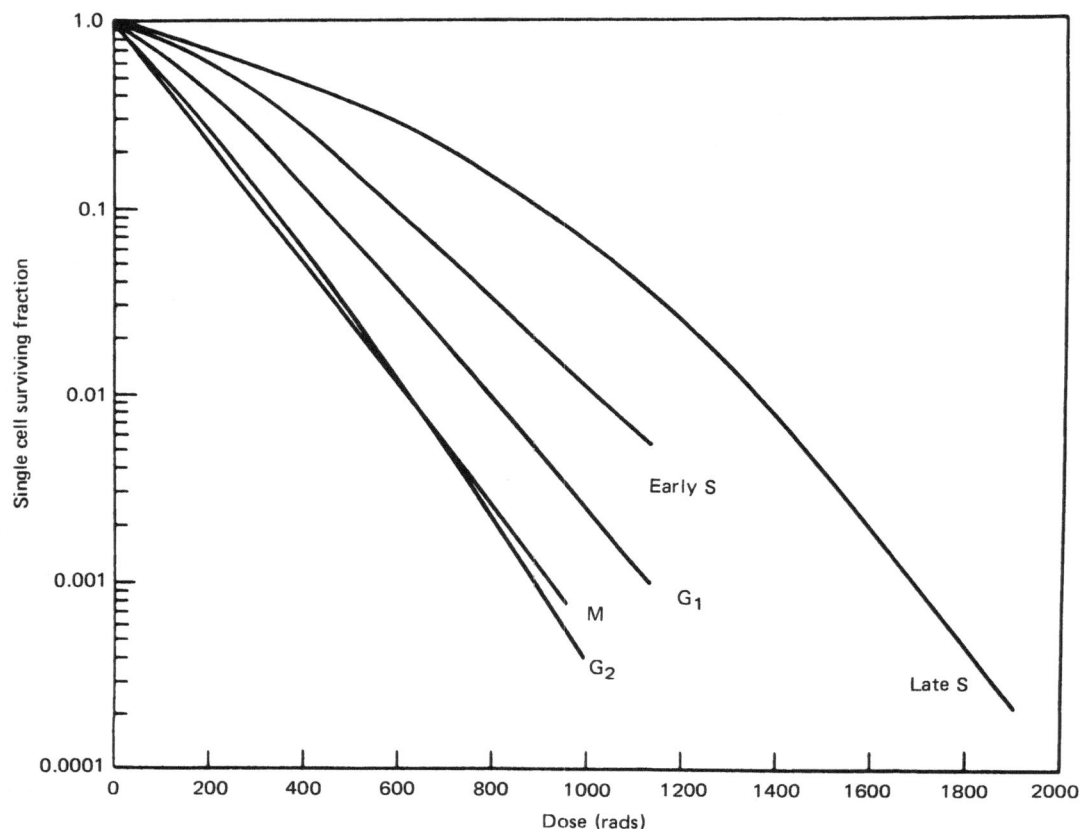

Figure 3-1. X ray survival curves for synchronized cultures of Chinese hamster cells irradiated during various stages of the cell cycle. From Sinclair and Morton [68]. Courtesy of the authors and Academic Press, Inc.

ies. Attainment of only partial cell synchrony at best has been a significant problem in the in vivo studies, although maximum radiosensitivity in *M* phase and radioresistance in late *S* phase have been confirmed. With respect to skin and appendages, investigations in hair matrix cell populations suggest that partial synchrony increases radiation sensitivity (as measured by hair loss) when x rays are administered during, or shortly after, release of a hydroxyurea-induced G_1/S block [47].

Resting cells, or cells which have left the proliferative pool and are undergoing maturation and differentiation, are usually more radioresistant than are actively dividing cells. In mouse skin, for example, the radiosensitivity of dividing anagen hair matrix cells is 2 times greater than that of G_0 telogen cells, as demonstrated by slowed incorporation of isotope-labeled amino acids [46]. Mouse follicle melanocytes are also more radiosensitive when the cells are actively proliferating [57]. In other mammalian cell lines in culture, cells in exponential growth phase are more radiosensitive than are stationary phase cells [28]. Cellular repair of radiation damage, however, appears to be more rapid and efficient in proliferating cells than in nondividing or differentiating cells. This phenomenon is also demonstrable in hair matrix cell populations [46].

G_0- or arrested G_1-phase cells comprise a special subpopulation of more radioresistant, nonproliferating cells which can be recruited back into the stem cell pool following appropriate stimuli. These G_0 cells, of importance in the repair of injury in normal tissues and in tumors, show increased radiosensitivity when they are stimulated to divide.

Division Delay

Tissue culture experiments conducted 50 years ago first revealed that onset of mitosis is delayed in cells exposed to ionizing radiation [13]. Division delay is characterized by reversible blocks in the postradiation progression of dividing cells through the cell cycle. The most significant block occurs in G_2, with cell division inhibited before the onset of prophase. To produce progression delay, radiation must be delivered in G_2 prior to a specific time interval preceding prophase [15]; later exposure to radiation has little or no effect in retarding mito-

sis. Since cells irradiated in *S* and G_1 phases continue to progress through the cell cycle—although at slowed rates in many cell lines—cell population "build-ups" occur in G_2 phase. Consequently, as the radiation block is dissipated, the mitotic index not only returns to normal, but briefly increases above normal levels ("mitotic overshoot").

The duration of division delay increases with increasing dosage. In Chinese hamster cells irradiated at doses of 200 to 1000 rads, delays of 1 hr/100 rads were recorded [22]. Much longer delays, up to 10-fold or more per rad, have been found with synchronized G_2 mouse L cells [77], HeLa cells [59], and mouse leukemia cells [9]. In vivo studies using dose ranges of 100 to 200 rads have demonstrated G_2 division delays of about 1 hr/100 rads in mouse hair matrix cells [48]. Additional in vivo studies have confirmed the in vitro observations of radiation-induced division delay [26,55].

Other phases of the cell cycle are also sensitive to division delay. Irradiation of G_1 or *S* cells induces a later G_2 block, though in most cell lines G_2 delays for given radiation dosages are greatest for cells irradiated in G_2. In addition, G_1- and *S*-phase delays have also been described for a number of cell lines [6,10,37,-40,44]. In one study, passage of G_1 cells into *S* phase has been found to be the most radiosensitive stage for division delay [41], and in other cell lines maximum delay occurs during *S* phase. Lastly, a number of experiments, including observations with time-lapse photography, have demonstrated that mitosis itself may be greatly prolonged by radiation, and that some of these mitoses are abortive [30]. Interestingly, division delay occurs both in cells destined to survive radiation and in cells subsequently killed, indicating that division delay and reproductive failure (see below) result from different pathomechanisms [23].

Various explanations for postradiation division delay have been advanced. Experiments with several cell lines have shown that impaired protein synthesis may be an important factor in the postradiation delay of cell cycle progression [21,61,74]. This delay has been linked to requirements for excess protein synthesis needed to repair cell damage [1]. Breakdown of preformed protein or structures related to imminent cell division might also account for this radiation effect [62]. Cellular target sites for radiation-induced progression delay appear to reside in the nucleus or in the immediately contiguous perinuclear cytoplasm [53].

Reproductive Failure and Interphase Death

Perhaps the most dramatic consequence of cell irradiation is the loss of reproductive capacity. Postradiation survival curves have been established for several mammalian cell lines by investigators utilizing quantitative techniques to study colony-forming ability [58,76]. Most cells are incapable of sustained proliferation after dose exposures of a few hundred rads. The D_0 or mean lethal dose (dose required to reduce the cell population to 37% of the initial value on the linear part of the survival curve [Fig. 3-1]) usually falls within a range of 100 to 150 rads for a variety of mammalian cell lines, normal or malignant [31].

Most lethally irradiated cells do not die immediately following irradiation, but undergo one or more division cycles first. This phenomenon is dose-dependent: the higher the dose the smaller the number of postradiation divisions, which seldom exceed 5 or 6 [22]. Ultimately, these cells undergo disintegration during or after an abnormal mitosis often characterized by sticky chromosomes, chromosome aberrations, cytoplasmic bridges, or cell fusion [34,-50]. In recent studies of HeLa cell populations it was shown that at doses of 500 rads all cells completed the first postradiation mitosis [73]. Three-fourths of the cells that subsequently died did so in mitotic arrest, either in the second postradiation mitosis (25%) or in a later one. The remaining cells died in interphase. Although division delay could no longer be detected in the first postmitotic, postradiation cell generation, subsequent generations again showed some delay in cell cycle progression, as well as an increased duration of mitosis [73].

Some irradiated, doomed cells ultimately survive for months despite reproductive failure. Continued synthesis of DNA and protein in these cultured cells results in formation of giant cells which may be polyploid and contain huge nuclei and nucleoli. Such cells range in size up to 50 times their original diameters. Similar cells have also been found in vivo in previously irradiated tissues.

Cells surviving irradiation are those capable of repairing sublethal damage, thereby retaining the capacity for unlimited proliferation. Some descendants of surviving cells may show delayed growth ("small colony formation") up to a year or longer in cell culture [66], apparently resulting in part from prolonged cell cycle times [50]. This change in cell growth is unrelated to cell cycle age at the time of irradiation [66].

The mechanism of postradiation reproductive failure is unclear. Tolmach et al have found that for HeLa S3 cells, deficient DNA synthesis occurs in the immediately following cell generations [73]. These workers have postulated that replicon synthesis is initiated normally but is not completed, and that unrepaired or malrepaired single-strand breaks in DNA are involved in mitotic death. The molecular basis for this effect remains unknown.

Combined postradiation effects of division delay and of reproductive failure occurring only after completion of one or more additional cell cycles are the principal factors accounting for gradual reductions in cell populations occurring over several days' time after single radiation exposures. A much more rapid form of cell destruction, ie, interphase death, occurs within a few hours in cells that die during the same division cycle in which they are irradiated. This phenomenon affects increasing numbers of cells at progressively higher radiation doses (especially at several thousand rads), but is a much less important factor in cell death within the therapeutic dose range. Interestingly, however, there are a few cell lines, proliferative and nonproliferative, which regularly display interphase death even after very low dose radiation. These include small lymphocytes [63], young oocytes, and spermatogonia. Cells undergoing interphase death show microscopic changes of necrosis, pyknosis, and karyorrhexis. The mechanism of interphase death is not clearly understood, but Klouwen et al have implicated inhibition of nuclear and mitochondrial oxygen-dependent ATP synthesis [38].

Chromosomal Damage

Muller's pioneering work with the fruit fly first established that x rays can produce mutational changes [52]. It is now well recognized that radiation-induced genetic damage may occur at the molecular level in the gene (point mutation) and at the cellular (microscopic) level in the chromosome. Some chromosomal changes produced by irradiation may be perpetuated in descendant cells, resulting in permanent genetic alterations. In certain cell lines, such as human leukocytes, radiosensitivity is exceedingly high, with visible damage appearing after exposure of only a few rads [7]. Radiation-induced chromosomal aberrations result from breaks in single- or double-stranded chromosomes, depending upon cell cycle age at the time of irradiation. Irradiation during G_1 phase results in chromosomal damage, since the strands are so closely wound together. In S or G_2 phases, paired chromatids present two distinct radiation targets, so that single chromatids of a pair may be broken. Postradiation chromosomal aberrations become visible in the following metaphase; changes induced during mitosis do not appear until the next metaphase.

In general, for chromosomal and chromatid aberrations, the G_1 period is relatively radioresistant, but sensitivity increases in S and G_2 phases [78]. In some cell lines, S phase is more sensitive than is G_2 phase [16]. Radiosensitivity appears to decrease again just before the onset of cell division. Mitosis itself is a highly radiosensitive phase for aberrations, perhaps because the more condensed chromatin fibers in this stage of the cell cycle provide the highest probability for interaction between chromosomal lesions [19]. As is the case with reproductive failure, "fine structure" variations in radiosensitivity for chromatid aberrations appear within specific cell cycle stages: early S phase is more sensitive than is late S phase, for example [42,79].

Noncycling cells are far more resistant to radiation-induced chromosomal aberrations than are cycling cells. In a study of mouse liver cells, the D_0 for chromosomal aberrations in G_0 cells was found to be 1228 rads, compared to 300 rads for partial posthepatectomy cells in G_1 or early S phase [12].

The frequency of chromosomal breaks is proportional to the radiation dose but may vary with dose rates [60]. However, most primary breaks are repaired in their original configuration without permanent genetic alteration, especially in low dose ranges. Protein synthesis, ATP production, and probably DNA and RNA synthesis are all required functions for chromosomal rejoining. However, the effectiveness of this restitution process may vary in different stages of the cell division cycle [17].

Irreparable genetic damage must contribute substantially to postradiation cell death, and there is generally good correlation between cell killing and gross chromosomal aberrations. Nonetheless, other factors appear to be involved as well, since sensitivity to mitotic inhibition may differ significantly from sensitivity to chromosomal aberrations (at least, point mutations), for example, in certain cell lines [18]. (For a review of repair processes, the morphology of chromosomal aberrations, and the contribution of such aberrations to malignant change in surviving cells see [54]).

DNA Synthesis

De Hevesy and his associates, studying normal and sarcomatous tissues of the rat, were the first to demonstrate radiaton-induced inhibition of DNA synthesis [14]. Other investigators found that ionizing radiation inhibits uptake of a variety of DNA precursors such as ^{32}P, ^{14}C-adenine, ^{14}C-thymidine, and ^{14}C-glycine. In mouse hair follicles, for example, ^{32}P incorporation into matrix cell DNA fell about 50% within a few minutes after exposure to radiation doses of 200 to 2000 rads; reduced uptake, at lower rates, continued for several hours [11].

Current concepts suggest that radiation effects on DNA pathways are diverse and, in part, indirect. Specific primary blockages in ongoing DNA synthesis have not been satisfactorily demonstrated within therapeutic dose ranges, and it appears that the process of DNA synthesis per se is moderately radioresistant. Radiation effects on precursor and enzyme synthesis, and on cellular metabolic processes, however, contribute significantly to impaired DNA formation, particularly at low dose levels.

In some irradiated tissues, notably regenerating liver, marked impairment of DNA formation results from inhibited synthesis of both kinase and DNA polymerase in late G_1 phase [4,8]. Irradiation *after* enzyme induction but prior to the onset of DNA synthesis also impairs DNA formation [5], suggesting blockage of another step in the preparation for DNA synthesis. During S phase, however, even high dose radiation has little effect on DNA synthesis in regenerating liver cells. But in other cell lines, ongoing DNA synthesis may be slowed by moderate to high radiation dosages [39]. Studies with HeLa S3 cells irradiated during G_1 phase have shown marked, dose-dependent reductions in DNA synthesis in the following cell generation [32]. Cells destined to survive irradiation synthesized about 80% of the normal amount of DNA, in contrast to 30% for cells permanently arrested in the next mitosis [32]. These quantitative differences suggest that reduced incorporation of labeled precursors into DNA may have predictive value for survival or demise in the next cell generation.

The studies of Lajtha and associates [39] and those of Ord and Stocken [56] led these investigators to propose that radiation-induced impairment of DNA synthesis depends on two factors, one of which is relatively radiosensitive and the other much more radioresistant. (In Lajtha's studies the D_0 for the former was 500 rads and for the latter 13,000 rads in bone marrow cells irradiated in vitro.) The radiosensitive component reflects damage to the biochemical pathways of precursor synthesis, while the radioresistant component is associated with damage to the DNA template [39,56].

The well-known effect of radiation in inducing division delay may also temporarily influence DNA synthesis. A G_1 block impairs DNA formation fairly rapidly. A G_2 delay will affect DNA synthesis only after several hours, since most M and G_1 cells continue to progress into S phase until the G_2 block depletes these compartments. It should be emphasized that reductions in DNA synthesis resulting from division delay occur largely because of reduced cell numbers in S phase. When the irradiated cells finally progress into S phase, however, they usually synthesize DNA at normal rates. The same observation has been made for cells irradiated during the stage of DNA synthesis. For example, a dose of about 500 rads delivered to synchronous HeLa cell populations in S phase reduced DNA synthesis by 50% with prolongation of S phase [72]. Very little effect on DNA synthesis occurred after irradiation in other phases of the cell cycle. Overall, total DNA synthesis was essentially normal [72].

After lengthier postradiation intervals, a significant incidence of mitotic failure or interphase death is followed by a general reduction in DNA synthesis, resulting specifically from smaller numbers of cycling cells.

Following initial depression of DNA synthesis by irradiation, a faster than normal synthetic rate may occur temporarily [75], perhaps on a compensatory or facilitated basis. Repair of damaged DNA ("nonscheduled" synthesis) may also contribute to the increase, but this is an unimportant factor after low or moderate dose radiation [69].

Space limitations preclude discussion of several additional topics concerning radiation and cell kinetics, including radioprotective agents and radiosensitizers; repair of sublethal or potentially lethal damage; cell proliferation kinetics after split (multiple) dose fractionation or continuous irradiation; and effects of radiation on the duration of the cell cycle.

Radiation and Cell Kinetics: Therapeutic Implications

The critical factors determining radiation response relate to radiation dose and its fractionation, cellular damage and repair processes, tissue oxygen tensions, stem cell repopulation potential, and vascular and nutritional supplies. In addition, cell kinetics parameters such as "age" in the division cycle at the time of irradiation and DNA damage and repair mechanisms also affect the severity of tissue damage. Although our understanding of the effects of radiation currently surpasses our knowledge of the mechanisms by which these effects are produced, further radiobiologic studies may help to elucidate the normal molecular changes which characterize cell proliferation and differentiation, as well as the critical biochemical "targets" that mediate radiation injury.

In the past, techniques developed for the administration of radiation therapy have been largely empirically derived. More recently, studies of radiation and its effects on cell kinetics have provided an important scientific basis for radiotherapy and for the combined use of ionizing radiation and chemotherapy. Although many of these investigations have been of more theoretical interest than of practical value to date, it seems likely that significant new treatment advances will result from continuing radiobiologic studies, especially those involving concomitant use of pharmacologic agents. Three examples will be briefly considered.

As described previously, cellular radiosensitivity varies significantly in different phases of the cell cycle. Partially synchronous cell populations, produced by prior exposure to radiation (eg, by reversible division delay in G_2) or by selected chemotherapeutic agents exhibiting phase-specific effects (eg, hydroxyurea arrest at the G_1/S boundary), should show enhanced response to radiation delivered during the radiosensitive phase of the cycle. This effect is illustrated experimentally for hydroxyurea and hair matrix cells in Fig. 3-2. Similar effects produced by hydroxyurea and vinca alkaloids combined with irradiation have been shown for other cell systems [43,67]. Analogous cyclic effects on hair matrix cells produced by other pharmacologic agents and radiation may also be inferred from older studies with colchicine and actinomycin D (Fig. 3-3 and 3-4) [29,49]. The main problem in the practical clinical situation is that effective cell synchrony induced by a variety of measures is seldom maintained beyond one or two division cycles. To date, all attempts to produce sustained cell synchrony have been ineffective or accompanied by intolerable side effects. Where chemotherapeutic agents have been used to produce cell synchrony in clinical trials, treatment results from drug–radiation therapy for tumors have often been unimpressive, because cell kinetics parameters have been inadequately studied or because little consideration has been given to the optimum sequence and time relationships of the agents used. Hope-

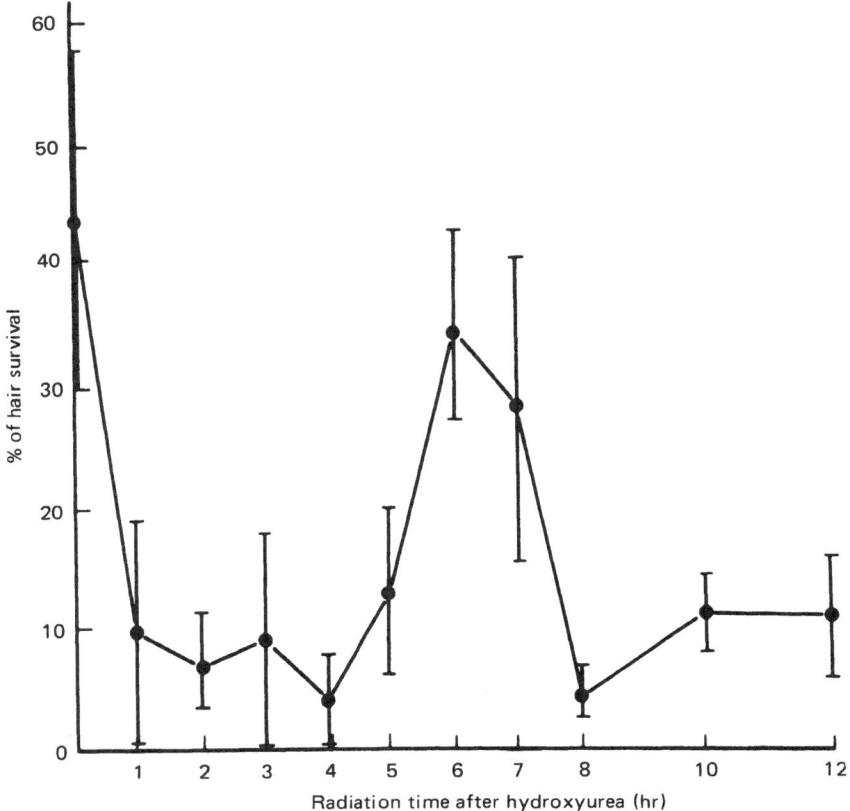

Figure 3-2. Anagen hair survival (%) in different groups of mice, 7 days after administration of hydroxyurea 1200 mg/kg, followed by 650 rads radiation given at varying time intervals after the drug. The increased alopecia (reduced hair survival) in the early time intervals probably reflects increased radiosensitivity of G_1/S cells "blocked" by hydroxyurea. Later decrease and subsequent increase in radiosensitivity also suggest drug-induced cyclic responses. From Malkinson et al [47]. Courtesy of Blackwell Scientific Publications.

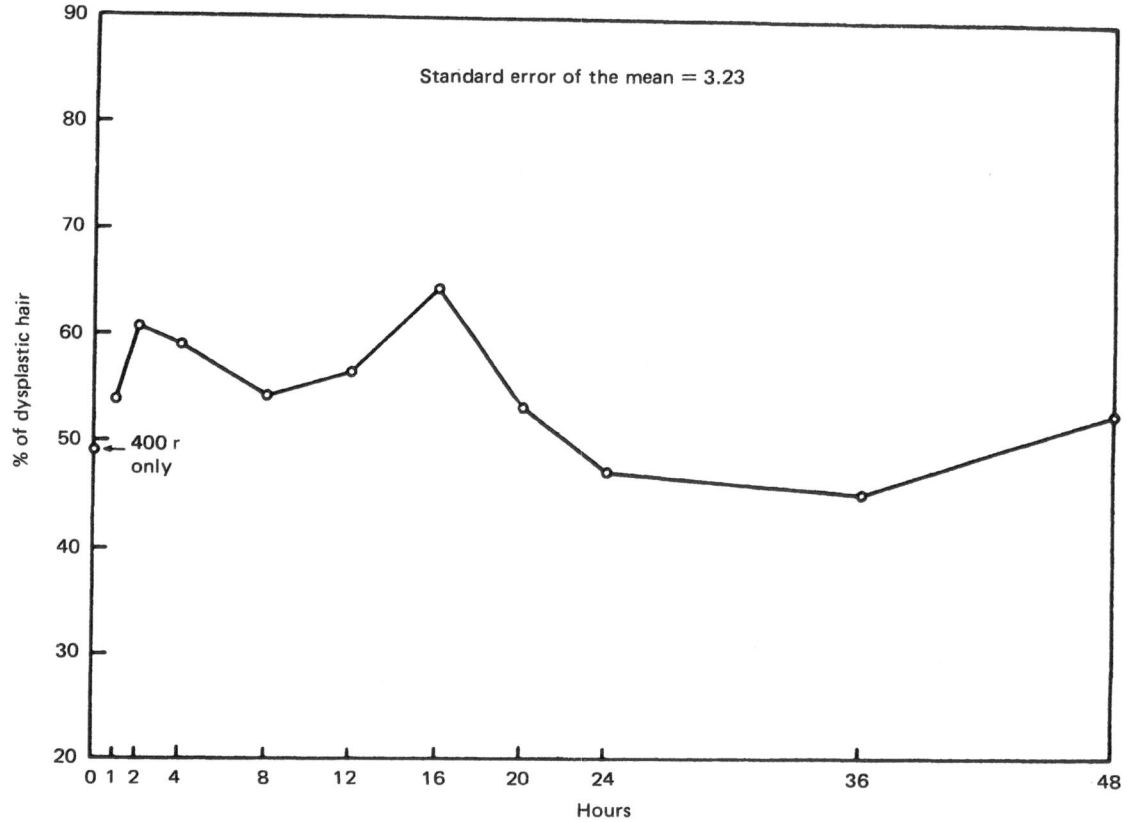

Figure 3-3.   Effects of varying the time interval (hr) between injection of colchicine 1 mg/kg and administration of x rays (400 rads) on production of dysplastic anagen hairs in different groups of mice. Enhanced dysplasia was found at the 2- to 4-hour intervals, presumably when many cells were arrested in the radiosensitive stage of mitosis. The increased response at the 16-hour interval may also reflect cyclic radiosensitivity. Colchicine alone (1 mg/kg) produced no hair damage, and reversed (radiation–colchicine) treatment sequence produced the same effect as radiation alone. From Malkinson et al [49]. Courtesy of Williams and Wilkins Company.

fully, improved treatment results will follow the development of more effective measures for induction of cell synchronization and more intensive correlative laboratory investigations of tumor cell responses to combined-agent therapy.

The effects of radiation in producing chromosomal damage and the contribution of such damage to cell death have been considered above. Certain compounds such as caffeine, chloroquine [27], and actinomycin D [24], among others, potentiate killing effects in vitro when added to culture media after irradiation. Some of these compounds act by blocking repair of single-strand breaks, presumably through inhibition of the required enzymatic action [27]. Other compounds, such as actino-

mycin D, inhibit repair of radiation-induced sublethal damage [24]. Suitable demonstrations of similar inhibitory effects on radiation repair processes in vivo might hold promise for the design of more practical and effective therapeutic regimens.

Halogenated pyrimidines (analogs of thymidine) potentiate the lethal effects of radiation on cells [20] by increasing the number of irreparable double-strand breaks [35], and by reducing the cell's capacity to accumulate sublethal radiation damage [64]. Since these compounds are active only after incorporation into cellular DNA, their combined use with radiotherapy can be effectively achieved only when there are strikingly different tumor versus normal cell kinetics [2]. Further exploration of the use of these compounds may be promising, especially for malignancies arising in tissues characterized by little or no proliferation in normal cells.

In conclusion, the clinical applications of radiation therapy could be further exploited by enhancing our understanding of the basic mechanisms producing radiobiologic and cell kinetics responses to ionizing radiation. For treatment purposes, practical applications of our current knowledge are most promising in areas where these responses can be modified or enhanced, ie, in areas involving varying radiosensitivity in different phases of the cell cycle, damage to DNA, and radiation repair pro-

cesses. These factors; the solutions to several basic radiobiologic problems, especially those of radiation-resistant anoxic cells; an increased understanding of the effectiveness of dose fractionation; better knowledge of normal and abnormal cell kinetics in benign and malignant disorders; and possible utilization of heavy particle radiation all appear to hold promise for the more effective use of radiation therapy in the future.

References

1. Bacchetti S, Sinclair WK: The relation of protein synthesis to radiation-induced division de-

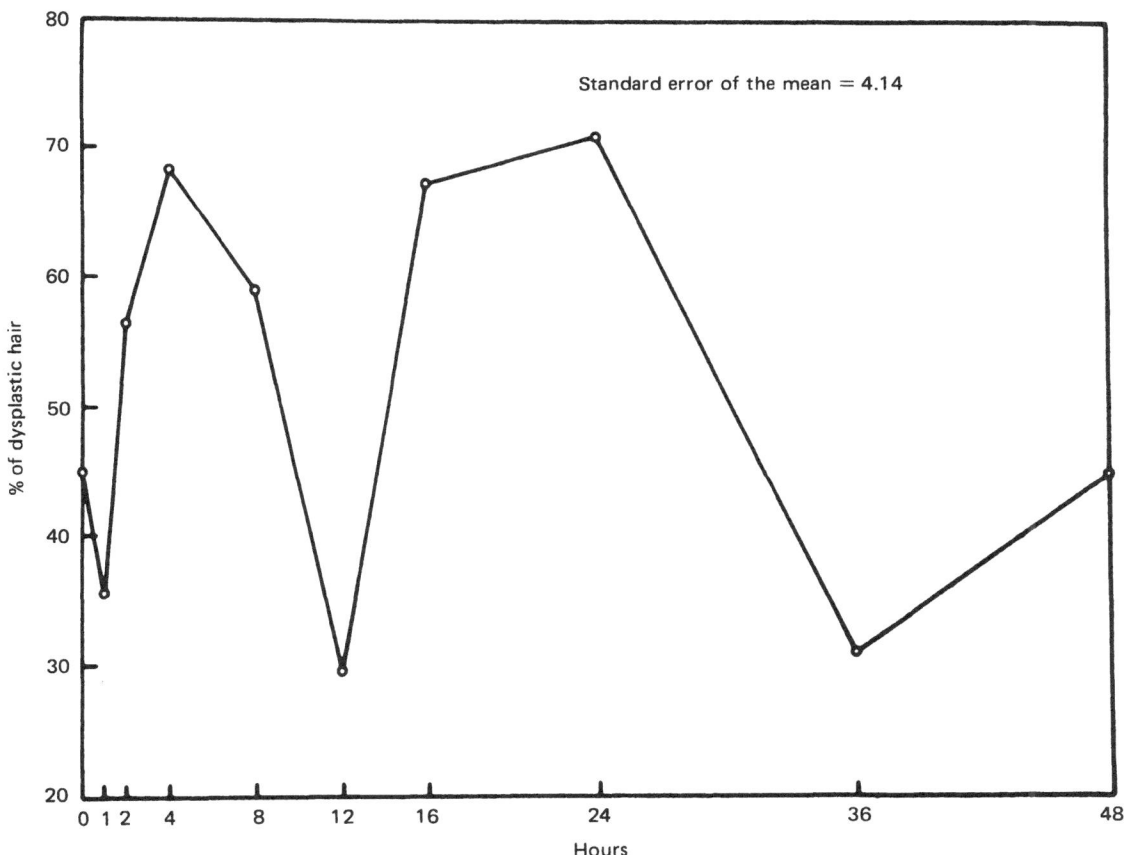

Figure 3-4. Effects of varying the time interval (hr) between injection of actinomycin D 150 μg/kg and administration of x rays (400 rads) on production of dysplastic anagen hairs in different groups of mice. Cyclic synergistic hair damage appeared at the 4- and 16- to 24-hour intervals, with relative protection occurring at the 12-hour period. Actinomycin D 150 μg/kg alone produced no dysplastic anagen hairs. X rays alone (400 rads) damaged 45% of hairs. From Griem and Malkinson [29]. Courtesy of S. Karger, Basel.

lay in Chinese hamster cells. Radiat Res 44:780, 1970

2. Bagshaw MA, Doggett RLS, Smith KC, et al: Intraarterial 5-bromodeoxyuridine and x-ray therapy. Am J Roentgenol 99:886, 1967
3. Baserga R: A radioautographic study of the uptake of C^{14}-leucine by tumor cells in desoxyribonucleic acid synthesis. Biochim Biophys Acta 61:445, 1962
4. Beltz RE, Applegate RL: X-ray inhibition of enzyme changes associated with DNA synthesis of liver regeneration. Biochem Biophys Res Commun 1:298, 1959
5. Beltz RE, Van Lanker J, Potter VR: Nucleic acid metabolism in regenerating rat liver. IV. The effect of x-radiation of the whole body on nucleic acid synthesis in vivo. Cancer Res 17:688, 1957
6. Bergonié J, Tribondeau L: Interprétation de quelques résultats de la radiothérapie et effets de fixation d'une technique rationnelle. C. R. Ste Biol 143:983, 1906
7. Blood AD, Tijo JH: In vivo effects of diagnostic x-irradiation on human chromosomes. N Engl J Med 270:1341, 1964
8. Bollum FJ, Anderegg JW, McElya AB, et al: Nucleic acid metabolism in regenerating rat liver. VII. Effect of x-radiation on enzymes of DNA synthesis. Cancer Res 20:138, 1960
9. Caldwell WL, Lamerton LF, Bewley DK: Increased sensitivity of in vitro murine leukemia cells to fractionated x-rays and fast neutrons. Nature 208:168, 1965
10. Cater DB, Holmes BE, Mee LK: Cell division and nucleic acid synthesis in the regenerating liver of the rat. Acta Radiol 46:655, 1965
11. Cattaneo SM, Quastler H, Sherman FG: DNA synthesis in x-irradiated hair follicles. Radiat Res 11:437, 1959
12. Coggle JE: Effect of cell cycle recovery from radiation damage in the mouse liver. Nature 217:180, 1968
13. Conti RG, Spear FG: The effect of gamma irradiation on cell division in tissue culture in vitro. Proc R Soc B 102:92, 1927
14. De Hevesy G: Radioactive Indicators. New York, Interscience, 1948
15. Dewey WC, Humphrey RM: Relative radiosensitivity of different phases in the life cycle of L-P59 mouse fibroblasts and ascites tumor cells. Radiat Res 16:503, 1962
16. Dewey WC, Humphrey RM: Relative radiosensitivity of different phases in the life cycle of L-P59 mouse fibroblasts and ascites tumor cells. Radiat Res 16:503, 1962
17. Dewey WC, Humphrey RM: Restitution of radiation-induced chromosomal damage in Chinese hamster cells related to cells' life cycle. Exp Cell Res 35:262, 1964
18. Dewey WC, Humphrey RM: Radiosensitivity and recovery of radiation damage in relation to cell cycle. In Cellular Radiation Biology: 18th Symposium on Fundamental Cancer Research, M.D. Anderson Hospital and Tumor Institute. Baltimore, Williams and Wilkins, 1965, pp 340–375
19. Dewey WC, Noel JS, Dettor CM: Changes in radiosensitivity and dispersion of chromatin during the cell cycle of synchronous Chinese hamster cells. Radiat Res 52:373, 1972
20. Djordjevic B, Szybalski W: Genetics of human cell lines. III. Incorporation of 5-bromo- and 5-iododeoxyuridine into the deoxyribonucleic acid of human cells and its effect on radiation sensitivity. J Exp Med 112:509, 1960
21. Doida Y, Okada S: Radiation-induced mitotic delay in cultured mammalian cells (L 5178 Y). Radiat Res 38:513, 1969
22. Elkind MM, Han A, Volz KW: Radiation response of mammalian cells grown in culture. IV. Dose dependence of division delay and postirradiation growth of surviving and nonsurviving Chinese hamster cells. J Natl Cancer Inst 30:705, 1963
23. Elkind MM, Han A, Volz KW: Radiation response of mammalian cells grown in culture. IV. Dose dependence of division delay and postirradiation growth of surviving and nonsurviving Chinese hamster cells. J Natl Cancer Inst 30:705, 1963
24. Elkind MM, Whitmore GF, Alescio T: Actinomycin D. Suppression of recovery in x-irradiated mammalian cells. Science 143:1454, 1964
25. Erikson RL, Szybalski W: Molecular radiobiology of human cell lines. IV. Variation in ultraviolet and x-ray sensitivity during the division cycle. Radiat Res 18:200, 1963
26. Frindel E, Tubiana M, Vassort F: The generation cycle of mouse bone marrow. Nature 214:1017, 1967
27. Gaudin D, Yielding KL: Response of a "resistant" plasmacytoma to alkylating agents and x-ray in combination with the excision repair inhibitors caffeine and chloroquine. Proc Soc Exp Biol Med 131:1413, 1969
28. Goldstein R, Okada S: Further studies of radiation-induced interphase death of cultured mammalian cells. Radiat Res 51:685, 1972
29. Griem ML, Malkinson FD: Some effects of radiations and radiation modifiers on growing hair. Progress review. In Vaeth JM (ed): Frontiers of Radiation Therapy and Oncology, Vol. 4. Basel, Karger, 1969, pp 24–45
30. Harrington H: The effect of x-irradiation on the

progress of strain V-12 fibroblasts through the mitotic cycle. Ann NY Acad Sci 95:901, 1961

31. Hewitt HB, Wilson CW: Survival curve for mammalian leukemia cells irradiated in vivo. Br J Cancer 13:69, 1959

32. Hopwood LE, Tolmach LJ: Deficient DNA synthesis and mitotic death in x-irradiated HeLa cells. Radiat Res 46:70, 1971

33. Howard A, Pelc SR: Synthesis of desoxyribonucleic acid in normal and irradiated cells and its relation to chromosome breakage. Heredity (suppl) 6:261, 1953

34. Hurwitz C, Tolmach LJ: Time-lapse cinematographic studies of x-irradiated HeLa S3 cells. II. Cell fusion. Biophys J 9:1131, 1969

35. Kaplan HS: DNA strand scission and loss of viability after x-irradiation of normal and sensitized bacterial cells. Proc Natl Acad Sci 55:1442, 1966

36. Kim JH, Evans TC: Effects of x-irradiation on the mitotic cycle of Ehrlich ascites tumor cells. Radiat Res 21:129, 1964

37. Kim JH, Evans TC: Effects of x-irradiation on the mitotic cycle of Ehrlich ascites tumor cells. Radiat. Res 21:584, 1964

38. Klouwen HM, Appelman AWM, Betel I: The biochemical basis of cell death in interphase. In The Cell Nucleus. Metabolism and Radiosensitivity. London, Taylor and Francis, 1966, pp 295–303

39. Lajtha LG, Oliver R, Berry R, et al: Mechanism of radiation effect on the process of synthesis of DNA. Nature 182:1788, 1958

40. Lajtha LG, Oliver RP, Kumatori T, et al: On the mechanism of radiation effect on DNA synthesis. Radiat. Res 8:1, 1958

41. Little JB, Parups D: Radiation effects on DNA synthesis and cell division in human cell cultures with long generation time. Radiat Res 31:606, 1967

42. Lozzio CB: Radiosensitivity of Ehrlich ascites tumor cells. I. Variation in x-ray sensitivity during the cell cycle. Int J Radiat Biol 14:133, 1968

43. Madoc-Jones H, Mauro F: Age responses to x-rays, vinca alkaloids, and hydroxyurea of murine lymphoma cells synchronized in vivo. J Natl Cancer Inst 45:1131, 1970

44. Mak S, Till JE: Effects of x-rays on progress of L-cells through cell cycle. Radiat. Res 20:600, 1963

45. Malkinson FD: Epidermal cell kinetics. Some general considerations and implications in skin disease and therapy. In Year Book of Dermatology. Chicago, Year Book Medical, 1972, pp 5–37

46. Malkinson FD, Griem ML: Radiation injury and recovery in anagen and telogen rodent hairs. Radiat Res 33:554, 1968

47. Malkinson FD, Griem ML, Marianovic R: Effects of hydroxyurea and radiation on hair matrix cells. Cell Tissue Kinet 6:395, 1973

48. Malkinson FD, Griem ML, Marianovic R: Follicle squash preparations. Uses in studies of cell kinetics following irradiation. J Invest Dermatol 57:382, 1971

49. Malkinson FD, Griem ML, Morse PH: Colchicine synergism of mouse hair root changes produced by x-ray irradiation. J Invest Dermatol 37:337, 1961

50. Marin G, Bender MA: Radiation-induced mammalian cell death. Lapse-time cinematographic observations. Exp Cell Res 43:413, 1966

51. Michison JM: The Biology of the Cell Cycle. Cambridge, Cambridge Univ Press, 1971, pp 25–57

52. Muller HJ: Artificial transmutation of the gene. Science 66:84, 1927

53. Munro TR: The site of the target region for radiation-induced mitotic delay in cultured mammalian cells. Radiat Res 44:748, 1970

54. Newcombe HB: The genetic effects of ionizing radiations. Adv Genet 16:239, 1971

55. Odartchenko N, Cottier H, Feinendegen LE, et al: Mitotic delay in more mature erythroblasts of the dog, induced in vivo by sublethal doses of x-rays. Radiat Res 21:413, 1964

56. Ord MG, Stocken LA: Radiobiological lesions in animal cells. Nature 182:1787, 1958

57. Potten CS: Some observations on melanin synthesis anomalies in mouse hair follicles after treatment with x-rays or actinomycin D. Radiat Res 51:167, 1972

58. Puck TT, Marcus PI: Action of x-rays on mammalian cells. J Exp Med 103:653, 1956

59. Puck TT, Steffen J: Life cycle analysis of mammalian cells. I. Method for localizing metabolic events within life cycle, and its application to action of colcemide and sublethal doses of x-irradiation. Biophys J 3:379, 1963

60. Russell WL, Russell LB, Kelly, E: Dependence of mutation rate on radiation intensity. Int J Radiat Biol (Suppl) 1:311, 1960

61. Rustad BC, Burchill BR: Radiation induced mitotic delay in sea urchin eggs treated with puromycin and actinomycin D. Radiat Res 29:203, 1966

62. Schneiderman MH, Dewey WC, Leeper DB, et al: Use of the mitotic selection procedure for cell cycle analysis. Exp Cell Res 74:430, 1972

63. Schrek R: In vitro sensitivity of normal human lymphocytes to x-rays and radiomimetic agents. J Lab Clin Med 51:904, 1958

64. Shipley WU, Elkind MM, Prather WB: Potentiation of x-ray killing by 5-bromodeoxyuridine in Chinese hamster cells. A radiation incapacity

for sublethal damage accumulation. Radiat Res 47:437, 1971

65. Sinclair WK: Cyclic x-ray responses in mammalian cells in vitro. Radiat Res 33:620, 1968

66. Sinclair WK: X-ray induced heritable damage (small-colony formation) in cultured mammalian cells. Radiat. Res 21:584, 1964

67. Sinclair WK: The combined effect of hydroxyurea and x-rays in Chinese hamster cells in vitro. Cancer Res 28:198, 1968

68. Sinclair WK, Morton RA: X-ray sensitivity during the cell generation cycle of cultured Chinese hamster cells. Radiat Res 29:450, 1966

69. Smets LA, Dewaide H: A reparative synthesis of DNA after x-irradiation. Naturwissenschaften 53:382, 1966

70. Taylor JH: Nucleic acid synthesis in relation to the cell division cycle. Ann NY Acad Sci 90:409, 1960

71. Terasima T, Tolmach LJ: Variations in several responses of HeLa cells to x-irradiation during division cycle. Biophys J 3:11, 1963

72. Terasima T, Tolmach LJ: Variations in several responses of HeLa cells to x-irradiation during the division cycle. Biophys J 3:11, 1963

73. Tolmach LJ, Weiss BG, Hopwood LE: Ionizing radiations and the cell cycle. Fed Proc 30:1742, 1971

74. Walters RA, Peterson DF: Radiosensitivity of mammalian cells. II. Radiation effects on macromolecular synthesis. Biophys J 8:1487, 1968

75. Watanube I, Okada S: Deoxyribonucleic acid synthesis during the first postirradiation life cycle of lethally irradiated cultured mammalian cells (L5178Y). Radiat Res 35:202, 1968

76. Whitmore GF, Till JE: Quantitation of cellular radiobiological responses. Ann Rev Nucl Sci 14:347, 1964

77. Whitmore GF, Till JE, Gulyas S: Radiation-induced mitotic delay in L cells. Radiat Res 30:155, 1967

78. Wolff S: Chromosome aberrations and the cell cycle. Radiat Res 33:609, 1968

79. Yu CK, Sinclair WK: Division delay and chromosomal aberrations induced by x-rays in synchronized Chinese hamster cells in vitro. J Natl Cancer Inst 39:619, 1967

4

Radiation Protection

Arthur H. Gladstein

The dermatologist is responsible for the radiation protection of the geographic vicinity, the patient, and, of course, himself and the office personnel. The following assumptions will be made: (1) Very deep, bone-fixed lesions are not treated, and therefore only relatively short exposures are used. (2) Voltages do not routinely exceed 100 kV (100 kV; HVL, 1.0 mm Al; $D_{1/2}$, 20 mm).

Radiation Protection of the Geographic Vicinity

The dermatologist becomes involved in radiation protection of his immediate environment the moment he turns on his x-ray machine. Three kinds of radiation are produced during x-ray therapy (Fig. 4-1). The *direct* or *useful* beam is the only one in which he is interested. However, there is always some leakage and scattered radiation which bounces off the patient, table, walls, and so forth. The amount of scattered radiation is a function of the kilovoltage. The dermatologic radiotherapist should always use the lowest effective kV, HVL, and $D_{1/2}$. For benign conditions, he should begin therapy with nonradiologic methods. He should resort to radiation only if these other methods fail. If grenz rays (14 kV; HVL, 0.03 mm Al; $D_{1/2}$, 0.6 mm) will suffice, conventional superficial radiation (100 kV; HVL, 1.0 mm Al; $D_{1/2}$, 20 mm) should not be used.

The relationship between scatter and kilovoltage is shown in Fig. 4-2. Scattered radiation reaching the patient can be minimized by covering the patient with lead–rubber sheeting, or leaded plastic sheeting of equivalent protective value. If the dermatologist is using an ordinary examining table as his x-ray table, this too should be covered by a suitable leaded material.

The use of cones will substantially help to reduce scatter. Proper technique mandates the use of cones in most conditions (for further discussion, see below). Open-field therapy is the rare exception rather than the ordinary rule.

Leaked radiation cannot be completely eliminated. However, it has been substantially reduced since the time when x-ray tubes were not properly shielded. The only practical solution is to obtain and use a machine with a therapeutic-type housing (see Glossary). The manufacturers of such machines must meet government standards. Handbook No. 76 of the National Council on Radiation Protection and Measurements [4a] states that a therapeutic-type protective tube housing shall be "so constructed that leakage radiation at a distance of 1 m from the target cannot exceed 1 R in 1 hr, and at a distance of 5 cm from any point on the surface of the housing accessible to the patient, cannot exceed 30 R in 1 hr, when the tube is operated at any of its specified ratings."

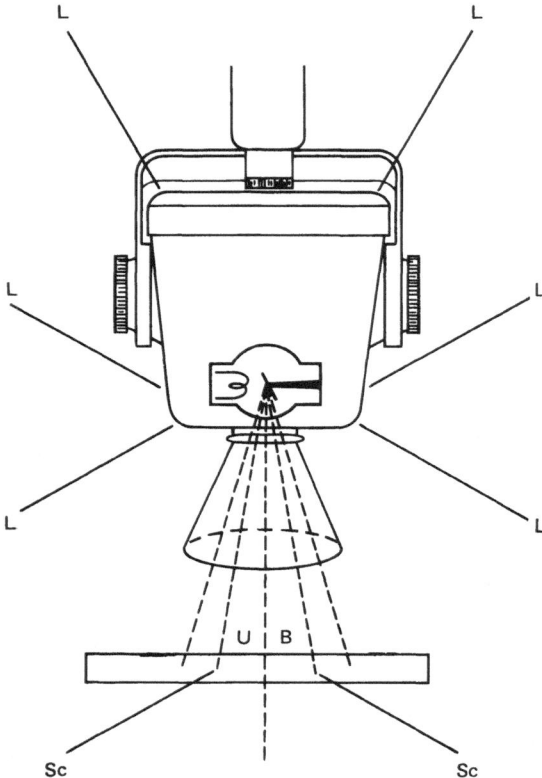

Figure 4-1. Types of radiation produced by an x-ray machine. UB, useful beam primary radiation; L, leakage radiation; Sc, scattered radiation. Modified from [4].

Proper placement of the x-ray tube head is important to the protection of both the environment and the patient. Except during teleroentgen therapy, the x-ray tube head should be perpendicular to the lesion(s) on the patient, who is best positioned horizontally and comfortably on the table. Only hands and arms may be treated with the patient in a sitting position. Foolish as it may sound, many errors are made because of improper placement of the x-ray tube head. Many dermatologists starting in practice frequently place their x-ray machines in the smallest room available. This may cause difficulties in treatment. For example, if a tall person is placed on a table in a tiny room, the tube frequently must be angled to treat the feet (Fig. 4-3). Some radiation so directed will permeate walls and may reach persons in other rooms. It must be possible to center the x-ray tube so that it is over the table and so that all radiation falls within the confines of the table.

Principles of teleroentgen protection will be discussed below.

Distance, time, and structural shielding are the main factors in protection from external sources of radiation.

Let us take a simple hypothetical example to demonstrate the manipulation of these factors. Assume we have a 3-room office with an x-ray machine in room *B* (Fig. 4-4). Room *A* is the waiting room with a receptionist seated at her desk at *O*. The x-ray machine is 3 m away in room *B*. What sort of protection is needed on the wall between rooms *A* and *B* to provide the receptionist with safe working conditions? To make this determination we must take into account the three kinds of x-rays that have to be considered in radiation protection, ie, useful, leakage, and scattered. It is estimated that the x-ray machine will be used a maximum of 2 hr per week.

Useful Radiation

Calibration shows that our x-ray machine produces 120 R at a 20 cm TSD in 3 min at 100 kV (HVL, 1.0 mm Al; $D_{1/2}$, 20 mm). We assume the beam will be directed at the wall one-third of the time. How many roentgens will reach *O*,

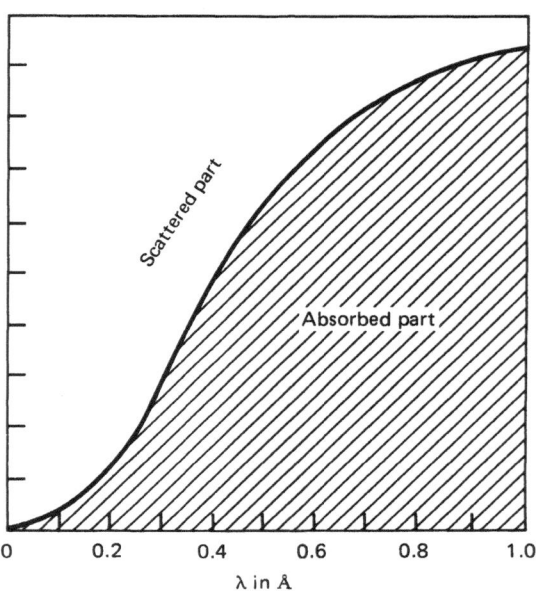

Figure 4-2. Scattered and absorbed parts of radiations of different wavelengths in water or tissue. From Fuhs H, Konrad J: Grenzstrahl Hauttherapie. Berlin, Urban & Schwartzenberg, 1931 [3].

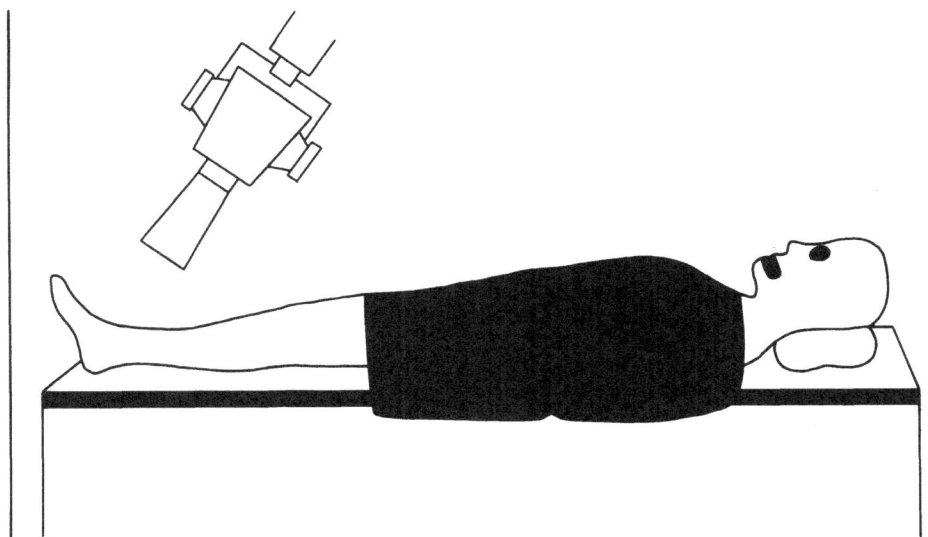

Figure 4-3. Improper shielding technique for treatment of a tall person. Modified from [4].

3 m distant? Using the inverse square law and converting meters to centimeters, we have the following:

$$40 \times (20/300)^2 = 0.177 \text{ R in 3 min,}$$
which is equivalent to 3.54 R per hr

Leakage Radiation

The leakage is 1 R at 1 m in 1 hr. If the machine were used for 1 hr, how much radiation would "leak" into room *A*? Again, using the inverse square law, the value will be:

$$1 \times (1/3)^2 = 0.11 \text{ R}$$

Scattered Radiation

If a lesion is treated by open-field therapy, 0.1% of the perpendicularly directed radiation (useful beam) is scattered at right angles to that direction.

$$3.54 \times 0.001 = 0.003 \text{ R}$$

If we now add the three components, the following is obtained:

Useful radiation	3.54
Leakage radiation	0.11
Scattered radiation	0.003
Total	3.653 R/hr

Thus, the total radiation reaching *O* in 1 week (2 hr use) equals 7.2 R.

Referring to standard lead-attenuation curves for 100-kV x rays, we find that to reduce 7.2 R to 0.01 R per week (maximum permissible dose (MPD) for an average person), the lead necessary will be about 1.4 mm in thickness. This is a large amount of lead and would be quite expensive to obtain and install. A better solution to the problem would be to change the arrangement of the office (Fig. 4-5). *A* should remain as the waiting room, with *B* as the consultation room and *C* as the x-ray room. The x-ray room should preferably be an end room away from the flow of traffic. Ideally, there should be no occupancies below or around it. The control panel for the machine should be in a hallway. Most physicians them-

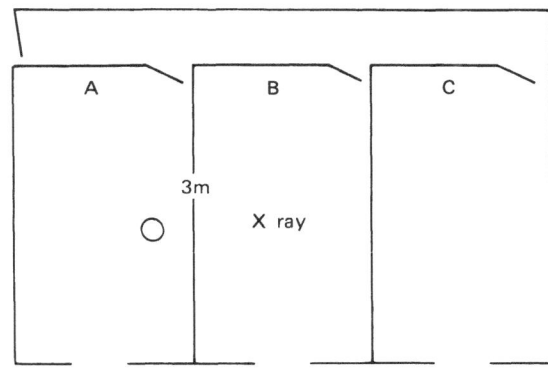

Figure 4-4. Diagram of hypothetical office layout. Distance from x-ray machine in room *B* to where receptionist sits in room *A* is 3 m.

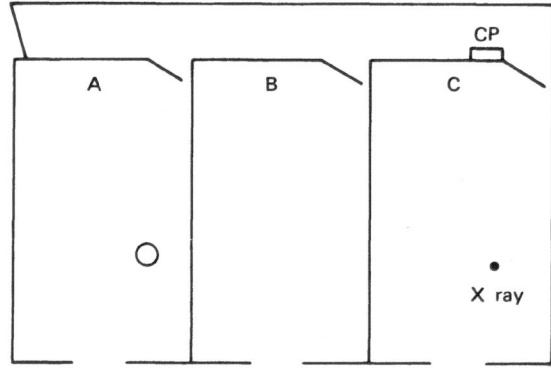

Figure 4-5. Suggested layout for good radiation protection. Room *B* is used for consultation.

selves operate their x-ray machines. This is another reason for placing the consultation room in the center. Only one person other than the patient, ie, the physician himself, could then be exposed to stray radiation.

It must be strongly emphasized that the aforementioned suggestions are highly oversimplified. The actual calculations necessary in particular instances may be quite involved and complicated. It is recommended that the doctor *not* do them himself. A registered physicist or health safety officer *must* be consulted for this purpose.

Radiation Protection of the Patient

If a combination superficial x-ray–grenz-ray machine is purchased, it will undoubtedly have a beryllium window. Such units are capable of delivering extremely high (and potentially dangerous) dosages. It is because of the possibility of such a tremendous output that serious accidents have occurred with the use of combination machines. If a controlling filter is not inserted, there may be two possible sources of error. First, the number of roentgens received by the patient may be many times the amount

planned; second, the depth dose may be less than contemplated, ie, too many roentgens may be delivered to the topmost layers of the skin and thus too few will penetrate to the desired depth. For proper radiation protection, a combination machine should have an automatic interlock system. For any kilovoltages about 15 kV, the machine should be automatically inoperable unless the filter has been inserted. Table 4-1 shows the actual calibration of a beryllium-window x-ray tube. It illustrates the changes in percentage depth dose and $D_{1/2}$ when appropriate filters are used.

Cones are essential to good radiation technique and should be used wherever possible. They are indispensable for good radiation protection for several reasons (Fig. 4-6).

1. They limit the exposure to the area of clinical interest only.
2. They firmly hold shielding in place.
3. They facilitate accuracy in measurement of distance.
   a. This is quite important because the dose rate varies inversely with the square of the distance.
   b. The x-ray machine must be calibrated with the exact cone in place. The physician should not use the measurement for distance without the cone, assuming that the same dose will obtain with the cone. It is not unusual to have a 5% or greater difference in dose rates with and without cones.
4. Cones are most effective in reducing scattered radiation.

For radiation energies used in dermatologic radiotherapy, lead, either in the form of sheets, or incorporated into rubber or other plastics, is the shielding material of choice. Lead is used for the following reasons.

1. Lead is a good absorber of x rays. Table 4-2 [4] shows the thickness of lead necessary to

Table 4-1 *Calibration Data for a Beryllium-window Tube (100 kV; 15 cm TSD)*

mA	Filter	HVL (mm Al)	$D_{1/2}$ (mm tissue)	R/min in Air	% Dose (5 mm below surface)
5	none	0.08	2.2	6500	20
	0.5	0.75	11	380	72
	1.0	1.3	16	200	80
	2.0	2.1	24	137	86
	3.0	3.0	32	100	90

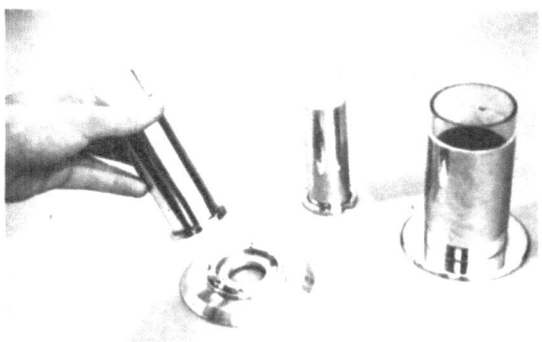

Figure 4-6. Cones for dermatologic radiation therapy.

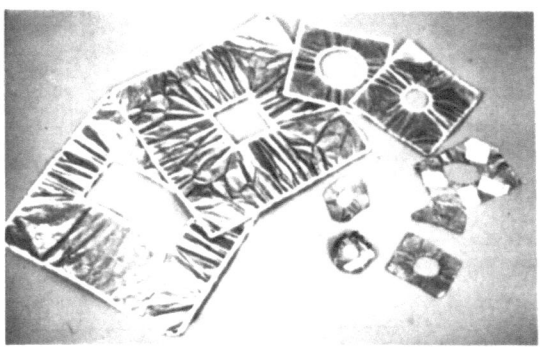

Figure 4-7. Lead shields prepared from rolls.

Table 4-2 *Thickness of Lead Necessary to Reduce Useful Beam to 5% [4]*

Tube potential (kVp)	HVL (mm)	Lead (mm)
60*	1.2 Al	0.10
100	1.0 Al	0.15
100	2.0 Al	0.25
100	3.0 Al	0.35
140	0.5 Cu	0.70

*The radiation produced at 60 kVp is filtered in order to give a HVL of 1.2 mm Al. Although the useful beam has a higher HVL than that produced at 100 kVp, the hardest rays produced at 60 kVp are not as hard as those produced at 100 kVp. Therefore, less lead is required to reduce the useful beam to 5% of its original value.

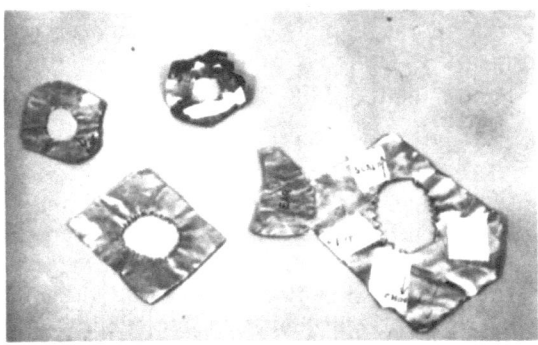

Figure 4-8. Close-up of Fig. 4-7 showing serrations and markings.

reduce the useful beam to 5% of its original intensity. Note that lead of 0.3 to 0.5 mm thickness should suffice for most dermatologic therapeutic situations.

2. Lead sheeting, since it is not rigid, can be molded and bent to fit body contours.

3. Lead sheeting can be cut easily with ordinary scissors, thus assuring accurate shielding and exposure. For areas such as the forehead, the opening in a shield may be serrated in order to blend depigmentation and thus improve the final cosmetic result. After the lead is cut, one must smooth the edges of the shield, because a jagged edge may gouge the patient when the weight of the machine through a cone is brought to bear on the area. Figure 4-7 illustrates various types of lead shielding. Note that each shield is so identified that it can be placed in exactly the same position for each treatment (Fig. 4-8).

4. Lead can be coated with other materials such as copper, silver, cadmium, and wax. This forms the basis of the "tongue" eye shield which will be discussed in the chapter on Radiotherapy of Cutaneous Malignancies.

Principles of X-ray Protection

There are four simple principles which, if followed, should properly protect the patient during x-ray therapy.

1. Whenever possible use a cone instead of an open field.
2. The x-ray tube should be perpendicular to the area treated.
3. The tube should be directed away from the gonads.
4. The eyes, thyroid, and gonads should always be protected when treating head and neck areas or using an open field.

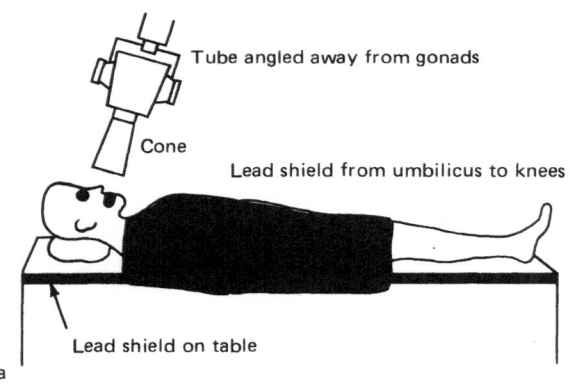

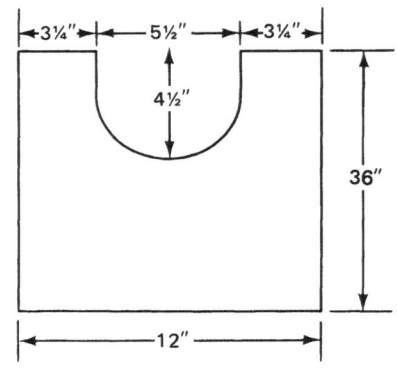

Figure 4-9a,b. Shielding technique for treatment of face. Modified from [4].

Let us apply these principles to treatment of various areas of the body. (Radiation protection measures for grenz-ray techniques are discussed in Chapters 14 and 15.)

Head

The head must be placed on a sandbag to be able to angle the target away from the gonads (Fig. 4-9). In treating diffuse, crudely separated lesions an open field may be necessary because the cone may not be sufficiently large. In such a case, the lips and hair line would also have to be protected (note shielding of lips in Fig. 4-9a).

A lead–rubber (or equivalent) shield (Fig. 4-9b) should extend from the neck (to protect the thyroid) to the knees (to protect the gonads). The top of this shield should be cut to fit securely around the neck.

Upper Extremity

A sandbag is used to elevate the hand. This allows the tube to be angled away from the gonads (Fig. 4-10). Note lead–rubber shield covering gonads and eyes directed away from the target in Figure 4-12.

Special Situations

For detailed shielding procedures utilized in treating malignancies of the ear, eye, nose, lip, and canthus see Chapter 9. Shielding techniques for radiotherapy of other body areas are illustrated in Figs. 4-11–4-16.

Gonads

One aim of dermatologic radiation therapy is to keep the gonadal dose to the lowest levels possible. With the proper understanding and use of those factors that influence the go-

nadal dose during x-ray therapy, it is not difficult to approach acceptable levels of exposure [8].

Using the new lithium fluoride disks, Petratos et al [5] measured exposure to the breasts, thyroid, and genital area during the course of treatment of basal cell carcinomas of the face using a standard technique. Their results are shown in Table 4-3 [2]. Note that the dose to the gonadal area was extremely small. Indeed, the highest exposure of only about 2 R

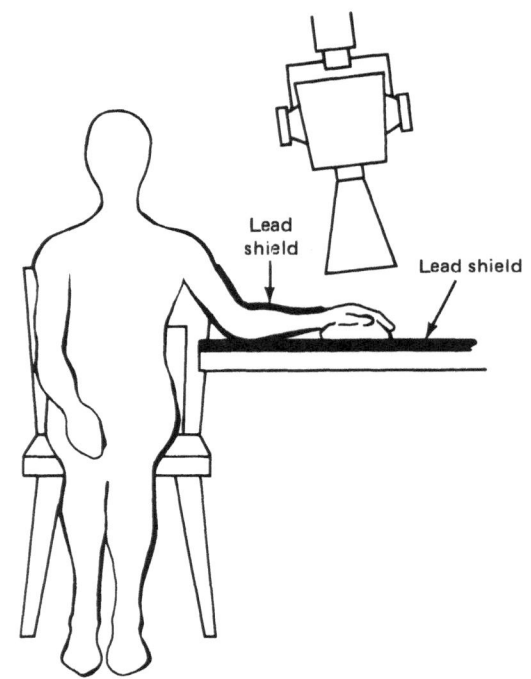

Figure 4-10. Shielding technique for treatment of hand. Note that all radiation falls within the confines of the table. Modified from [4].

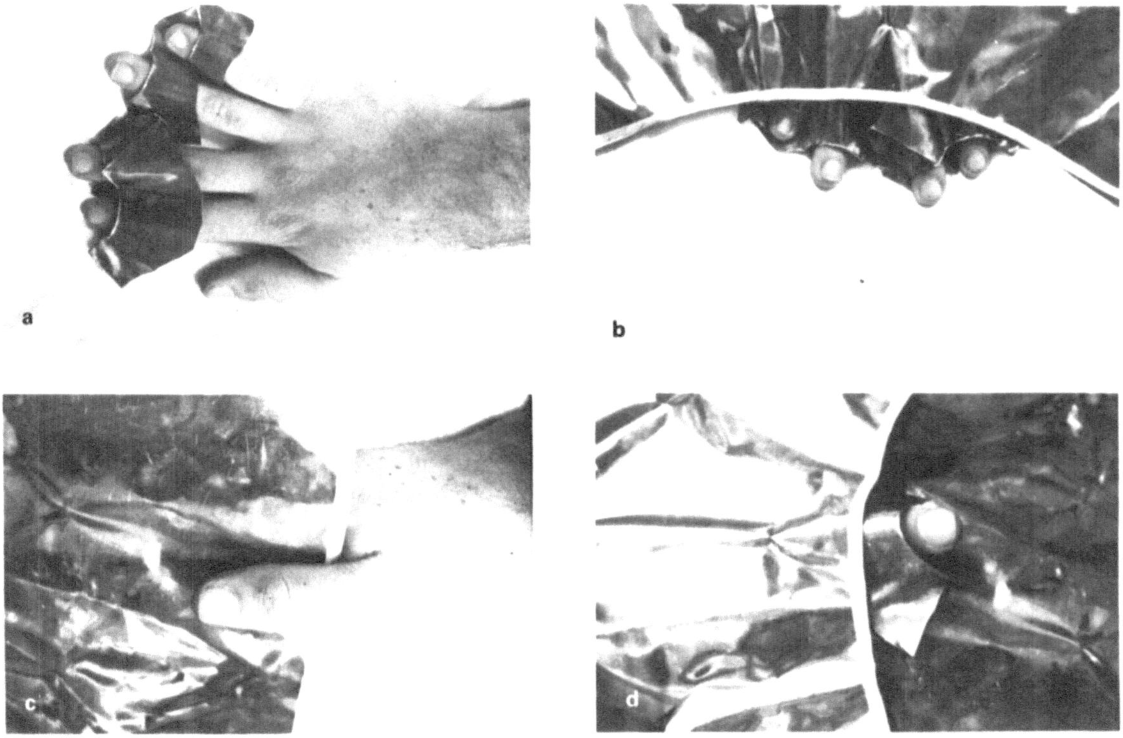

Figure 4-11a–d.   Shielding technique for treatment of finger nails (paronychia).

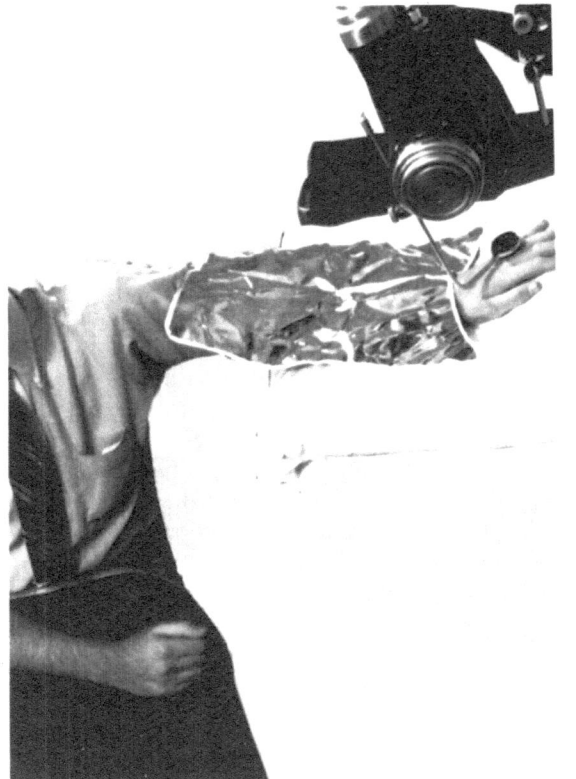

Figure 4-12.   Shielding technique for treatment of hand. Open field (compare with Fig. 4-10).

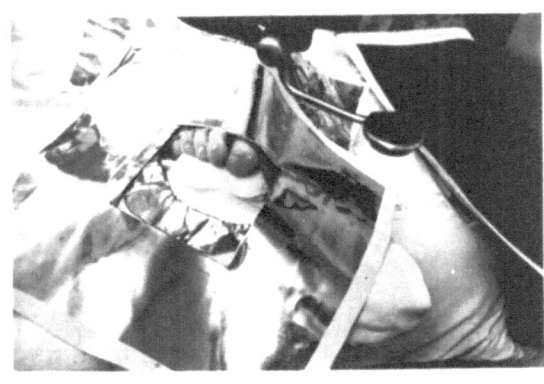

Figure 4-13.   Shielding technique for treatment of toe nails. Open field.

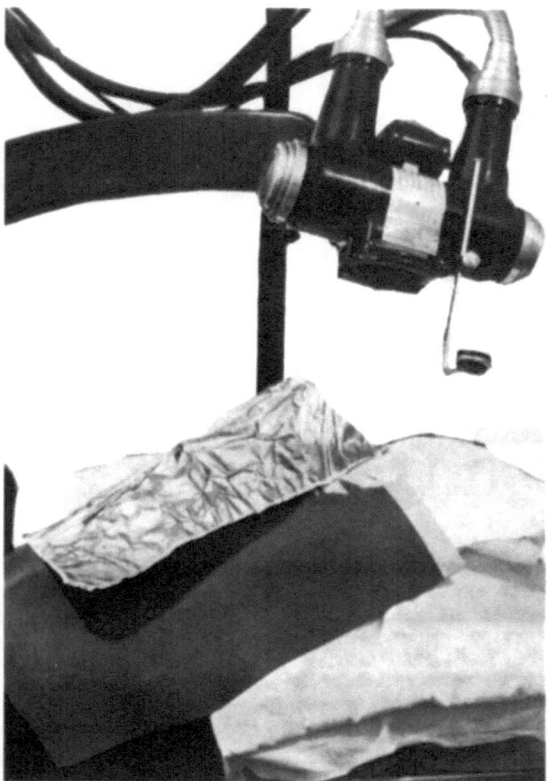

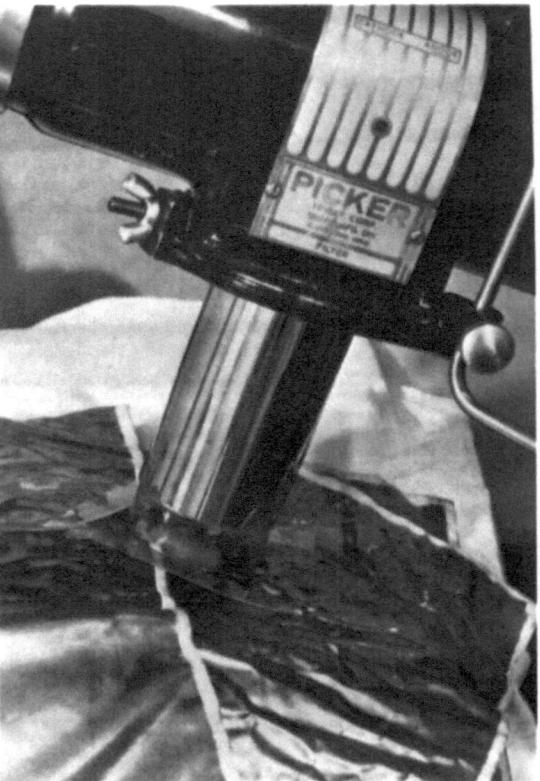

Figure 4-14. Shielding technique for treatment of sole. Open field (compare with Fig. 4-15).

Figure 4-15. Shielding technique for treatment of plantar wart. Wherever possible, cones are preferred to open fields.

was to the thyroid area. Considering that the average dose to the face was 3400 R, the described manner of irradiation resulted in minimal scatter.

Lowest Effective kV (HVL, $D_{1/2}$)

Current concepts of dermatologic radiation therapy have recently undergone profound changes. In the not too distant past, radiation therapy seemed to have been used for almost everything. Shelley [6] wrote: "Here was a

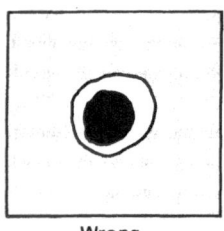

Wrong

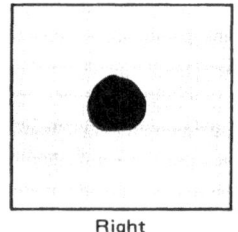

Right

Figure 4-16. Shielding technique for radiotherapy of plantar wart.

modality which removed unwanted hair, provided palliation for chronic eczema, shrunk hemangiomas, and cleared psoriasis as well as warts. It even fit shoes!" Fortunately, this is no longer the rule. For benign lesions, radiation should not be the initial method of choice. Nonradiologic modalities should be employed first. Radiation should be considered only if these fail—provided the condition is radiosensitive and the dosage required is not excessive or dangerous. To ascertain a safe dosage of radiation in benign conditions, Sulzberger et al [7] examined 1000 patients irradiated for benign conditions at the New York University Skin and Cancer Unit and compared them to 1000 control patients. Based upon the large sample so investigated and the findings on reexamination, they inferred:

There is no evidence that any sequelae are produced by totals of 1000 R or less of superficial x-ray treatment in the fractional doses and in the qualities employed for the treatment of benign dermatoses

TABLE 4-3 *Stray X-Radiation**

		Skin-Surface Dose in Roentgens at:					
		Thyroid	*Breast*	*Pubis*	*Iliac Crest*	*Coccyx*	*Inner Thigh*
Men	Average	0.85	0.24	0.20	—	0.29	0.23
(8 Subjects)	Range	0.09–2.4	0.04–0.5	0.04–0.52	—	0.04–1.17	0.02–0.52
Women	Average	0.72	0.32	—	0.09	0.12	—
(8 Subjects)	Range	0.13–2.3	0.09–0.9	—	0.04–0.21	0.04–0.32	—

*When 3400 R ("Standard Schedule") were delivered to facial basal-cell epitheliomas.

such as acne vulgaris, eczema, neurodermatitis, and psoriasis.

These findings are the basis of our rule at the Skin and Cancer Unit limiting the *total lifetime dosage to any single area to 1000 R* for benign conditions.

For malignant lesions such as basal cell carcinoma, squamous cell carcinoma, mycosis fungoides, Kaposi's sarcoma, Bowen's disease, and intraepidermal basal cell epitheliomatosis, radiation therapy is used extensively and very successfully. See Chapters 9 and 10 for a detailed discussion of dosages and techniques.

For both benign and malignant conditions, the proper kind of radiation must be employed. Its penetration should correspond to the depth of the process. For example, if lichen planus will respond to radiation with a $D_{1/2}$ of 20 mm or 3 mm, the latter should be preferentially used. Similarly, for the ordinary basal cell carcinoma which does not extend deeply, 140-kV radiation is not the modality of choice (Chapter 6).

In general, the use of the lowest effective radiation qualities will provide patients with the best radiation protection available today.

Radiation Protection of Office Personnel

It is assumed that the physician has consulted a physicist or radiation health officer to ensure that his office conforms to current standards.

The x-ray machine must be calibrated for all distances, filters, cones, and half-value layers that will be used. There must be no guesswork in the use of radiation. It is the dermatologist's responsibility to inform the physicist of all the factors necessary to treat a patient prop-

erly. It is not enough merely to instruct the physicist to calibrate the machine. A useful procedure for the novice dermatologist is to obtain a copy of the calibrations used at his teaching center, and have the physicist duplicate these as closely as possible. The dermatologist will then be dealing with a familiar set of calculations.

The screen behind which the operator stands must be radioopaque and sufficiently wide and long so that the operator is adequately protected.

The window in the screen must be composed of lead glass, and be of sufficient thickness to absorb the energies employed. The x-ray machine should be so wired that it will automatically shut off if the door to the room is opened during treatment; the x-ray machine should not be operable if the door is not completely closed. In addition, there should be a light above the outside of the door which stays on while treatment is being given.

Preferably, the screen on which the control panel is located should be placed outside the room. If the patient should move during treatment, the machine must be shut off before the operator comes out from behind the screen to readjust the patient.

If an infant or an elderly person is to be treated and if the patient cannot remain still, a member of the family, preferably one past the child-bearing age, protected by a fluoroscopic apron and lead gloves, should hold the patient still. This task should not be done by the operator or an office assistant.

One of the main disadvantages of contact therapy is the amount of stray radiation reaching the operator. To be properly protected, the operator should wear a lead fluoroscopic apron and lead gloves.

A film badge, a necessary item of radiologic equipment, is essentially a piece of film enclosed in a suitable holder. It is worn by x-ray personnel to measure their exposure to radiation. It is the cheapest, most practical means of accomplishing this purpose.

The film, after being exposed to an unknown amount of radiation (new badges are usually issued monthly), is developed under standard conditions. Its density is compared to that of a sample of the same film, processed in a similar manner, but exposed to a known amount of radiation. Film badges may also be placed on walls and in corridors as an aid in radiation surveys. The film badges are sent monthly to a laboratory and a "film badge dosimetry report" is returned.

Glossary

"Useful" beam. The useful beam is defined as the radiation that passes through the window, cone, or other collimating device of the tube housing.

Scattered radiation. This is radiation which, during its passage through matter, has been deviated from its original direction. It may also have been reduced in energy. Radiation may be scattered by the patient, the shield, the table, objects in the room, or the floor, walls, and ceiling of the room itself. The penetrating power of scattered radiation from dermatologic installations is approximately the same as that of the useful beam. The amount of scattered radiation, measured at an angle of 90° and 1 m from the scatter material, is about 0.1% of that of the useful beam.

Leakage radiation. Leakage radiation is all radiation passing through the tube housing with the exception of the useful radiation. The penetrating power of leakage radiation is greater than that of the useful beam because it has passed through the protective barrier around the tube, which filters out all but the hardest rays. Handbook 76 [1] states that a therapeutic-type protective tube housing shall be "so constructed that leakage radiation at a distance of 1 m from the target cannot exceed 1 R in 1 hr, and at a distance of 5 cm from any point on the surface of the housing accessible to the patient, cannot exceed 30 R in 1 hr, when the tube is operated at any of its specified ratings."

Lead equivalent. The thickness of lead affording the same attenuation, under specified conditions, as the material in question.

Maximum permissible dose (MPD). The maximum RBE dose that the body of a person or specific parts thereof shall be permitted to receive in a stated period of time. For the radiations considered herein, the RBE dose in rems may be considered numerically equal to the absorbed dose in rads and the exposure dose in roentgens numerically equal to the absorbed dose in rads.

Roentgen (R). The unit of exposure dose of x or γ radiation. One roentgen is an exposure dose of x or γ radiation such that the associated corpuscular emission per 0.001293 g of air produces, in air, ions of either sign carrying 1 electrostatic unit of electricity.

References

1. American Academy of Dermatology: Radiation Protection. A Guide for Dermatologists. p 7
2. Bart RS, Lopf AW, Petratos MA: X-ray therapy of skin cancer. Evaluation of a "standardized method for treating basal cell epitheliomas. In Proceedings of the Sixth National Cancer Conference, Lippincott, 1970
3. Bucky G, Combes FC: Grenz Ray Therapy. New York, Springer, 1954
4. Cipollaro AC, Crossland PM: X Rays and Radium in the Treatment of Diseases of the Skin, 5th ed. Philadelphia, Lea & Febiger, 1967
4a. National Council on Radiation Protection and Measurements: Structural Shielding Design and Evaluation for Medical Use of X-Rays and Gamma Rays of Energies up to 10 Me V. Report No. 49, Washington, D.C., 1976
5. Petratos MA, Grisewood EN, Wingate C: Measurement of scattered radiation to body areas during radiotherapy of basal cell epitheliomas. Dermatologica Internationalis 8:10–13, 1969
6. Shelley WB: Consultations in Dermatology. Philadelphia, Saunders, 1972, p 100
7. Sulzberger MB, Baer R, Borota A: Do roentgen-ray treatments as given by skin specialists produce cancers or other sequelae? Arch Dermatol (Suppl) 65:639, 1952
8. Witten VH: Physical methods of protection against ionizing radiation in dermatologic therapy and its importance in relation to gonadal radiation exposure. Proceedings of the XII International Congress, Washington, DC, 1962, Vol 1. Amsterdam, Excerpta Medica, 1962, p 594

5

Radiodermatitis and Other Adverse Sequelae of Cutaneous Irradiation

Robert I. Rudolph and Herbert Goldschmidt

Radiodermatitis may be defined as any deleterious effect produced in the skin and its appendages by radiation which either has been administered in therapeutic applications or received as a consequence of accidental overexposure. The effects may range from an acute inflammatory reaction to a noninflamed chronic condition.

Shortly after the discovery of roentgen rays, it was noted by many workers that both reversible and irreversible effects could be produced in the skin. These early investigators were unaware, of course, of the hazards inherent in long and improperly protected use of ionizing radiation, and quite often the early cases of radiodermatitis reported concerned themselves. In the ensuing years increased awareness of the hazards of radiation; far greater protection for both patient and therapist; correct and frequent calibration of machines; and vast improvements in the design, shielding, and operation of the radiation-producing equipment have dramatically reduced the incidence of untoward effects. At present, however, the cumulative, long-term effects of radiation administered in the last 70 years are becoming increasingly evident.

Until the advent of the roentgen (R) as an accurate measurement of radiation exposure, the delivered dose of radiation could only be crudely expressed in terms of the threshold *erythema dose.* This dosage was the amount of radiation necessary to produce a barely noticeable erythema, and was quite different from person to person and from treatment to treatment, varying according to the voltage, filtration, and type of apparatus being used. Even after the introduction of improved methods for quantifying the dose of radiation, however, most therapists were not aware of the long-term effects of the small, but frequently administered, doses of radiation that they were giving, in as much as the period of developing postirradiation complications is now recognized to be as long as 20 to 60 *years* after treatment. Furthermore, most therapists used only their experience to guide them in determining both the length of an individual treatment and the total number of treatments to be administered. Very often they had no idea at all of the precise physical quality or quantity of radiation their machines were delivering. The availability of modern dermatologic therapy units and the enormous amount of information concerning radiation production and protection are rapidly reducing the untoward effects of radiation.

Primary Effects of Cutaneous Radiation

Several types of effects on skin produced by ionizing radiation have been categorized [21]. These include the following:

1. The *reversible* changes such as erythema, sebaceous gland and eccrine sweat gland suppression, and temporary epilation
2. The *conditional reversible* effects such as long-term pigmentation
3. The *irreversible* manifestations such as radiodermatitis and radiation-induced malignancies
4. *Rare cutaneous reactions* such as erythema multiforme–like eruptions [7]

Radiation (Roentgen) Erythema

Clinical Aspects

The longest-observed and most intensively studied radiation-induced effect is the so-called *roentgen erythema*. Within several minutes of receiving a sufficiently high single dose of radiation,* the skin will show a light pink color in the area of irradiation. This color change is believed to be due to an immediate vascular dilation caused by released histamine or serotonin [61], and persists for about 2 to 3 days as the result of a continued, but decreasing, output of the vasoactive amines. A delayed erythema (the main erythema) then develops at about the eighth to tenth day postirradiation and continues to darken for about 7 to 8 days, sometimes turning a deep violet hue. After this period the erythema slowly fades away. It is now felt that this second type of erythema is due to the release of proteolytic enzymes (lysozymes) from damaged epithelial cells [32]. The erythema subsides, presumably, as the number of damaged cells diminishes and as the amount of enzymes released decreases. It has been found that this erythema can be reduced by prior ^{60}Co high-energy irradiation of the area [33,34]. In addition, the ingestion of large doses of ε-aminocaproic acid or trihydroxyethylrutoside has been shown experimentally to decrease the intensity of the main erythema [35]. Pigmentation usually occurs by the third week after irradiation. Occasionally, another very delayed erythema can occur, sometimes noted about 6 to 7 weeks after the initial dose has been administered, which can last for 2 or 3 weeks.

*Usually about 300 to 400 R, depending on the quality of the x rays used for irradiation.

Histology

During the first erythema there is histologically marked dilation of the capillaries and blood vessels in the upper dermis and a mild lymphocytic and neutrophilic perivascular infiltrate. Thereafter, during the main erythema, degenerated nuclei in the epidermis are noted along with an occasional abnormal mitosis. After the first week mitotic activity in the epidermis ceases for a time, but eventually the components of the epidermis regenerate and the histologic picture returns to normal.

The pigmentation which occurs approximately 20 days after irradiation is manifested histologically by a large number of chromatophores in the dermis and also by an increased number of dopa-positive cells [23]. The dropping down of the pigment presumably is secondary to the liquefaction degeneration of the basal cell zone sometimes noted in histologic sections. A similar process occurs in such diseases as lichen planus and fixed drug eruptions.

Chemical Modification of Cutaneous Irradiation Reactions

Other chemicals, in addition to those mentioned above, have been investigated for their irradiation "sparing effects." Malkinson utilized intravenous cysteamine in mice and noted clear-cut protective effects of the drug on the hair matrix cells of mice given 200 to 16,000 R [44]. More recently, Chung and associates studied 7 potent antiinflammatory drugs to assay their effectiveness in suppressing the signs of acute radiodermatitis [15]. The drugs were administered intraperitoneally, topically, and orally after the test animals received 3000 to 4000 R of β-irradiation. In this test situation, chloroquin diphosphate, meclofenamic acid, and indomethacin given systemically were most effective in suppressing the dermatitis produced up to the third week posttreatment. The effective compounds slowed the onset of irradiation ulcers, but did not prevent their occurrence. Also, the drugs did not prevent the occurrence of chronic radiodermatitis in the test animals (although one experimental compound [S-2-(3-aminopropylamino) ethyl-phosphorothioic acid] did appear to offer some protection against the occurrence of chronic radiodermatitis). Several comprehensive reviews on the irradiation sparing effects of various chemical compounds have recently been published [6,13,26,38]. Finally, it has recently been found that some drugs *enhance* the effects of irradiation on skin and other organ systems; a good example is adriamycin, an agent used in treating bronchial small cell carcinoma [28].

The Maximum Permissible Dose for Benign Skin Disease

As mentioned before, in the past many therapists used radiotherapy to the skin in a very casual way. Accurate dosage records were seldom kept. The older machines, moreover, were often poorly calibrated and the actual dose delivered to the skin or the quantity of emissions as a whole from the apparatus was not appreciated. Consequently, many patients received enormous doses of radiation over the course of many years.

Sulzberger and associates in 1952 analyzed the clinical courses of 763 patients who had received intermittent, low-dose radiation [68]. Their most important finding was that about 1.5% of patients, when followed for between 5 and 23 years, developed a chronic radiodermatitis, but only if they had recieved more than 1000 R. This figure has since been the accepted upper limit for the total cumulative dose of irradiation for benign conditions. More recently, however, an attempt has been made to revise the figure upward. In an important investigation conducted in Britain, 136 patients who had received intermittent low-dose radiation for benign conditions were studied by Rowell [62]. The follow-up period was from 9 to 34 years. There were excellent records kept for all of the patients concerning individual and total dosages. The treatments were given in doses of 100 R for 3 doses (60 to 90 kV at 0.75 mm Al) at 3- or 4-week intervals. It was found that in patients receiving 2000 R or more to the hands, keratoses and telangiectasia developed in about 20% of patients, respectively, while atrophy occurred in about 10%. When the patients received from 1500 to 1975 R, keratoses were the only sequelae noted, and these occurred in only 18% of the cases. The skin of the face and neck was found to be more sensitive: lower doses of radiation produced about twice the number of changes as were produced on the hands. In 25 patients who had received 1600 R or more to the face and neck, 50% developed telangiectasia, 45% exhibited atrophy, and 8% developed keratoses. The atrophy that occurred on the face was noted to be mild. Rowell recommends that the upper limit for the total lifetime dose of radiation for benign conditions can be revised upward to 1200 R. Of interest in this study was the fact that in some patients up to 2750 R had been given with *no* clinically detectable changes. As will be discussed below, only 5% of the patients developed a malignancy (4 had basal cell cancers of the face and 1 developed a squamous cell cancer on the dorsum of the hand [NB, in areas where actinic damage is higher]). All of these afflicted patients had received more than 2000 R, varying from 2090 to 3170 R.

Acute Radiodermatitis

Acute radiodermatitis is characterized by intense local inflammation at the site of irradiation. It is the unavoidable consequence of therapy designed to destroy a malignancy (Fig. 5-1), but it may also occur because of an error of technique, such as overlapping of irradiation fields [24]; use of the wrong filter, kilovoltage, or target–skin distance; or miscalibration of the apparatus. An acute radiodermatitis may also occur as a result of a malfunction of the protective devices surrounding a large radiation generator, such as a nuclear reactor or a Van de Graaff generator.

Clinical Aspects

The course of acute radiodermatitis following excessive radiation exposure has been divided into four stages [73]. The first stage consists of initial erythema and edema which peaks at 48 hr and then subsides quickly. The second stage is a period varying from 2 to 5 days in which there is a relative absence of symptoms and physical findings. This is followed by the third stage in which an intense erythema develops, sometimes with hemorrhage. Vesiculation occurs at about the tenth day postirradiation, and for the next week or so there is a spread of the erythema and formation of many vesicles and bullae. The color of the skin by this time is an intense violet. The bullae rupture and secondary infection often supervenes. Pain is usually

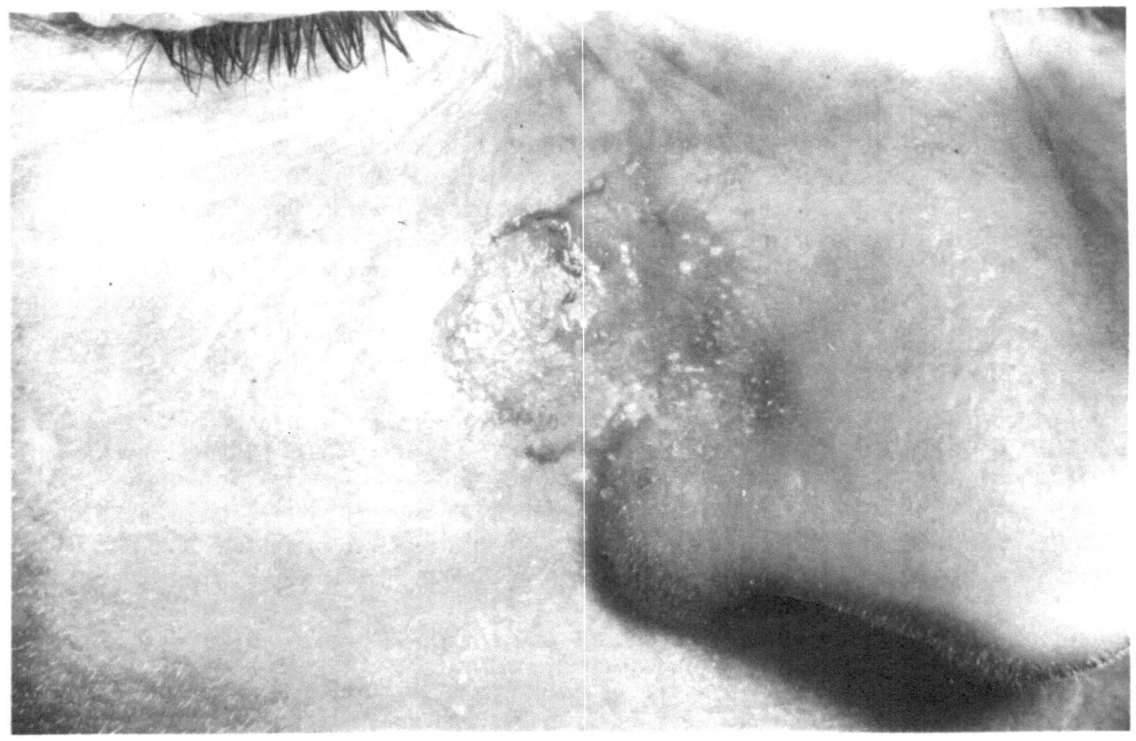

Figure 5-1.   Acute radiodermatitis 2 weeks after treatment of a basal cell carcinoma of the nose. This is a necessary reaction in cancer therapy (and not an indication of overdosage).

very severe. The process of inflammation and bulla formation ceases on about the fourth or fifth week after irradiation, and then repair (the fourth stage) occurs. The healing process may take a few weeks to several months. Eventually, the afflicted area becomes atrophic, with deep pigmentation and many telangiectasias. Sweet reported on 11 patients exposed accidentally to single doses of 6000 R or more, and noted that their clinical courses were very similar to those produced experimentally [69].

Therapy

In some cases acute radiodermatitis is associated with pain and may require narcotic analgesics. Too frequent or vigorous washing is prohibited, as these activities may lead to infection, and infection and trauma predispose an already severely damaged skin to necrosis. Some workers have stated that in very severe reactions systemic steroids may be used to control the inflammatory changes and reduce the permanent sequelae [76].

Histology

The pathologic picture of acute radiodermatitis has been well described [23,49]. There is usually marked spongiosis of the epidermis, with basal cell liquefaction, many pyknotic nuclei, and intense intracellular edema. There may be loss of the epidermal rete ridges. The most marked changes occur in the dermis, with a large accumulation of edema fluid in the upper portion of the dermis. This massive accumulation of fluid combined with loss of the attaching fibers in the dermis leads to the formation of subepidermal vesicles and bullae. The endothelial cells of the blood vessels are swollen, the smaller vessels are markedly dilated, and the larger vessels may exhibit intense edema of their walls. Very often thromboses are present, and extravasated red blood cells are usually conspicuous. The elastic fibers have been noted to be decreased in number and fragmented. As healing occurs, there is a return to a more normal arrangement of the epidermis, which often shows some thickening of the stratum corneum and the stratum granulosum, combined with thinning of the epidermis as a whole. The dilation of the blood vessels becomes permanent, leading to the telangiectasia seen clinically. Fibrosis around nerve elements and adnexal structures may occur and the presence of large numbers of chromatophores is noted. The sebaceous glands and hair follicles are affected by the same inflammatory patterns as is the epidermis and often undergo atrophy as healing supervenes. Complete fibrosis and occlusion of blood vessels can occur with consequent changes in the surrounding collagen.

In the experimental irradiation of rats with varying dosages of x rays, deRay and Cabrini noted that after 24 hr (as viewed under the electron microscope) the number of keratinosomes decreased markedly, the tonofibrils often formed retracted bundles around the cell nuclei, desmosomes were split apart, and discontinuities were seen in the cell membranes. [20]. In addition, there were many microvesicles of various sizes scattered throughout the cytoplasm and the mitochondria were swollen with holes in their membranes. These findings were noted to increase up to 72 hr after the initial dose. Special stains for both DNA and RNA have recently shown changes in these molecules as early as the third day after exposure [39].

Except for the *unavoidable* damage to normal tissue which occurs in the attempt to destroy malignancies on the skin, with the aid of modern machines and dosage schedules the occurrence of acute radiodermatitis has been (and should remain) a phenomenon of the past.

Chronic Radiodermatitis

Types of Radiodermatitis

There are two types of chronic radiodermatitis. The first type follows the short but intensive fractionated courses of irradiation utilized in the treatment of cutaneous malignancies. The second variety is that which has been produced by the application of relatively low dosages of radiation over long periods, leading to large, and occasionally enormous, cumulative doses. This type occurs either as the result of occupation or excessive past irradiation for such be-

nign conditions as nevi, acne, hirsutism, lichen simplex chronicus, and tinea capitis.

Clinical Manifestations

Chronic Radiodermatitis Following Treatment of Malignancies

Following the standard treatment for a cutaneous malignancy with 3000 to about 6000 R, sloughing of the irradiated skin occurs, with an intense erythema, occasionally associated with pain (Fig. 5-1). This acute radiodermatitis heals gradually in about 6 weeks. Over the ensuing years, the irradiated area may look inconspicuous or may show progressive atrophy of the skin, marked hypopigmentation (often associated with areas of hyperpigmentation), development of telangiectasia, and increased sensitivity to minor trauma, leading in rare instances to slow-healing ulcerations.

Chronic Radiodermatitis Following Overirradiation of Benign Conditions

Long-term treatment of benign dermatoses with repeated small doses at weekly or longer intervals (with total doses far exceeding 1000 R per area) may also be followed by chronic radiodermatitis. In contrast to radiodermatitis secondary to treatment of malignant skin tumors (which is considered unavoidable to a certain degree), chronic radiodermatitis following radiotherapy of benign skin conditions cannot be condoned.

When the radiodermatitis occurs on the face (eg, following epilation at the "Tricho Institutes"—where excessive facial hair growth was treated by lay persons—or after overzealous treatment of acne or eczema) a characteristic clinical picture emerges. There is a masklike facies and the nose becomes thin and pointed. Furrows radiating from the mouth occur, along with diffuse hyper- and hypopigmentation, atrophy, and many prominent telangiectasias. There is an almost total absence of both sebaceous glands and hair in the affected areas. Similar changes can be observed following excessive radiation doses for benign disorders in other regions. (Figs. 5-2 and 5-3).

Chronic Radiodermatitis as a Consequence of Occupational Overexposure

Similar clinical features are evident in persons with the "occupational type" of

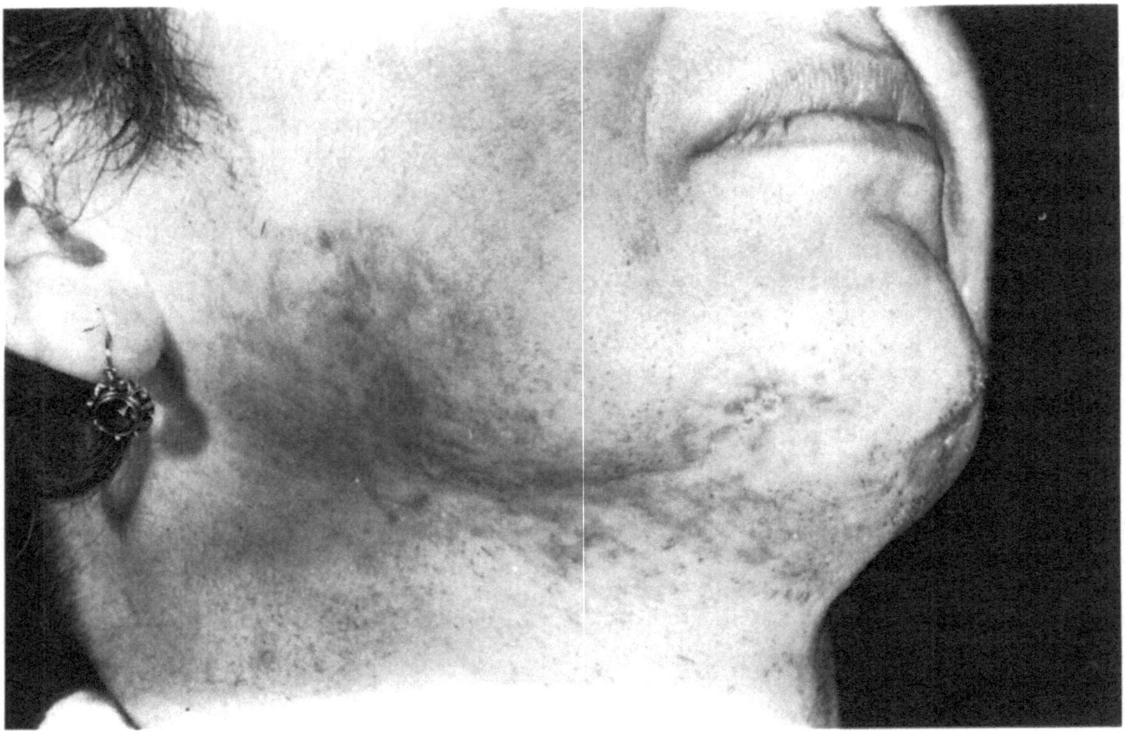

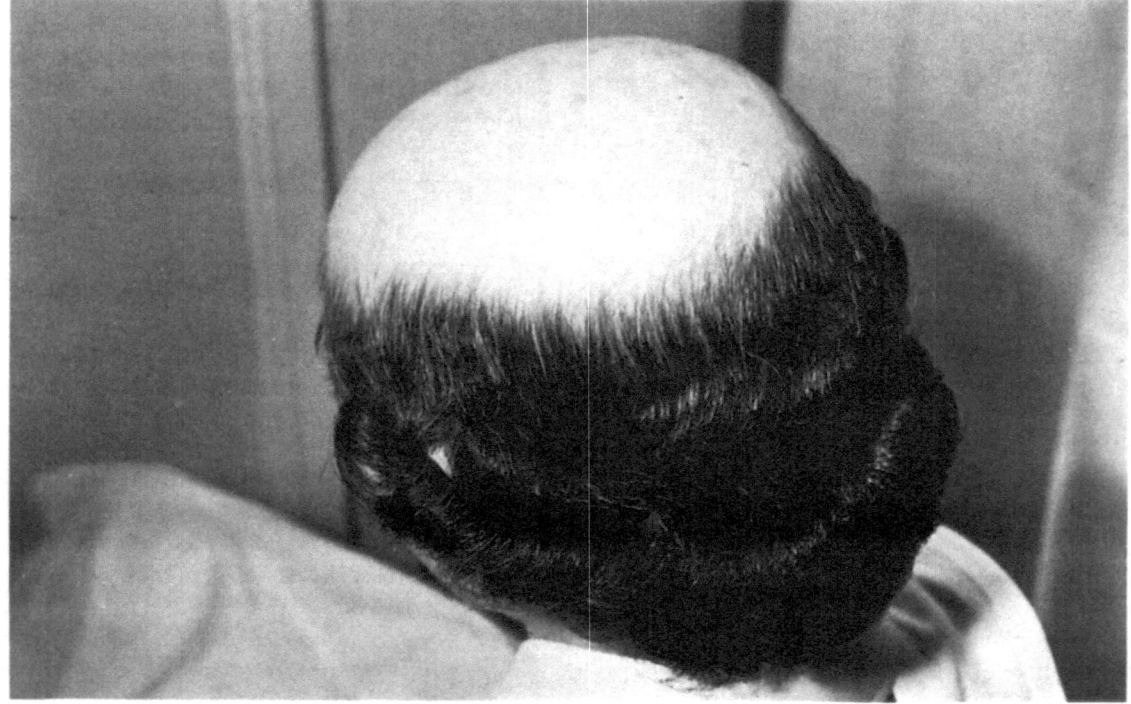

Figure 5-2.   Chronic radiodermatitis with marked atrophic and pigmentary changes following radiotherapy for hirsutism with unknown dose.

Figure 5-3.   Chronic radiodermatitis with permanent alopecia following accidental excessive epilation dose for tinea capitis.

chronic radiodermatitis [11]. These patients have been exposed over long periods to very low doses (50 to 100 R) leading to a large total exposure. The affected skin (often on the hands) first becomes red-violet in color and then thickens. The epidermal ridges flatten and many warty keratoses appear. There is loss of all hair, and the nails (if included in the irradiated area) become friable and exhibit longitudinal striations. There may be severe pain, and quite often indolent, exquisitely tender ulcers develop, leading to loss of function of the affected part. This type of radiodermatitis was reported early in the use of ionizing radiation, and has been frequently seen in dentists, veterinarians, workers in industry, and physicians (especially dermatologists, internists, and family practitioners). The point has been made that the incidence of radiodermatitis seems much lower in radiologists because these physicians have been more aware of the hazards for a longer period of time [11].

Histologic Findings

The pathologic changes of chronic radiodermatitis have been studied for many years [23,41,-48]. The epidermis is very often irregular, being thickened in some areas and thinned in others. There is usually marked hyperkeratosis but only a few areas of parakeratosis. The prickle cell layer may show spongiosis, a disorderly progression, and individual cell keratinization. Nuclear atypicality is seen. The epidermis may show a downward proliferation of the rete ridges, which may eventually surround blood vessels in the upper portion of the dermis. The collagen bundles are swollen and often show irregular staining. The changes in the dermal blood vessels comprise the major pathologic findings, with the vessel walls being markedly thickened so that the lumen may be partially or totally occluded. Thromboses are found in many of the larger vessels and dilated lymphatic channels are frequently seen. The blood vessels lying most superficially in the dermis are widely dilated. The number of normal elastic fibers is markedly diminished, and elastotic fibers predominate. These abnormal fibers have a distinct appearance under the electron microscope [40]. Appendages such as sebaceous glands and hair follicles are entirely absent, but the eccrine sweat apparatuses are usually

found, being absent only if the radiation injury was quite severe. Ulceration occurs when there are many vessels that are completely occluded. The pathologic changes may closely resemble those of severe actinic damage, but the basophilic degeneration of the collagen extends much deeper into the dermis in radiodermatitis, and usually the marked parakeratosis of actinically damaged skin is absent.

Effects of Grenz Radiation

Benign Changes Following Grenz Irradiation

It has long been known that both acute and chronic dermatoses can result from grenz irradiation. If an erythema dose is administered (usually about 150 to 300 R) there is redness and some edema. Fine scaling then ensues and hyperpigmentation can result after several months. If the dose is sufficiently large there may be intense pigmentary changes, telangiectasia, and atrophy. Lewis, in a review of over 40,000 patients treated with grenz ray therapy for actinic keratoses, describes an acute, although mild, dermatitis occurring after administration of 1300 to 1800 R to the face or 1500 to 2800 R elsewhere [42]. These doses were usually given in a single treatment and were never fractionated. No adverse reactions have been noted in over 20 years of follow-up. Epstein is of the opinion that grenz rays, in very low doses of about 75 R, can be given in weekly, 3-month courses every 6 months apparently indefinitely without any sequelae [22]. Rowell mentioned that there were no clinically detectable residua in 5 patients who had received fractionated doses of between 6400 and 12,800 R of grenz radiation many years earlier [62].

Malignant Changes Following Grenz Irradiation

Although it has been shown experimentally in animals that large doses of grenz rays (30,000 R) will produce malignancy [66], there have been only a few fully substantiated reports of malignancies arising in humans in areas previously irradiated by grenz rays. Kalz reported a squamous cell cancer arising on the thumb of a physician who had received a total dose of about 18,000 R over 15 years [36]. Cipollaro and Crossland reported on two cancers developing after grenz irradiation [16]. The first case was that of a man who had received grenz irradiation for low back pain for several years, and who 23 years later developed a basal cell cancer on the lower back. The second case had a nevus flammeus treated with grenz rays for about 4 years, and after a number of years developed several basal cell carcinomas in the irradiated area. Finally, Sagher [63] mentions a case in which a squamous cell cancer developed on the finger of a dermatologist who used his finger to hold patients' eyelids apart during radiotherapy. It was estimated that in 4 years he received between 60,000 and 70,000 R to his finger. The squamous cell cancer had developed more than 14 years after the treatment techniques were altered. The development of radiation angiokeratoma following grenz irradiation has been reported [1]. It appears that if given in low doses, even for very large cumulative exposures, grenz irradiation will apparently rarely cause radiodermatitis or carcinoma. Pillsbury, however, does suggest a total cumulative dose of *no more* than 5000 R, particularly in skin regions exposed to solar radiation [56].

The Roentgen Ulcer

The roentgen ulcer is an uncommon complication of radiation overdosage following in the wake of an acute or chronic radiodermatitis [71]. The radionecrosis is characterized by extreme pain, an undermined border, and a beefy base. Such areas take a long time to heal, and in fact may never do so completely, breaking down intermittently instead. This type of ulceration is most likely to occur on the neck, back, anogenital area, and the dorsum of the hand (Fig. 5-4). When healing does occur the area is atrophic, pigmented at its margins, and contractures with deformities sometimes result. Rarely, this type of indolent, painful ulceration may also be observed in areas of chronic radiodermatitis which are inflamed by secondary factors, such as trauma or thermal injuries. Montgomery et al noted that this type of delayed, very painful necrosis is quite characteristic of the plantar radiodermatitis following overtreatment of plantar warts [50]. The only effective treatment of such ulcerated areas is

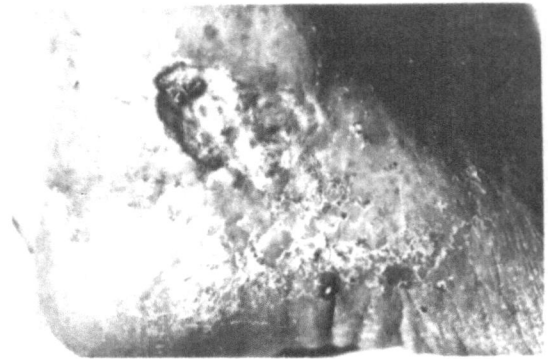

Figure 5-4.   Squamous cell carcinoma developing in chronic radiodermatitis of foot following numerous radiation treatments for recurrent "eczema" over a period of 10 years.

surgical excision and grafting, taking a wide and deep margin to insure that there is relatively healthy tissue on which the graft can take and in which sutures can be placed without fear of the area degenerating.

Radiation-Induced Skin Carcinoma

Skin cancer developing after radiation treatment has always been a pervasive and vexing problem. In the early 1900s many cases of carcinoma occurring in irradiated sites had been cited in the literature. By 1914 at least 94 cases had been tabulated (50 in radiologists) [30]. Epstein stated that by 1922 more than 100 radiotherapists had died as the result of overexposure [23]. The incidence of malignant tumors arising in areas of chronic radiodermatitis or in areas previously irradiated has been determined in several patient populations. Epstein noted that in his series of 368 patients malignant changes developed in 13.9%, and Cannon et al mentioned a rate of malignant change of 22% [12].

Carcinomas Arising After Superficial Radiotherapy

There have been two recent series of importance which have attempted to show the long-term effects of irradiation with respect to the development of carcinomas following therapy for benign dermatoses. The first study is that of Rowell in which 5 patients developed carcinomas in previously irradiated sites [62]. This represented a 5% incidence in a clinic population that received carefully measured and delivered dosages of radiation. Four of the patients developed basal cell cancers, all of which were located on the face. These patients received fractionated doses of between 2090 and 3075 R and the lesions were noted to occur from 8 to 34 years after the treatments had been given. The remaining patient developed a squamous cell cancer on the hand 23 years after receiving a total dose of 3170 R.

The other important study was by Martin et al and involved 368 patients seen in a plastic surgery clinic [45]. All of these patients had received, at some previous time, radiation for a variety of benign conditions such as hirsuitism, acne, "barber's itch," greasy skin, hemangiomas, psoriasis, and other unspecified conditions. Reliable data on the number and frequency of the treatments could not be obtained, however, and the information was derived solely from the patients' memories. It can be assumed, however, that the total doses greatly exceeded the safe doses discussed above. The patients had most often been treated at nonmedical facilities. In this series, there were 227 basal cell cancers, 41 basosquamous cell carcinomas, 63 squamous cell cancers, and 11 malignancies of the spindle cell and adenoid cystic types. The lesions were most often found on the cheek, nose, lip, and chin, being located on other areas of the face and neck with less frequency. Many of the patients had extensive, often mutilating, involvement by the cancer. In about 20% of the cases in this series the skin cancers appeared after a latent period of 31 to 64 years, the median latency for all patients being 21 years. In 3 young patients, however, cancers developed within 5 years after treatment. In this large series, 85% of the lesions developed in skin which was atrophic, hypopigmented, keratotic, and telangiectatic. This is to be contrasted to Rowell's series in which, despite chronic radiation changes, only 5% of the patients developed radiation cancers. The critical and unobtainable information in the second series, of course, is the amount, frequency, and type of radiation received. This latter study documents the fact that carcinomas occurring in irradiated areas are not at all uncommon, especially when the radiation has been administered in an apparently unregulated and haphazard manner.

It should be carefully noted that the malignancies discussed in these two series developed in areas subjected to actinic damage. The question then arises as to whether these lesions were induced by long exposure to solar radiation, by the dermatologic irradiation, or by the combined cumulative and synergistic effects of both types of radiation. Since both varieties of radiation are well known to induce cutaneous malignancies, such as interaction must always be kept in mind when evaluating results of such investigations and surveys as discussed above.

Other studies have reported on the occurrence of carcinomas in areas previously irradiated, and all have agreed that basal cell cancers predominate over squamous cell cancers [5,-60]. Such cancers have been reported on the scalps of children [60] as the result of irradiation for lupus vulgaris [53], and have been observed in areas over the spine which had been previously irradiated [64]. A recent study mentioned by Urbach demonstrated that in irradiated patients basal cell epitheliomas are now being seen almost exclusively on the head and neck, while squamous cell cancers are found predominantly on other body areas (Fig. 5-5) [72]. This observation was noted also by Rowell. Of interest is the fact that in the large series observed by Martin et al, there were more than 100 squamous cell and basosquamous cell cancers occurring on the face (ie, almost one-third of all the malignancies in this patient population). This very high incidence of

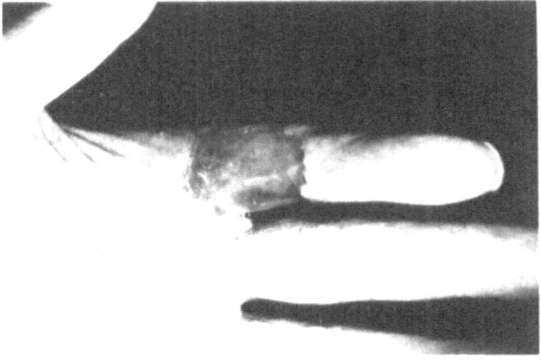

Figure 5-5. Chronic radiodermatitis and radiation ulcer in a 74-year-old dentist. Radiation protection was not used routinely during dental x-ray studies.

squamous cell cancers appearing on the face and neck has not been found in other studies.

Incidence of Metastases from Radiation-Induced Skin Cancers

Lund reported that carcinomas arising in sun-damaged areas have only a 0.5% chance of metastasizing [43], while it has been noted that the incidence of metastases from a radiation-induced skin cancer was much higher [64]. In the series of patients surveyed by Martin et al, there was a 20% incidence of metastases to the cervical nodes in 110 persons who had either pure squamous cell or basosquamous cell carcinomas. One case is also reported where a pure basal cell cancer, on the ear of one man who had received irradiation to the ear years previously, metastasized to the cervical lymph nodes and eventually killed him. In 10 patients, the squamous cell cancer was found in areas below the level of the clavicles. Of the total number of patients surveyed in this series 35 (or 10%) died as a result of disseminated radiation-induced skin cancer. Park and Davis reported a mortality rate of 12% in 59 patients with radiation-induced skin cancers [52]. It is thus quite apparent that any suspicious lesions that develop in an area which had previously been irradiated must be treated adequately, vigorously, and as soon as possible in view of the high statistical incidence of metastasis.

Treatment

The treatment of skin carcinomas arising in previously irradiated areas, if the lesions are not extensive, is the same as that for sun-induced cancers, and any number of accepted dermatologic methods may be utilized for their removal (eg, electrodesiccation and curettage, cryosurgery). For larger, sometimes mutilating carcinomas, extensive and radical surgical procedures (both chemosurgical and plastic) may be resorted to for eradication of the tumor and an acceptable cosmetic appearance. Further radiotherapy for removal of the tumor is absolutely contraindicated.

Persistence of Risk

A most important point made by Martin et al is that the risk of cancer formation in previously irradiated skin evidently persists for the life of the patient (eg, sometimes over 60 years), and that because of this hazard and the lifetime propensity for developing new lesions, the conventional estimations of cure rates for carcinomas are meaningless. In their opinion, once a person has had a radiation-induced cancer removed there is a distinct probability that new lesions will develop. They feel that such patients, furthermore, cannot be said to be cured even after the commonly accepted 5-year interval, because of the enormous latent period over which new cancers can emerge, either in new locations or in sites of previous removal.

Other Cutaneous Tumors Arising After Skin Irradiation

The list of tumors arising after irradiation for dermatologic purposes is not as long as that found after treatment with deeper radiation (vide infra), but instead has been limited essentially to rare cases of cylindromas [10], malignant melanomas [70], and fibrosarcomas, in addition to the more common (and usually more benign) basal and squamous cell cancers.

Fibrous Reactions and Tumors After Skin Irradiation

Some fibrosis occurs in every case of radiodermatitis, but occasionally a more exuberant and diffuse fibromatosis arises. A series of cases has been reported in which a red, granulomatous, sometimes ulcerating lesion has occurred on the ears and cheeks of elderly patients who had received irradiation to these areas [57]. Histologically, the lesions were characterized by many large and atypical fibroblasts and histiocytes along with dilated blood vessels and multinucleated giant cells. Such lesions bore a strong resemblance to a connective tissue malignancy, but were in fact benign and never metastasized. These peculiar growths have been termed "pseudosarcoma of the skin" or "paradoxical fibrosarcoma." They can be distinguished from true fibrosarcomas (which incidentally, have been noted on occasion in areas which had been irradiated repeatedly many years previously [latent period about 26 years]) [54]. Such malignant sarcomas may also occur in scars of burns, lupus vulgaris, late syphilis, and xeroderma pigmentosum. The lesions are nodular, may be either firm or soft, and occasionally ulcerate. Histologically, the malignant tumors are characterized by large, atypical fibroblasts which are pleomorphic in appearance and contain abnormal mitoses. They may be either well differentiated or appear quite anaplastic. Such tumors may occasionally metastasize. There has recently been agreement among pathologists, however, that most, but certainly not all, of the postirradiation fibrosarcomas which had been reported were in fact merely expressions of a benign fibroplastic process. Some of the sarcomas which had been reported, moreover, were in reality spindle cell carcinomas as demonstrated by the presence of horn pearls and epidermal attachments. The treatment for both of the above conditions is wide and deep excision.

Noncutaneous Effects of Skin Irradiation

Thyroid Cancers and Other Cephalic Tumors

There has recently been an enormous amount of interest and concern, both in the medical literature and in the lay media, regarding the long-term effects of irradiation in infancy and childhood on the thyroid and other glands. The association of thyroid irradiation with x rays and radionuclides with the development of benign and malignant thyroid neoplasms has been conclusively established in experimental animals. Recently, there have been many elaborate studies on populations which had received varying doses and types of radiation to the head and neck as infants and children. All of these investigations indicate a very strong correlation between such childhood irradiation and risk of neoplasm development in adulthood [14,18,25,-58,65,67]. These studies, and many others, clarify several points. (1) The thyroid glands of children (and, particularly, infants) are much more sensitive to radiation effects than are those of an adult. (2) The interval in which a malignancy or benign tumor may develop is often 20 to 25 years after the irradiation. (3) The tumors engendered by this irradiation in childhood are not more malignant than are those occurring in nonirradiated patients.

Of great concern to dermatologists, naturally, are those populations which have received irradiation to the face and neck in the past few decades for a variety of benign conditions, such as acne and hirsutism. Unfortunately, many of the studies implicating such dermatologic radiation as a cause for thyroid neoplasia are found lacking in one very important area, ie, the precise quality and quantity of the irradiation given. Many simply state that the patients received an unknown quantity and type of radiation in childhood [3,18]. In the few studies where specific dosages are mentioned (without specifying the quality of the radiation), the dosages are usually either very high, or included with treatments for other, deeper processes, such as tonsillitis or abscesses [9,58].

Within the past several years considerable attention has been given to determining the minimum dose to the thyroid gland necessary to induce later neoplasia. About 15 years ago—and until recently—it was felt that thyroid carcinomas would only develop in a gland which had received at least 90 R (and usually more than 167 R) [8]. Recently, however, this figure has been revised down to 6.5 R, based on the large study by Modan et al [47]. These workers conducted a follow-up study on over 10,000 Israeli children who had received the Adamson–Kienböck treatment for ringworm of the scalp, and found a much higher incidence of benign and malignant thyroid, parotid, and brain tumors in the irradiated children. For example, there were 12 thyroid malignancies in the treated group, with only 2 in the untreated group. Modan et al estimated that the dose to the thyroid gland (as measured with a phantom) was only 6.5 R, and they cautiously associated this low dose—along with other factors—with the increased incidence of malignancy. The figure of 6 R has been accepted by many workers as the minimum dose necessary to induce thyroid cancer in a very small percentage of patients [51,67].

The concept of a threshold dose is now abandoned and it is assumed that any dose of radiation, even the smallest, may be hazardous in a proportionately small number of exposed patients. This "linear hypothesis" is explained in the 1974 BEIR report of the National Academy of Sciences (51).

A dose of 6 R to the thyroid gland has also been estimated in a study by Albert et al of irradiation for tinea capitis [2,29]. These authors report an increased incidence of thyroid adenomas among 2000 children with ringworm of the scalp treated at New York University. Thyroid cancers were not observed in this large group. This latter study reports doses produced by a treatment schedule of 5 fields of 300 to 400 R, with 100 kV, unfiltered. The Modan group, on the other hand, used 5 fields of 350 to 400 R at 75 to 100 kV, but with a filter of 3.5 mm Al.

The Modan study also noted that the children who had received irradiation had a significantly increased incidence of both benign and malignant tumors of the brain and parotid glands. There were twice as many malignant, cranial tumors as there were benign tumors. There were 4 malignant parotid tumors versus 3 benign tumors. A recent report describes malignant salivary gland tumors following excessive doses of x rays [59]. Acne irradiation has recently been implicated as a cause of breast cancer.[67] However, the author himself admits that "the evidence for the relation of radiation for acne to the subsequent occurrence of carcinoma of the breast is circumstantial."

Kirk et al measured thyroid doses of 6 R during acne therapy with a HVL of 0.7 mm Al and a fractionated total dose of 760 R [37]. Petratos et al [55] showed that the thyroid dose can be markedly reduced in the treatment of cutaneous neoplasms. They determined the dose delivered to the thyroid gland during actual treatment for basal cell cancers of the upper face in 15 patients. In these individuals the treatment schedule consisted of 3400 R in fractionated doses with the following factors: HVL, 0.9 mm Al; 100 kV; 10 mA; and TSD, 20 cm. Using standard protection measures these investigators found a radiation dose over the thyroid gland of between 2.0 and 0.1 R, with the average around 0.52 R.

Developments in the last two decades in dermatologic therapy have made radiotherapy of tinea capitis and most other dermatologic conditions in younger age groups obsolete. The only remaining indication for radiotherapy of the head and neck region with superficial x ray qualities is acne vulgaris resistant to other forms of treatment.

Studies of current importance for dermatologists—which have yet to be done—involve measuring the dose to the thyroid gland during modern, properly administered and protected acne therapy and following such patients for several decades, or initiating large-scale retrospective investigations of patients treated under modern conditions. Only then will there be a firm basis for implicating (or exonerating)

properly done dermatologic radiation therapy as a cause of thyroid cancer. Field size, direction of the useful beam, age of the patient, radiation quality, fractionation of dosage, and application of radiation protection standards are among several factors affecting the dose reaching the thyroid gland and other important organs.

Other Effects of Skin Irradiation

Finally, one other consequence associated with skin irradiation must be mentioned. This is the finding that, in a follow-up study of 2043 patients who had received irradiation to the scalp for the treatment of tinea capitis, there was a 2.5-times greater incidence of confirmed mental illness than in 1413 control subjects (2). The mental illnesses were of both the neurotic and psychotic (schizophrenic) categories. The authors were unable to offer any readily apparent reasons for these findings, which were refuted by Epstein [22].

Gonadal Exposure and Protection During Dermatologic Irradiation

One of the major concerns of any radiotherapist is to minimize the amount of radiation delivered to the gonads during treatment. The amount of exposure to the gonads during irradiation for dermatologic problems has been monitored several times. One group treated tinea capitis with radiation (HVL, 0.7 ml Al; 100 kV) and measured the gonadal dose [17]. The total dosage to the scalp was 1600 R. With this therapy it was noted that when thin lead foil was used alone for gonadal protection the gonadal dose was about 2.6 to 6.3 mR, but that if the thickness of the lead apron was increased, the machine angulated away from the pelvic area, and the machine fitted with a cone, the gonadal dose was essentially zero.

Even when the perianal areas are irradiated the dose to the gonads can be kept quite low with careful attention to machine placement and patient protection [4]. Witten et al noted that in patients who received about 170 R to the face the measured gonadal dose was between 2 and 13 mR, and if the axillae were irradiated (with doses of about 300 R) the gonadal dose was about 125 to 200 mR [75]. All of these investigations show that sufficient radiation can be administered to the skin without causing any undue gonadal exposure. Witten emphasized that with proper techniques the gonadal dose during any irradiation session can be reduced by more than 99% [74].

It is important to note that exposure to seemingly very low doses of ionizing radiation can cause chromosomal aberrations, such as breaks and aneuploidy. A recent study, using men who worked in a nuclear submarine, found that the subjects had a somewhat higher incidence (6%) of chromosomal abnormalities than did controls not exposed to radiation [19]. The cells studied were peripheral leukocytes and the whole body doses received ranged from 4.7 to 0.027 R. Changes in gonadal cell populations were not assessed. Careful attention to dermatologic radiation techniques will keep the gonadal dose within the range of the normal yearly background radiation (see table 5-1), and thus ensure that gonadal chromosomal abnormalities are not higher in patients receiving dermatologic radiotherapy than in the normal population.

Cataract Production

It should also be mentioned that irradiation can cause cataract formation. Merriam and Focht determined that the minimum cataractogenic

Table 5-1 *Annual Whole Body Dose Rates in the United States (1970)*

Source	Dose (mrem/year)	
Environmental		106
Natural background radiation		
Cosmic radiation	44	
Terrestial radiation		
External (eg, radioactive materials in earth)	40	
Internal (eg, inhaled radon or ingested, ^{40}K)	18	
Global fallout	4	
Nuclear power	0.003	
Medical		73
Diagnostic	72	
Radiopharmaceuticals	1	
Occupational		0.8
Miscellaneous		2
Total		182

From Rice et al [59].

Table 5-2 *Dose-limiting Recommendations of the National Council on Radiation Protection (NCRP)*

Type of Exposure	Dose (rems/year)
Occupational exposure	
Combined whole body	
Prospective annual limit	5
Retrospective annual limit	10–15
Long-term accumulation	$(N - 18 \times 5)$*
Skin	15
Hands	75 (25/qtr)
Forearms	30 (10/qtr)
Other organs, tissues, and organ systems	15 (5/qtr)
Pregnant women	0.5†
Public, or occasionally exposed individuals	0.5
Occasionally exposed medical students	0.1
Population	
Genetic	0.17
Somatic	0.17
Emergency	
Life saving	
Whole body (older than 45 years)	100
Hands and forearms	<u>200</u>
Total	300‡
Less urgent	
Whole body	25
Hands and forearms	<u>75</u>
Total	100‡
Family member of radioactive patients	
Under age 45	0.5
Over age 45	5

From National Council on Radiation Protection and Measurements: "Basic Radiation Protection Criteria." NCRP Report No. 39. Washington, DC, NCRP, 1971.
*Where N is age in years.
†Rem/gestation period.
‡Dose limit at time of emergency.

dose was about 400 R [46]. With adequate eye protection, even during therapy for such problems as cancers near the eye that require administration of thousands of roentgens, the dose of radiation reaching the eye will certainly be far less than this cataractogenic dose.

Appendix

Many dermatologists and other physicians have encountered, or probably will encounter in the future, questions from patients and other persons concerning the proper thyroid investigative examinations and tests for patients who had received head and neck irradiation as children. Two recent papers summarizing the current recommendations for handling such patients have appeared, and should be consulted if any questions or difficulties arise regarding this vexing problem [27,31].

Table 5-3   *Summary of Dose Limits for Individuals as Recommended by the International Commission on Radiologic Protection (ICRP) (rem/year)*

Organ or Tissue	Adults Occupationally Exposed	Members of the Public
Gonads, red bone-marrow	5	0.5
Skin, bone, thyroid	30	3*
Hands and forearms; feet and ankles	75	7.5
Other single organs	15	1.5†

From ICRP: Protection Against Ionizing Radiation From External Sources. ICRP Publ. 15. Oxford, Pergamon Press, 1970
*1.5 rem/year to the thyroid of children up to 16 years of age.
†In any 1 year the maximum permissible doses (MPD) should not be exceeded, but in a period of a quarter of a year up to one-half of the annual MPD may be accumulated. If necessary, the quarterly quota may be received as a single dose, but the commission believes that it would be undesirable for doses of this magnitude to be repeated at close intervals.

In benign diseases, indications for radiotherapy should be reduced substantially in order to limit administration of potentially hazardous radiation to various important organs.

Therapeutic radiation is not the only important source of potentially hazardous radiation levels. Table 5-1 lists estimates of contributions of various factors to annual whole body dose rates in the United States (excluding medical therapeutic radiation). Obviously, most of the background radiation cannot be limited under any circumstances.

Various radiation protection agencies have published recommended dose limits (formerly known as maximum permissible doses) for workers in radiation facilities. The dose limits are usually expressed in rem ("roentgen equivalent, man"), the "dose equivalent," based on the concept of relative biologic effectiveness (RBE). This term is usually reserved for radiation protection purposes; in dermatologic radiotherapy, 1 rem corresponds roughly to 1 rad (Tables 5-2 and 5-3).

References

1. Abe T, Sugai T, Saito T: Radiation angiokeratoma following grenz irradiation. Arch Dermatol 100:294, 1969
2. Albert RE, Omran AR: Follow-up study of patients treated by x ray for tinea capitis. Arch Environ Health 17:899, 1968
3. Albright EC, Allday RW: Thyroid carcinoma after radiation therapy for acne vulgaris. JAMA 199:128, 1967
4. Alden HS, Weens HS, Yoamans HD: Observa-

tions on radiation exposure in dermatologic x-ray therapy. Arch Dermatol 79:159, 1959
5. Anderson LP, Anderson HE: Development of basal cell epithelioma as a consequence of radiodermatitis. Arch Dermatol 63:586, 1951
6. Arena V: Ionizing Radiation and Life. St Louis, Mosby, 1971, pp 446–457
7. Arnold HL Jr: Erythema multiforme following high voltage roentgen therapy. Arch Dermatol Syph 60:143, 1949
8. Beach SA, Dolphin GW: A study of the relationship between x-ray dose delivered to the thyroid of children and the subsequent development of malignant tumors. Phys Med Biol 6:583, 1962
9. Becher FO, et al: Adult thyroid cancer after head and neck irradiation in infancy and childhood. Ann Inter Med 83:347, 1975
10. Black MM, Jones EW: Dermal cylindroma following x-ray epilation of the scalp. Br J Dermatol 85:70, 1971
11. Braasck NK, Nickson MJ: A study of the hands of radiologists. Radiology 51:719, 1949
12. Cannon B, Randolph JG, Murray JE: Malignant irradiation for benign conditions. N Engl J Med 260:197, 1959
13. Carr C, et al: Protective agents modifying biological effects of radiation. Arch Environ Health 21:88, 1970
14. Carroll RG: The relationship of head and neck irradiation to the subsequent development of thyroid neoplasms. Semin Nucl Med 6:411, 1976
15. Chung J, Song CW, Yamaguchi T, et al: Effects of anti-inflammatory compounds on irradiation induced radiodermatitis. Dermatologica 144:97, 1972
16. Cipollaro AC, Crossland PM: X Rays and Radium in the Treatment of Diseases of the Skin, 5th ed. Philadelphia, Lea & Febiger, 1967, pp 394–395

17. Cipollaro AC, Kallos A, Ruppe JPJ: Measurement of gonadal radiations during treatment for tinea capitis. NY State J Med 59:30, 1959
18. DeGroot L, Paloyan E: Thyroid cancer and radiation. A Chicago endemic. JAMA 225:487, 1973
19. Depenbusch FL: Chromosomal aberrations in man due to low levels of ionizing radiation. A pilot study. Milit Med 137:436, 1972
20. deRay BM, Cabrini RL: Ultrastructural alterations in X-irradiated epidermis. J Invest Dermatol 60:136, 1973
21. Ellenger F: Medical Radiation Biology. Springfield, Ill, Thomas, 1957
22. Epstein E: Dermatologic radiotherapy 1973. Presented at Fifth Aspen Conference for Dermatologists. Dermatol News 6:8, 1973
23. Epstein E: Radiodermatitis. Springfield, Ill, Thomas, 1962, p 75
24. Epstein S: Importance of overlapping for the occurrence of roentgen late injuries in surface therapy. Arch Dermatol Syph 168:548, 1933
25. Favus MJ, et al: Thyroid cancer occurring as a late consequence of head and neck irradiation. N Engl J Med 294:1019, 1976
26. Foye WO: Radiation-protective agents in mammals. J Pharm Sci 58:283, 1969
27. Goldschmidt HG: Dermatologic radiotherapy and thyroid cancer. Cutis 18:551, 1976
28. Greco FA, Brereton HD, Kent H, et al: Adriamycin and enhanced reaction in normal esophagus and skin. Ann Intern Med 85:294, 1976
29. Harley NH, Albert RE, Shore RE, et al: Follow-up study of patients treated by x-ray epilation for tinea capitis. Estimation of the dose to the thyroid and pituitary glands and other structures of the head and neck. Phys Med Biol 21:631, 1976
30. Hesse O: Das Röntgenkarzinom. Fortschr Geb Röntgenstrahlen 17:82, 1911
31. Information for physicians on irradiation. Related thyroid cancer. CA 26:150, 1976
32. Jolles B, Harrison RG: Enzymic processes and vascular changes in the skin radiation reaction. Br J Radiol 39:12, 1966
33. Jolles B, Harrison RG: Radiation skin reactions and depletion and restoration of body immune response. Nature 198:1216, 1963
34. Jolles B, Harrison RG: Studies of the influence of wave lengths on biological effects. Time and dose differentials at "radiation action sites in the skin." Strahlentherapie 139:716, 1970
35. Jolles B, Harrison RG: Enzymic processes and vascular changes in the skin radiation reaction. Br J Radiol 39:12, 1966
36. Katz F: Observation on grenz rays reactions. Dermatologica 118:357, 1959
37. Kirk J, Worthley BW: Superficial radiotherapy in acne vulgaris. Australas J Dermatol 12:10, 1971
38. Klayman DL, Copeland ES: The design of anti-radiation agents. In Ariens EJ (ed): Drug Design, Vol 6. New York, Academic Press, 1975, pp 81–142
39. Kuban AK, Farah FS: Effects of irradiation on the skin. Acta Derm Venereol (Stockh) 49:64, 1969
40. Ledoux-Corbusie M, Achten G: Elastosis in chronic radiodermatitis. Br J Dermatol 91:287, 1974
41. Lever, WF, Schaumberg-Lever G: Histopathology of the Skin, 5th ed. Philadelphia, Lippincott, 1975, pp 196–198
42. Lewis HM: Twenty years experience with grenz rays. Bull Assoc Mil Dermatol 21:17, 1973
43. Lund HZ: How often does squamous cell carcinoma metastasize? Arch Dermatol 92:635, 1965
44. Malkinson FD, Griem ML: Cysteamine protection of x-ray induced dysplasia in mouse hair. A summary. In Pillsbury DM, Livingood CS (eds): Proceedings of the XII International Congress of Dermatology. Amsterdam, Excerpta Medica, 1962, pp 585–586
45. Martin H, Strong E, Spiro RH: Radiation-induced skin cancer of the head and neck. Cancer 25:61, 1970
46. Merriam GR Jr, Focht EF: A clinical study of radiation cataracts and relationship to dose. Am J Roentgenol 77:759, 1957
47. Modan B, et al: Radiation-induced head and neck tumours. Lancet 1:277, 1974
48. Montgomery H: Pathologic histology of radiodermatitis. In Cipollare AC, Crossland PM: X Rays and Radium in the Treatment of Diseases of the Skin, 5th ed. Philadelphia, Lea & Febiger, 1967, pp 411–545
49. Montgomery H: Burns and radiodermatitis. In Montgomery H (ed): Dermatopathology, 2nd ed. New York, Hoeber, 1967, pp 232–248
50. Montgomery AH, Montgomery RM, Montgomery DC: The problem of plantar radiodermatitis. NY State J Med 49:1664, 1949
51. National Academy of Sciences: The Effects on Populations of Exposure to Low Levels of Ionizing Radiation: Advisory Committee on the Biological Effects of Ionizing Radiations. Washington, DC, USGPO, 1974
52. Park GT, Davis J: Radiation cancer of the skin. Radiology 84:436, 1965
53. Pegum JS: Radiation-induced skin cancer. Br J Radiol 45:613, 1972
54. Petet VD, Chamness JT, Ackerman LU: Fibromatosis and fibrocarcoma following irradiation therapy. Cancer 7:149, 1954

55. Petratos MA, et al: Measurement of scattered radiation to body areas during radiotherapy of basal cell epitheliomas. Dermatol Int J Dermatol 8:10, 1969

56. Pillsbury DM, Shelley WB, Kligman AM: Dermatology. Philadelphia, Saunders, 1956, p 334

57. Rachmaninoff N, McDonald JR, Cook JC: Sarcoma-like tumors of the skin following irradiation. Am J Clin Pathol 36:427, 1961

58. Refetoff S, et al: Continuing occurrence of thyroid carcinoma after irradiation to the neck in infancy and childhood. N Engl J Med 292:171, 1975

59. Rice DH, et al: Postirradiation malignant salivary gland tumor. Arch Otolaryngl 102:699, 1976

60. Ridley CM: Basal cell cancer following x-ray epilation of the scalp. Br J Dermatol 74:222, 1962

61. Rook A, Wilkinson DS, Ebling FJG: Textbook of Dermatology, 2nd ed. Oxford, Blackwell Scientific, 1972, p 471

62. Rowell NR: A follow-up study of superficial radiotherapy for benign dermatoses. Recommendations for the use of x rays in dermatology. Br J Dermatol 88:583, 1973

63. Sagher F: Squamous cell carcinomas due to grenz rays. In Pillsbury DM, Livingood CS (eds): Proceedings of the XII International Congress of Dermatology. Amsterdam, Excerpta Medica, 1962, pp 638–639

64. Sarkany I, Fountain RB, Evans CD, et al: Multiple basal cell epitheliomata following radiotherapy of the spine. Br J Dermatol 80:90, 1968

65. Schneider AB, et al: Plasma thyroglobulin in detecting thyroid carcinoma after childhood, head and neck irradiation. Ann Intern Med 86:29, 1977

66. Shapiro EM, Knox JM, Freeman RG: Carcinogenic effects of prolonged exposure to grenz ray. J Invest Dermatol 37:291, 1961

67. Simon N: Breast cancer induced by radiation. JAMA 237:789, 1977

68. Sulzberger MB, Baer RL, Borota A: Do roentgen ray treatments as given by skin specialists produce cancers or other sequelae? Arch Dermatol Syph 65:639, 1952

69. Sweet RD: Acute accidental superficial x-ray burns. Br J Dermatol 74:392, 1962

70. Traenkle HL: X-ray induced cancer in man. Nat Cancer Inst Monogr 10:243, 1963

71. Traenkle HL, Mulay D: Further observations on late radiation necrosis following therapy of skin cancer. Arch Dermatol 81:908, 1960

72. Urbach F: Pathologic effects of ionizing radiation In Fitzpatrick TB, et al (eds): Dermatology in general medicine. New York, McGraw-Hill Book Co, 1971, p 1042

73. Wendeyer BW: Radiotherapy in its relation to dermatology. Br Med J 1:945, 1954

74. Witten VH: Physical methods of protection against ionizing radiation in dermatologic therapy and its importance in relation to gonadal radiation exposure. In Pillsbury DM, Livingood CS (eds): Proceedings of the XII International Congress of Dermatology, Vol 1. Amsterdam, Excerpta Medica, 1962, pp 593–596

75. Witten VH, Sulzberger MB, Stewart WD: Studies on the quantity of radiation reaching the gonadal areas during dermatologic x-ray therapy. Arch Dermatol 76:683, 1957

76. Zschunke E, Behrbohm P: Uber die behandlung des röntgenschadens an der haut mit prednisone. Dermatol Wochenschr 152:1417, 1966

6

Treatment Planning
Selection of Physical Factors and Radiation Techniques

Herbert Goldschmidt

A review of older publications in the field of dermatologic radiotherapy shows a bewildering array of recommendations concerning the proper selection of physical factors. Recent advances in the technology of dermatologic radiotherapy units made it possible to define more precisely which factors are most suitable for specific therapeutic purposes, resulting not only in greater therapeutic efficacy but also in a reduction of necessary variations. This simplification of modern therapeutic techniques has been a major factor in the elimination of potential technical or human errors, the main causes of unnecessary radiation sequelae. Standardization of therapeutic factors and the introduction of advanced x-ray units with sophisticated safety devices have largely eliminated these risks.

Basic physical considerations have been discussed in Chapter 1. Essential points will be repeated but special emphasis will be given to practical aspects of dermatologic radiotherapy and to specific recommendations concerning technical details. Some of these definitions have been discussed in greater detail elsewhere [2,11].

Physical Factors

Milliamperage

The milliamperage of an x-ray machine deter-mines its output. However, the quantity of radiation per unit time (dose rate) depends both on milliamperage (mA) and kilovoltage (kV). The penetrating power (quality) of an x-ray beam is not changed by altering the milliamperage alone if the kilovoltage remains constant. As the milliamperage of an x-ray tube is increased the intensity of the x-ray beam changes almost in direct proportion. The increased milliamperage means that more electrons strike the target per minute, producing more x-ray photons per minute and therefore increasing the quantity of radiation per minute (ie, its intensity). In modern dermatology the amperage of an x-ray unit is usually not changed; most modern dermatologic units are calibrated at one standard amperage only (eg, 5 mA or 25 mA). Older glass-windowed units often required two different settings (eg, 5 mA and 10 mA) in order to increase the relatively low output of these machines for special purposes, thus adding another potential source of error.

Target–Skin Distance

Target–skin distance (TSD), also known as focus–skin distance (FSD) or source–skin distance (SSD), indicates the distance between the target of the x-ray tube and the treated skin area. For hard x rays, the intensity or dose rate of radiation at a given point is inversely proportional to its distance squared as measured from the focal spot. In dermatology the inverse square law applies only in principle. It cannot be used instead of actual measurements since soft x rays and grenz rays are partially absorbed in air. Theoretically, all x-ray machines (except grenz-ray units) could be used at any distance, limited only by very low dose rates at long target–skin distances. Under practical conditions, however, the choice is usually reduced to only two different distances. Modern rules of radiation protection require the use of cones in most circumstances and most manufacturers supply cones in sets of only two different lengths. These metal cones confine the beam to the field to be treated and minimize direct and indirect exposure of other areas. Their sizes usually correspond to TSDs of 15 and 30 cm (or 20 and 40 cm). Consequently, calibration is necessary only for these two target–skin distances.

The selection of the target–skin distance depends almost exclusively on the size of the lesion to be treated. Longer TSDs are required when larger skin surfaces are treated; the dose at the periphery of the treated area is *relatively* higher and the radiation is more evenly distributed over the treatment area than with short TSDs. The periphery of an area 30 cm in diameter may receive only 50% of the dose at the center when the target–skin distance is 15 cm, while at a target–skin distance of 30 cm the periphery of the area may receive 80% of the dose at the center of the field. The main advantage of a short TSD (except when using contact therapy machines) is the increased dose rate for equal kV and mA factors. Since modern beryllium-windowed units yield a high dose rate even at long target–skin distances, some of them are now supplied with a set of cones of only one long target–skin distance (eg, 30 cm). This arrangement eliminates yet another source of error since only one set of calibrations (for only one TSD) is necessary.

Quality of Radiation

The heterogeneous beam produced by dermatologic x-ray units consists of x rays of varying wavelengths. The proportion of shorter wavelengths (hard x rays) versus longer wavelengths (soft x rays) determines the penetrating effect (quality) of radiation. X-ray qualities are commonly described by the term half-value layer

(HVL). This term has recently been replaced by a newer designation, half-value thickness (HVT), but most textbooks in dermatology and radiotherapy continue to use HVL as a standard definition of radiation quality [16,18].

Half-value Layer (HVL)

The half-value layer is defined as that thickness of a given filter material (in dermatology, usually aluminum) which reduces the intensity of a narrow beam of photons to 50% of the original exposure. A beam of hard quality requires a greater thickness of aluminum for 50% attenuation than does a beam of soft quality. Therefore, the more penetrating beam has a greater half-value layer. In dermatologic therapy the HVL usually varies from 0.01 (grenz-ray range) to 2.0 mm Al; more penetrating x-ray qualities are rarely indicated in skin disorders. The half-value layer of radiation is influenced by several factors. For practical purposes, however, only two of these are important: kilovoltage and additional filtration.

Kilovoltage Most dermatologic x-ray machines are operated within a range of 10 to 100 kV. When the kilovoltage applied to an x-ray tube is increased the intensity (quantity) of the radiation is increased. In addition, the speed and kinetic energy of the electrons are increased and the resulting x rays contain photons of higher energy. Consequently, an x-ray beam produced by higher kilovoltage has a shorter wave length and greater penetrating power. Depending on which window material is used in the x-ray tube, longer wave lengths can be absorbed by the inherent filtration of the window itself. For this reason, older glass-window (Pyrex) units are rarely used below 50 kV because their inherent filtration is approximately 0.5 mm Al. Modern beryllium-window tubes have an inherent filtration of only 0.1 mm Al, and allow utilization of a wider range of x rays of different penetration (10 to 100 kV).

Filtration A filter is a sheet of metal—in dermatologic therapy, usually aluminum—which is placed in the x-ray beam to change its quality. Cellulose acetate or polyethylene filters are occasionally used in grenz-ray therapy. The beam is attenuated by absorption and scattering so that its intensity is diminished by the filter. With a given kV and mA, the thicker the filter and the higher its atomic number the greater the reduction in beam intensity. Thus, 1 mm of copper reduces beam intensity more than does 1 mm of aluminum because copper has a higher atomic number, and 1.0 mm of aluminum reduces intensity more than does only 0.1 mm of aluminum. Since the x-ray beam is heterogeneous in wavelength and the lower-energy photons are more readily removed from the beam by the filter than are the higher-energy photons, there is a *relative* increase in the number of high-energy photons in the emerging beam and its average penetration power is increased.

Selection of a filter thickness that is suitable for the desired depth of penetration is an important step in treatment planning. The choice is limited by the fact that most manufacturers provide only 4 to 5 different thicknesses of aluminum filters (eg, 0.1, 0.25, 0.5, and 1 mm). In the interest of standardization this limitation is desirable to avoid confusion and error. Only a limited number of different combinations of filter and kV are needed in daily practice.

Quantity of Radiation

The intensity or dose rate of radiation is expressed in R/min; the dose rate increases when kilovoltage and/or milliamperage are increased. It decreases as the distance is increased, approximately in inverse-square proportion; it is also reduced as the thickness and atomic number of the filter are increased. The radiation dose is directly proportional to the exposure time if all other factors remain constant. The penetration of radiation is not influenced by the duration of exposure.

Dosage Definitions

The x-ray dose in roentgens (R) specifies the exposure to a certain quantity of radiation based on its ability to ionize air. It does not indicate the absorbed dose in the tissue (which is expressed in rads). Radiation doses can be expressed in several different ways.

Skin Unit Dose
The erythema dose was used in the past to express x-ray dosage in fractions or multiples of "skin units." Since it varies considerably depending on radiation quality, skin thickness, and other factors, this inaccurate biologic unit has been abandoned and replaced by measurements in R.

Air Dose
The air dose is now termed exposure and represents the ionization of air at a given distance from an x-ray tube. The unit of exposure is the roentgen (R).

Surface Dose
The skin surface dose is measured by a thimble chamber in the presence of a scattering medium (tissue or phantom). It represents the exposure (air dose) at a given point in the beam plus the backscatter dose. It is also expressed in roentgens. The amount of backscatter depends on the quality of the beam, the size of the field, and the thickness of the underlying tissue. In dermatology, the backscatter factor varies from almost zero (for grenz rays) to 30% (for penetrating radiation with a HVL of 2 mm Al in a 20×20 cm^2 field).

Absorbed Dose
The biologic effect of any radiation depends on the quantity absorbed, chiefly through the process of ionization. Only the absorbed radiation is capable of producing therapeutic or damaging effects on tissues. The unit of the absorbed dose (tissue dose) is the rad. One rad is the absorption of 100 ergs of energy/g of absorbing material. The rad is the most useful unit of dosimetry. Since experimental determination of the absorbed dose is still difficult and not available for all theoretical factors, the International Commission on Radiation Units and Measurements* has recommended "that the roentgen, in view of its long established usefulness, shall continue to be recognized as the unit of x-ray and γ-ray quantity." In dermatologic therapy, the difference between 1 roentgen and 1 rad is insignificant, although in orthovoltage therapy the values for roentgen and rad may be at great variance. The absorption of x rays by the skin has been measured for various physical parameters and published in the form of depth dose charts or curves and isodose curves. Depth dose curves

*International Commission on Radiation Units and Measurements Report No 10b: Physical Aspects of Irradiation, ICRV Publications, 1964

indicate the dose at various depths along the central axis of the beam, while isodose curves establish points at various depths of tissue at which the absorbed dose is the same. The depth dose is influenced by kilovoltage, filtration, target–skin distance, and field size.

Exit Dose

This is the amount of radiation that emerges from a part of the body after the beam has traversed its entire thickness. In dermatology it corresponds to the dose received by the skin on the side opposite to the irradiated surface. It is important in thin parts of the body, such as the hand, foot, nose, and ear, particularly when more penetrating types of radiation are used. The exit dose can be reduced to a minimum when soft x-ray qualities are employed.

Selection of Physical Factors

Since many physical factors can now be standardized, the basic decisions before treatment deal only with the quantity of radiation (dose) and its quality (half-value layer). The x-ray penetration should be correlated to the depth of the pathologic process. When very soft radiation qualities are used, there may be too great a difference between the doses received by the upper and lower levels of the lesion. Conversely, when the selected x rays are too penetrating, the normal tissue below the lesion may receive an excessive dose. A compromise is usually necessary so that the depth dose below the actual lesion falls off as rapidly as possible. Data on actual penetration of a given x-ray beam can be obtained from depth dose tables, which give the dose on the central axis of the beam as a percentage of the surface dose. In the past, the dose at the base of the lesion had to be computed arithmetically utilizing these sources in order to determine the exposure (air dose) which would result in the desired surface and depth dose [5].

Half-value Depth ($D_{1/2}$) in Treatment Planning

The selection of the appropriate combination of kilovoltage, filter, and half-value layer is the most important decision in treatment planning. The introduction of the half-value depth ($D_{1/2}$) as a guideline in the selection of radiation

qualities has simplified this process immensely. Its main advantage is that its routine application makes roentgen therapy safer and more effective; in addition, it eliminates confusing arithmetic computations. Instead of using several sets of depth dose charts for different combinations of radiation factors, followed by arithmetic computation of the dose at the base of the lesion, the modern radiotherapist takes advantage of calibrations based on the half-value depth. The half-value depth ($D_{1/2}$, or HVD) is the tissue depth (expressed in mm) at which the absorbed dose is 50% of the surface dose (Chapter 1). Proposed and elaborated by Jennings [15] and Wachsmann [20], this biologic term has achieved greater significance for the dermatologist than has the physical term, HVL. The logical term, half-dose depth (HDD, or $D_{1/2}$, was recently proposed by Kopf and associates (Chapter 9). The practical importance of the $D_{1/2}$ concept was emphasized by Schirren [17] for treatment of skin cancers (see also [10]) and by Goldschmidt [9] for benign dermatoses.

The basic consideration in dermatologic therapy is to give as large a dose as necessary to the lesion and as little as possible to the underlying normal tissues. Unfortunately, the absorption of radiation is exponential and it is not possible to deliver a uniform dose throughout the lesion without any radiation being absorbed below the lesion (except in electron beam therapy). The suggested compromise consists of giving 50% of the surface dose to the base of the lesion with as rapid an attenuation of the beam as possible beyond this region. The main significance of this concept is that most of the radiation is absorbed in the pathologic process and is therefore of greater therapeutic benefit. The deeper tissues are also more protected than in most other radiation methods and the possibility of undesirable radiation effects is reduced markedly. Of course, radiation can also be therapeutically effective when qualities are used which are either too superficial or more penetrating than the tissue depth would warrant. Traditionally, skin cancers have often been treated with very penetrating radiations. Yet only a small percentage of the surface dose is absorbed in the tumor itself and a disproportionately high percentage penetrates to deeper uninvolved tissues, thus increasing the possibility of undesirable radiation sequelae. On the

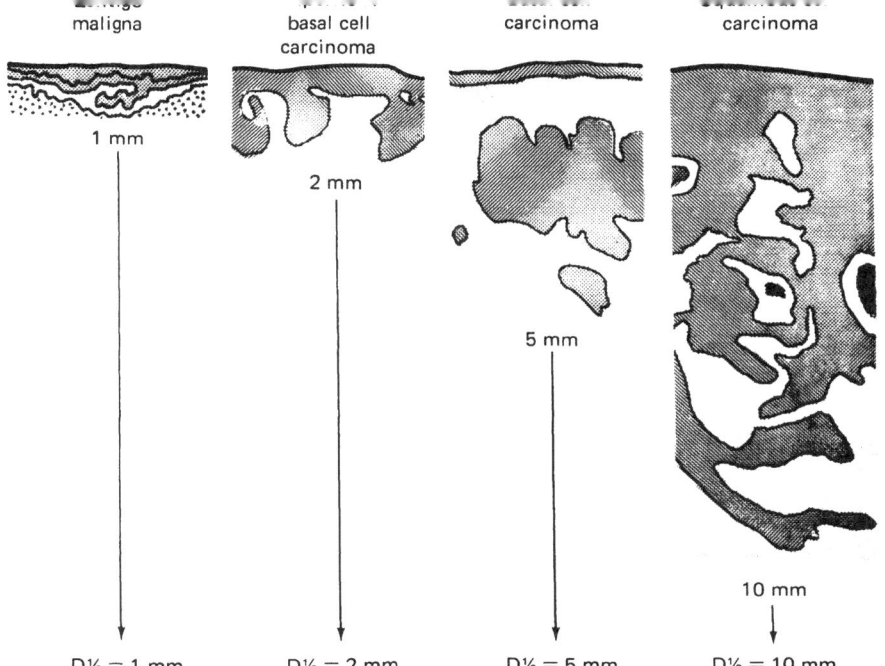

maligna | basal cell carcinoma | carcinoma | carcinoma

1 mm

2 mm

5 mm

10 mm

D½ = 1 mm   D½ = 2 mm   D½ = 5 mm   D½ = 10 mm

Figure 6-1. Selection of half-value depth for skin cancers and premalignant tumors. From Goldschmidt [11].

other hand, ultrasoft x rays have been found effective in some inflammatory cutaneous disorders of much greater tissue depth than the maximum $D_{1/2}$ of grenz rays (usually not more than 0.5 mm of tissue). This therapeutic response may be explained by the release of unknown factors from the epidermis and uppermost dermis which subsequently reduce the inflammatory reaction in tissue depths not reached by ultrasoft x rays.

It should also be noted that routinely used individual doses for grenz-ray therapy are 2 to 3 times higher than are individual doses recommended for superficial x rays; this also accounts for a relatively deeper effect. In either case, the selection of radiation qualities corresponding to tissue depth would seem to be a more reasonable choice. Figure 6-1 illustrates this concept for skin cancers and premalignant tumors. Figure 6-2 demonstrates the same for benign dermatoses. An example of a typical calibration based on the $D_{1/2}$ concept is given in Table 6-1. (Since the half-value depth is influenced by field size, target–skin distance, and half-value layer, different sets of calibrations should be available.) Table 6-1 shows calibration data for a beryllium-window machine with physical factors arranged according to their half-value depth. In our experience, these 5 standard combinations of kilovoltage and filtra-

Table 6-1 *Calibration Data: 50 kV Beryllium-window Unit (Siemens Dermopan 2)*

$D_{1/2}$ (mm tissue)	HVL (mm Al)	kV	Filter (mm Al)	mA	TSD (cm)	Dose Rate (R/min)
0.2	0.02	10	—	25	30	100
3.0	0.15	29	0.3	25	30	100
7.5	0.40	43	0.6	25	30	100
13.0	0.75	50	1.0	25	30	100
18.0	1.40	50	2.0	25	30	45

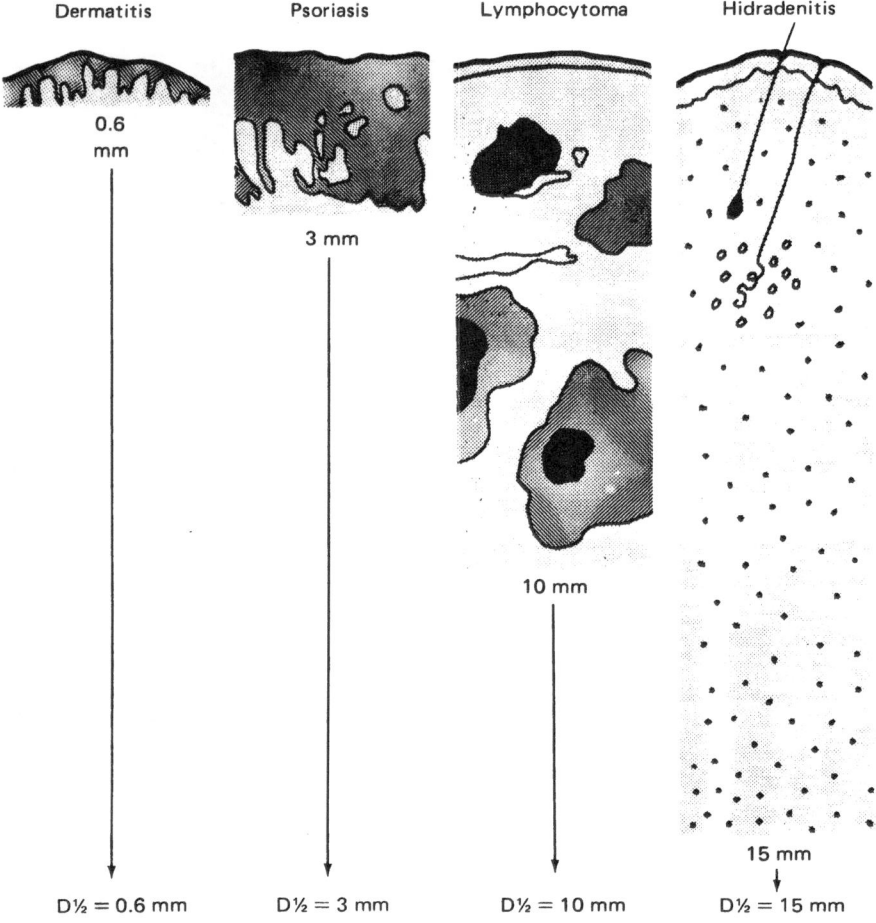

Figure 6-2.   Selection of half-value depth for benign dermatoses. From Goldschmidt [11].

tion have been satisfactory for 95% of routine dermatologic radiation treatments. Instead of calculating the dose which will reach the depth of the treated lesion, the physician consulting this set of data will easily locate the depth at which 50% of the surface dose is absorbed and select the other physical factors accordingly. Calibrations based on $D_{1/2}$ can easily be provided by a radiophysicist; detailed depth dose data have been published by several authors [16,19]. Since the dermatologist knows the depths of various skin disorders, he should advise his physicist which half-value depths would be useful in routine indications (Fig. 6-3). Accurate measurements of the actual depths of various skin diseases have been published by Zoon and Werz [22], and can serve as the basis for selection of adequate half-value depths which are needed frequently in a dermatologic

office (Table 6-2). Atkinson [1] has correlated depths of skin cancers and dose homogeneities.

Table 6-2   *Depth Dose Data*

	Depth (in mm)
Normal Skin	
Epidermis	0.03 – 0.25
Stratum corneum	0.015– 0.5
Corium	3.0 – 4.0
Hair papilla	2.5 – 3.5
Eccrine sweat glands	2.0 – 3.0
Benign Dermatoses	
Dermatitis, eczema	0.8 – 2.1
Psoriasis vulgaris	0.7 – 3.2
Lichen simplex chronicus	1.1 – 4.4
Lichen planus	0.4 – 2.1
Folliculitis, acne vulgaris	3.0 – 5.0
Cutaneous Tumors	3.0 –10 (rarely deeper)

After Zoon and Werz [22].

In addition to providing for an optimal tissue depth, the adoption of the $D_{1/2}$ concept offers practical advantages in the calculation of required surface doses for lesions of varying depth. When the $D_{1/2}$ is chosen properly, the base of the lesion receives exactly 50% of the surface dose; the necessary individual and total surface doses can then be computed easily for each required tissue depth by doubling the depth dose (eg, if the base of a skin cancer is to receive 2500 R, a surface dose of 5000 R will be required).

Radiation Techniques

Tables 6-3 and 6-4 present a summary of x-ray therapy methods and x-ray generators which are presently used in dermatology and radiol-

ogy. A systematic classification is difficult because different physical and technical aspects were emphasized when new radiation methods were developed. Consequently, these modalities can be arranged according to depth of penetration (ie, deep x-ray therapy, intermediate x-ray therapy, and superficial x-ray therapy), or according to the type of x-ray generator used. In dermatology, the type of window is particularly important and x-ray units have been classified accordingly as glass-window (Pyrex) machines (high-voltage or low-voltage units), beryllium-window machines (soft x-ray units and modern grenz-ray machines), or Lindemann-window machines (older grenz-ray machines). Most x-ray machines function at target–skin distances varying from 15 to 40 cm. The major exception is with the contact x-ray

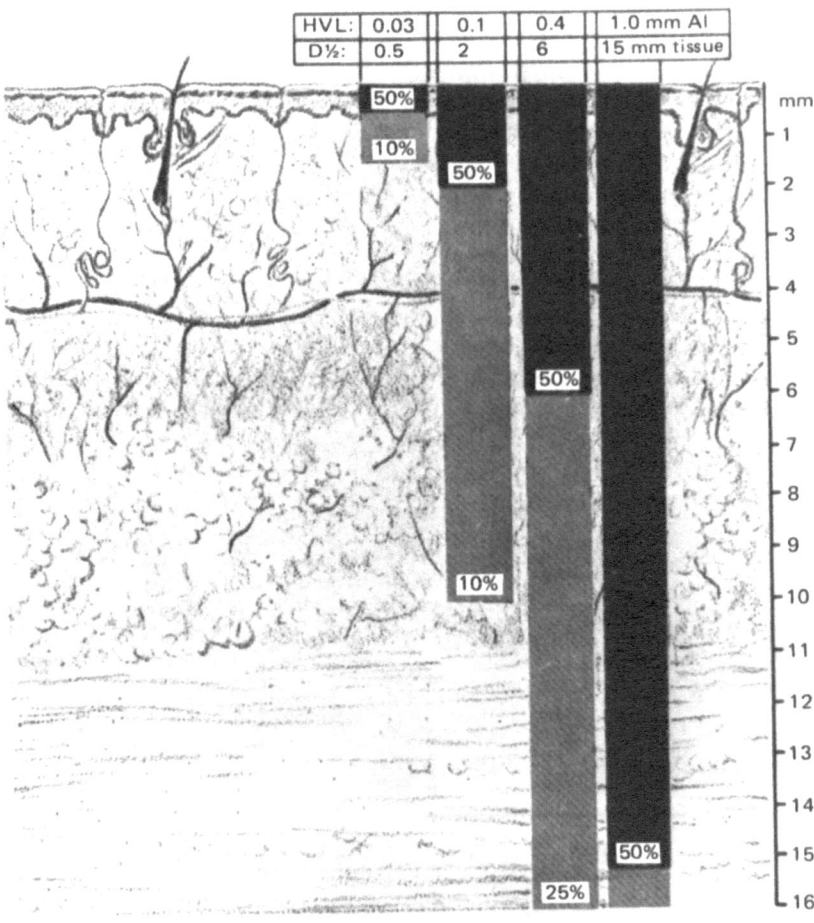

Figure 6-3. Depth of penetration (D½) of various x-ray qualities. From Goldschmidt [8].

Table 6-3   *Radiation Methods*

Type	Sources and Synonyms	kV	TSD (cm)	Wavelength (Å) (average)	HVL	$D_{1/2}$ (mm tissue)
Megavoltage therapy	Betatron, particle accelerators	>1000	80	0.001	>10 mm Pb	200
Supervoltage therapy	γ ray Telecurie sources	400–800	50–80	0.03	5–10 mm Pb	80–110
Orthovoltage therapy	Deep x-ray therapy Conventional x-ray therapy	200–400	50–80	0.14	2–4 mm Cu	50–80
Intermediate x-ray therapy	Half-deep therapy	110–130	30	0.1	4 mm Al	30
Contact therapy	Ultrashort distance (Chaoul)	50–60	1.5–3.0	0.8	2–4 mm Al	4–30
Superficial x-ray therapy	Low voltage, standard x-ray therapy Pyrex window	60–100	15–30	0.5	0.7–2.0 mm Al	7–10
Soft x-ray therapy	Beryllium window	20–100	10–30	0.15	0.1–2.0 mm Al	1–20
Grenz-ray therapy	Ultrasolf therapy Supersoft therapy	5–20	10–15	2	0.03 mm Al	0.2–0.8

From Goldschmidt [7].

technique, which is also known as ultra–short-distance therapy (Chaoul and Philips units). In radiotherapy modern therapy units have been subdivided into high-energy x-ray units, where x rays are produced with particle accelerators (eg, Van de Graaff accelerator, linear accelerator, betatron), and teleisotope machines (telecurie therapy machines), where γ rays are produced by isotopes (eg, radium teletherapy, ^{137}Cs teletherapy, ^{60}Co teletherapy).

Tables 6-3 and 6-4 also emphasize the obvious differences in radiotherapeutic as opposed to dermatologic concepts and objectives.

A chief aim of the newer techniques in radiotherapy has been the development of generators that produce more penetrating ionizing radiation in order to treat tumors at greater depth. At the same time, efforts have been made to reduce cutaneous side effects which often prevented the delivery of therapeutically effective doses to deeper tissues. Major achievements in this area are exemplified by the new megavoltage treatment units which combine great penetration with a "skin-sparing" effect, thereby reducing both the acute and chronic radiation reactions which had been

Table 6-4   *Terminology of Ionizing Radiations*

Energy	Classification	Commonly Used Voltages	Type of Generator
100 MeV			
	Megavoltage		
		20 MeV	Betatron
10 MeV	or	10 MeV	
			Linear Accelerators
		4 MeV	
	Supervoltage		Isotope teletherapy machines (^{60}Co)
		2 MeV	(^{137}Cs)
1 MeV		1 MeV	(γ rays)
(1000 kV)	Orthovoltage		
	or	250–600 kV	
	Deep x rays		
	Half-deep x rays	150–250 kV	
100 kV	Superficial x rays	50–100 kV	X-ray machines
	Soft x rays	20–50 kV	
10 kV	Grenz rays	10–20 kV	

a serious problem with previous techniques. It is obvious that the great penetration of modern x-ray generators as used by the radiotherapist makes them totally unsuitable for most dermatologic purposes. The radiotherapist tends to view radiation effects on the skin as undesirable secondary reactions, while the dermatologist sees them as objects of treatment. Dermatologists have been instrumental in developing x-ray units with less penetrating qualities, particularly when it became clear that only absorbed doses have any therapeutic effect and after it had been established that softer x rays have the same therapeutic effects as do harder x rays. Limited penetration was considered essential in order to achieve absorption in the skin itself instead of in deeper tissues. The first improvement in dermatologic x-ray therapy was the introduction of so-called superficial (low voltage) x-ray machines with Pyrex (glass) windows. These machines are still in use and are suitable for most dermatologic purposes. The designation "low voltage superficial x-ray units" derives from the fact that their effect on the skin was more superficial and that they employ a lower voltage than did previously used deep (orthovoltage) x-ray generators. Very low voltages with even more superficial radiation could be utilized when grenz-ray machines became available.

The construction of an x-ray tube with a window of lithium borate glass by Lindemann permitted the therapeutic use of very long wavelengths. The advantages of grenz-ray machines in dermatologic therapy were described by Bucky and other authors [3], starting in 1925. The grenz-ray technique was revived when beryllium windows became available; all modern grenz-ray machines are now supplied with beryllium windows.

If one uses the half-value depth as a criterion for the selection of x-ray machines for dermatologic purposes, a glance at Table 6-3 shows that there was still a large difference between the tissue depths which could be treated properly with superficial x rays or with grenz rays (ie, between 1 and 7 mm, where most skin diseases are located). An attempt to bridge this gap was the introduction of the contact x-ray technique by Chaoul [4], who used extremely short target–skin distances to simulate the fall-off ratio of radium corpuscular radiation. Its main limitation was the limited field size. The technologic gap between superfi-

cial x-ray units and older grenz-ray machines was finally closed with the introduction of modern beryllium-window tubes (10 to 100 kV), which made it possible for the first time to build x-ray machines for the intermediate range of penetration which are suitable for all dermatologic purposes.

Superficial X-ray Therapy

The superficial (ie, low voltage, standard, conventional) x-ray technique was the most widely used dermatologic radiation method before the advent of the beryllium-window machine. It was employed in the treatment of superficial lesions utilizing radiation produced by a tube with a Pyrex (glass) window at 60 to 100 kV with a HVL of 0.7 to 0.1 mm Al and a TSD of 15 to 30 cm. Normally, no additional filtration was used. The $D_{1/2}$ of this radiation varies from 7 to 10 mm of tissue and is satisfactory for most dermatologic conditions, even though it is more penetrating than necessary, since most dermatoses involve only the upper 3 to 5 mm of skin. The same treatment units have also been used in "filtered techniques" for deep skin lesions or skin cancers where radiations of 120 to 140 kV filtered through 3 mm Al with a HVL of 2 to 3 mm Al were used. The HVD of this radiation is 20 to 30 mm; it is indicated only in tumors which are extremely deep and rarely seen in dermatology.

Grenz-ray Therapy (ultrasoft x rays; supersoft x rays)

For many years grenz-ray machines have been considered the most suitable and safest x-ray units for use by the dermatologist [2,12,21]. Ultrasoft x rays are radiations of low energy, produced between 5 and 20 kV. Electromagnetic waves of very long wavelength (1 to 3 Å) occupy the portion of the electromagnetic spectrum between x rays and ultraviolet rays. Because of this position they were also called grenz ray or borderline rays (from the German *Grenze*, borderline). Originally, it was thought that they had special biologic properties, but it is now clearly established that these waves are x rays and can cause sequelae similar to those of x rays if applied improperly. Because of their low penetration, the incidence of radiodermatitis is lower than in superficial x-ray therapy.

There is no doubt, however, that radiodermatitis, especially severe telangiectasia, may result from excessive therapy with grenz rays, and in very rare instances (with tremendous total dosages given), radiation cancer has occurred after grenz-ray treatment. In the past, radiation sequelae were often due to improper calibration. Modern iontoquantimeters for the specific purpose of measuring soft radiation are now available, so that grenz-ray units can be calibrated with almost the same accuracy as can higher-voltage equipment.

The utilization of extremely long wavelengths was originally made possible by the construction of the Lindemann window, a thin lithium borate glass that permitted the passage of long-wavelength x rays which would have been absorbed by other types of glass. Physical properties and clinical indications were investigated by Bucky; for this reason ultrasoft x rays are also known as Bucky rays. Lithium borate windows were rather delicate and broke easily when higher voltages (over 15 kV) were applied. Modern grenz-ray machines use 0.5 to 1-mm thick beryllium windows with an inherent filtration of 0.1 mm Al HVL. Theoretically, many of these tubes could be used for higher voltages but the kV was deliberately restricted to usage in the grenz-ray range by the manufacturers. Most grenz-ray machines can be operated at different kilovoltages from 5 to 20 kV and allow for the use of additional thin aluminum filters. The resulting half-value layers vary from approximately 0.018 to 0.036 mm Al. Most dermatologists have tended to select radiations toward the upper limit of 0.036 mm Al HVL for routine use, taking advantage of slightly deeper penetration and higher dose rates. The average HVD is only 0.3 to 0.5 mm of skin; radiation effects are sharply limited to 2 to 3 mm in depth. This limited penetration accounts for the safety of grenz rays when properly used. The high dose rate (R/min) of modern grenz-ray machines makes careful attention to kV and exposure time necessary.

Small alterations in the applied kilovoltage cause much wider fluctuations in output than with conventional x rays. The inverse square law does not apply to changes in the target–skin distance since the absorption of grenz rays by air reduces the delivered dose considerably, limiting to a maximum of 20 to 30 cm the target–skin distance which can be used effectively with routine grenz-ray therapy. The same factors also limit the field size to approximately 20 × 20 cm; larger areas can only be treated by multiple overlapping exposures.

Contact X-ray Therapy

A new type of x-ray therapy suitable for the treatment of skin cancers was proposed in 1931 by Chaoul, who called it "ultra–short-distance therapy." It was developed to imitate the effects of radium, which was then widely used in the treatment of skin cancers; at the short target–skin distance employed, the dose fall-off closely approximated that of radium. The basis of contact x-ray therapy is a rapidly decreasing depth dose; this is achieved by shortening the target–skin distance, an application of the inverse square law. Two different units are presently in use. In the Chaoul Contact Therapy Unit, the anode is located at the end of the tube close to the treatment field; the anode transmits the x rays that are produced in it. The Chaoul tube is a transmission target tube; the x rays go through the target and are not reflected. Even though a very hard irradiation of 3.3 mm Al HVL is produced, the half-value depth is approximately 10 mm when operated at 60 kV and 3-cm TSD through a 3-cm port. This radiation is useful for skin cancers up to 2 cm in diameter in various body areas.

In the Philips Contact Therapy Unit, another modification of ultra–short-distance therapy, the x-ray beam does not pass through the target because the filament is placed between the target and the treatment area. The rays are actually reflected straight forward from the tungsten target. This is the reason why the HVL of the radiation emanating from the Philips tube is much smaller than that from the Chaoul tube. Older units utilize glass windows; newer units are equipped with beryllium windows.

The development of contact therapy units was an important advance over use of older radiation methods, particularly in the treatment of small skin cancers. The new method permitted treatment with a quantity of radiation that was fairly evenly distributed throughout the pathologic process, and was predominantly absorbed within the tumor with adequate protection of the underlying tissues. In comparison to older standard techniques with heavy additional filtration (HVL, 3 mm Al; HVD, 40 to 50 cm), therapeutic results were markedly im-

Table 6-5 *Dermatologic X-ray Machines: Advantages and Disadvantages*

X-ray Machine	Advantages	Disadvantages
Grenz-ray units (ultrasoft)	Relative safety	Useful only for very superficial dermatoses
Soft x-ray units (beryllium window)	Useful for all dermatologic purposes (including treatment of neoplasms and teleroentgen therapy)	May need shielded treatment room
Superficial (conventional) x-ray units	Useful for most dermatologic purposes	Often too penetrating; shielded treatment room required
Contact therapy units	Useful in cancer therapy	Field size very limited due to short TSD

proved for most skin cancers which are ordinarily not deeper than 3 to 10 mm. Domonkos [6] has described the special advantages of contact therapy in locations where injury to underlying tissue must be minimized, particularly in the eyelid region.

Contact therapy machines have now been largely superseded by modern soft x-ray units with beryllium windows. These newer units can also be used for other skin lesions but offer the same therapeutic advantages as do contact therapy machines for skin cancers, particularly that of absorption almost solely within the tumor tissue. Even large tumors can be treated with soft x rays, whereas contact therapy units require subdivision of large lesions into multiple contiguous fields where overlapping cannot be avoided completely. Soft x-ray techniques also yield a more even distribution of radiation over irregular surfaces, and eliminate potential damage to the operator by the hand-held contact therapy tube. They also reduce the possibility of accidental overdosage inherent in contact therapy machines with very high dose rates.

Soft X-ray Therapy With Beryllium-window Machines

The introduction of dermatologic x-ray units with beryllium windows in the late 1940s has strongly influenced cutaneous radiotherapy. Because of its low atomic number (4), beryllium possesses a very low absorption coefficient for x rays. When malleable beryllium became available, thin beryllium windows could be produced which were heat resistant and durable at kilovoltages between 5 and 100 kV.

Even very long wavelengths can penetrate this window material. The combination of lower inherent filtration and increased kilovoltage also made higher dose rates possible. Depth dose curves for beryllium tubes show that their range of penetration fills the gap between ultrasoft grenz-ray machines and standard superficial x-ray units [13,14]. Beryllium windows are currently utilized in modern grenz-ray units with kilovoltages up to 20 kV; all-purpose units with a range of from 10 to 50 (or 10 to 100) kV are now considered the most versatile x-ray machines for dermatologic therapy. A potential disadvantage is the extremely high output of the tube when filters are omitted at higher voltages by either human or technical error. This problem has been overcome by use of modern x-ray machines with fixed kV–filter combinations and interlock mechanisms. Some of these units have the added safety feature of delivering the same dose rate (eg, 100 R/min) for different radiation qualities. Other potential sources of error are eliminated by utilizing these beryllium units at only one TSD (eg, 30 cm) and one milliamperage (eg, 25 mA) for all radiation qualities used in dermatology.

Dermatologic X-ray Machines

Four basic types of x-ray machines are used in dermatology: superficial x-ray machines, grenz-ray units, soft x-ray machines, and contact therapy units. The advantages and disadvantages of these machines are summarized in Table 6-5.*

*The availability and usage of various types of dermatologic radiation equipment are discussed in Chapter 8.

Table 6-6 *Different Types of Ionizing Radiation Equipment Used in Dermatologic Offices*

Type of Equipment	No. of Replies	Offices with X-ray Equipment (%)
Grenz-ray units (5–20 kV)	1361	604 (44.4)
Beryllium-window units (soft x-ray machines; 10–50–100 kV)	1095	141 (12.8)
Superficial low-voltage machines (Pyrex window; 60–120 kV)	1589	984 (61.9)
Contact therapy units	1025	14 (1.4)
Other x-ray machines	1008	71 (7.0)
Radium	1063	102 (9.6)
Other radionuclides	933	12 (1.3)

From Goldschmidt[8].

Superficial X-ray Units

A recent survey of the Task Force on Ionizing Radiation of the National Program for Dermatology showed that superficial (Pyrex-windowed) x-ray machines are the most commonly used dermatologic radiotherapy units in the United States and Canada (Table 6-6) [8]. Only one firm is presently manufacturing this type of dermatologic unit (Fig. 6-4). Used superficial x-ray machines are available at reasonable prices. Table 6-7 lists physical specifications for superficial x-ray units sold and serviced in the United States.

Grenz-ray Units

Grenz-ray machines are the second most common type of x-ray equipment. They are manufactured by several firms (Fig. 6-5) and are the most widely available type of apparatus. Table 6-8 lists physical specifications for grenz-ray units sold and serviced in the United States.

Soft X-ray Units

Modern beryllium-window x-ray units are gradually replacing superficial x-ray machines because of their greater versatility and built-in safety factors (Figs. 6-6–6-9). Most of these units can also be operated at very low kilovoltages including the grenz-ray range. One soft x-ray machine can do the work of a superficial x-ray machine, a grenz-ray machine, and a contact x-ray unit. Table 6-9 lists the physical specifications for soft x-ray units sold and serviced in the United States.

These universal dermatologic radiotherapy units are the most useful but also the most expensive type of dermatologic x-ray equipment. Table 6-10 summarizes their advantages.

Contact X-ray Units

Only one manufacturer is presently distributing contact x-ray machines (Fig. 6-10). These ma-

Table 6-7 *Specifications for Superficial X-ray Machines (60–120 kV)*

Manufacturer	Model	Window	mA	kV	HVL Range (mm Al)	$D_{1/2}$ (mm tissue)	Safety Devices	Cooling Method	Remarks
Universal X-ray Products, Inc 4014 West Grand Avenue Chicago, Ill 60651	Treatmaster X-ray Unit	Pyrex	3–5	60–95	0.25–3.0	8–30	Color-coded filters	Air	
Picker X Ray 2880 Comly Road Philadelphia, Pa 19154	Zephyr	Pyrex	5–10	60–120	0.25–3.0	8–30	Color-coded filters	Air	Manufacture discontinued

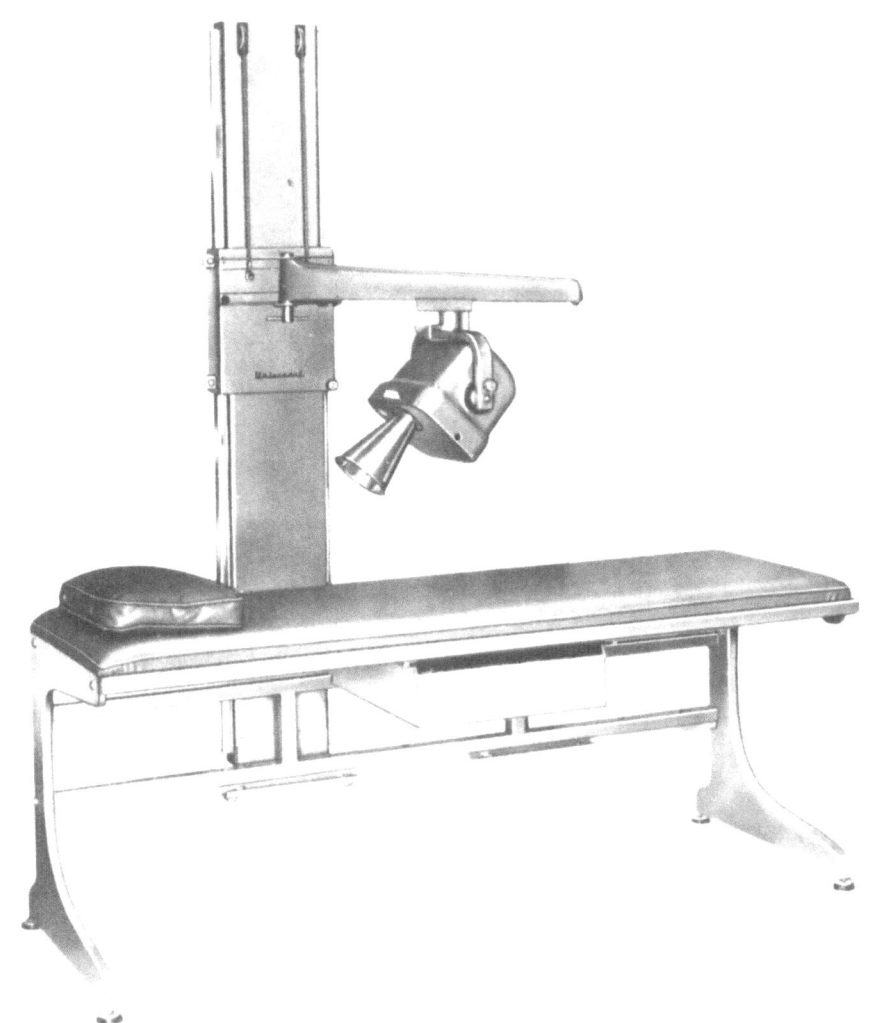

TREATMASTER DELUXE X-RAY   Cat. No. 3184

TREATMASTER DELUXE GRENZ   Cat. No. 3184-G

Figure 6-4.   Universal grenz-ray machine.

Table 6-8   *Specifications for Grenz-ray Machines (<20 kV)*

Manufacturer	Model	Window	mA	kV	HVL Range (mm Al)	$D_{1/2}$ Range (mm tissue)	Cooling Method
Universal X-ray Products, Inc 4014 West Grand Avenue Chicago, Ill 60651	Treatmaster Grenz-ray Unit	Beryllium	5	20	0.02–0.04	0.2–0.5	Air
J. J. Stark Equipment Co 29-28 41st Avenue Long Island City, NY 11101	Dermex G	Beryllium	5–10	12–15 (18)	0.02–0.04	0.2–0.5	Air

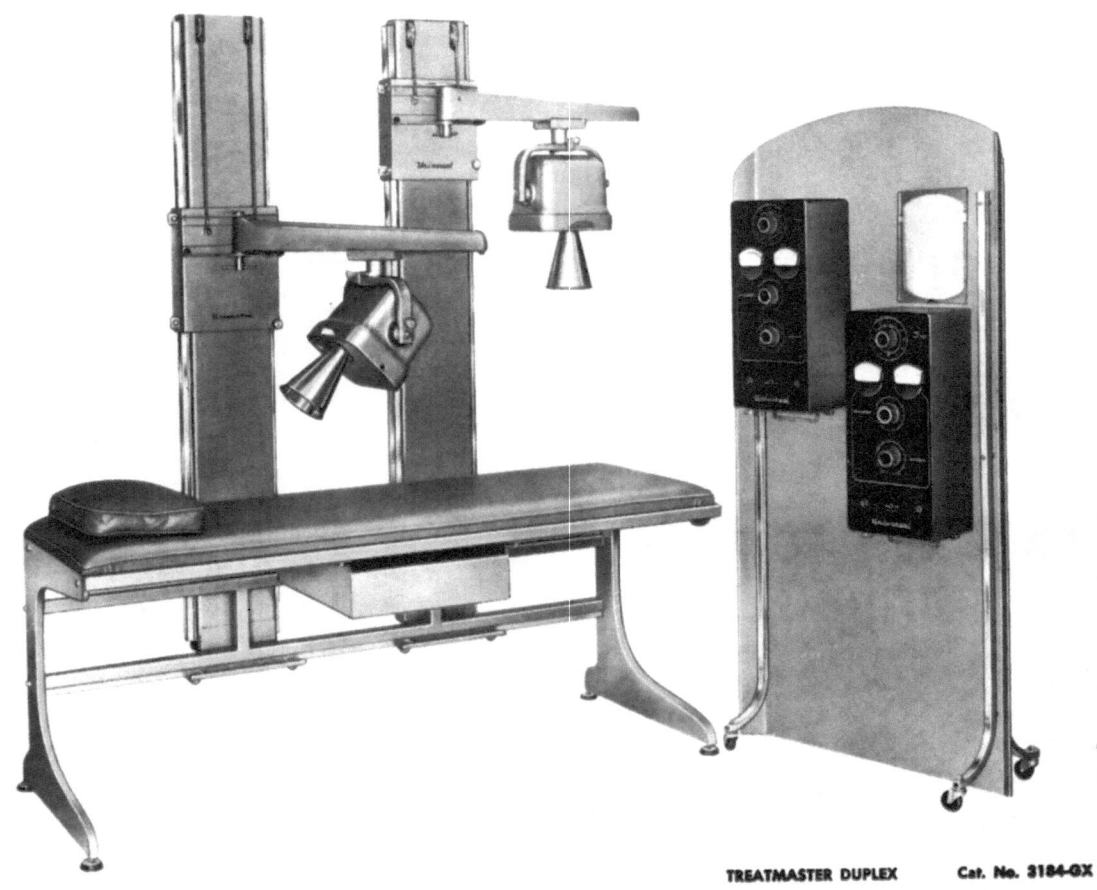

TREATMASTER DUPLEX   Cat. No. 3184-GX

Figure 6-5. Superficial x-ray machine: Universal Treatmaster x-ray unit. This unit is also available as the Universal Duplex Treatmaster (combined with Universal grenz-ray unit).

chines are most useful in the treatment of skin cancers. They are gradually being replaced by soft x-ray machines, which offer the same theoretical advantages that were originally associated with contact x-ray machines. Table 6-11 lists the physical specifications for contact x-ray units sold and serviced in the United States.

Table 6-9 *Specifications for Soft X-ray Machines (10–50 or 5–100 kV)*

Manufacturer	Model	Window	mA	kV	HVL Range (mm Al)	$D_{1/2}$ Range (mm tissue)	Safety Devices	Cooling Method	Remarks
Siemens Corp 186 Wood Avenue South Iselin, NJ 08830	Dermopan II	Beryllium	25	10–50	0.02–18	0.2–20	4 standard kV–filter combinations with automatic control	Closed water circulating system	
Philips Medical Systems Inc 710 Bridgeport Avenue PO Box 484 Shelton, Conn 06484	RT 100	Beryllium	8–10	10–100	0.025–2.5	0.3–30	10 standard kV–filter combinations with automatic control	Closed water circulating system	
General Electric Co Medical Systems Division PO Box 414 Milwaukee Wisc 53201	GE Maximar 100	Beryllium	5	30–100	0.3–2.0	1–30	Color-coded filters, flashing light without filter	Air	Manufacture discontinued
Bucky X-ray International Inc 30 East 81st Street New York, NY 10028	Dermatologic Combination Therapy machine	Beryllium	5–10	5–100	0.02–3.0	0.2–35	Automatic filter control above and below 15 kV	Air	

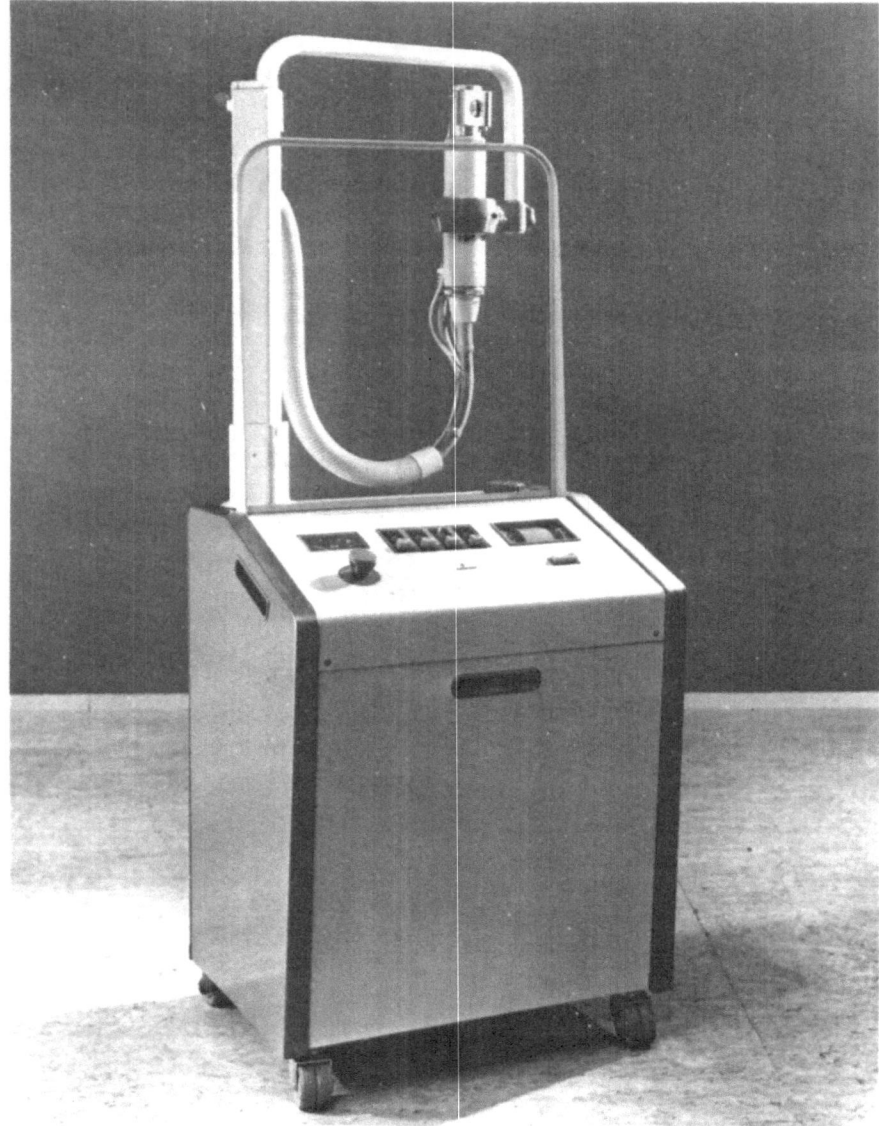

Figure 6-6.   Siemens Dermopan 2 soft x-ray unit.

Table 6-10   *Advantages of Beryllium-window Machines*

1. Utilization of long wavelengths
2. Proper correlation between radiation quality (penetration) and depth of pathologic process
3. Protection of underlying normal tissue
4. Higher dose rates permit the following:
    a. Longer target–skin distances (and more homogeneous irradiation)
    b. Treatment of large areas
    c. Shorter treatment times
    d. Selection of filter and kV combinations that yield same dose rate (eg, 100 R/min for different radiation qualities)

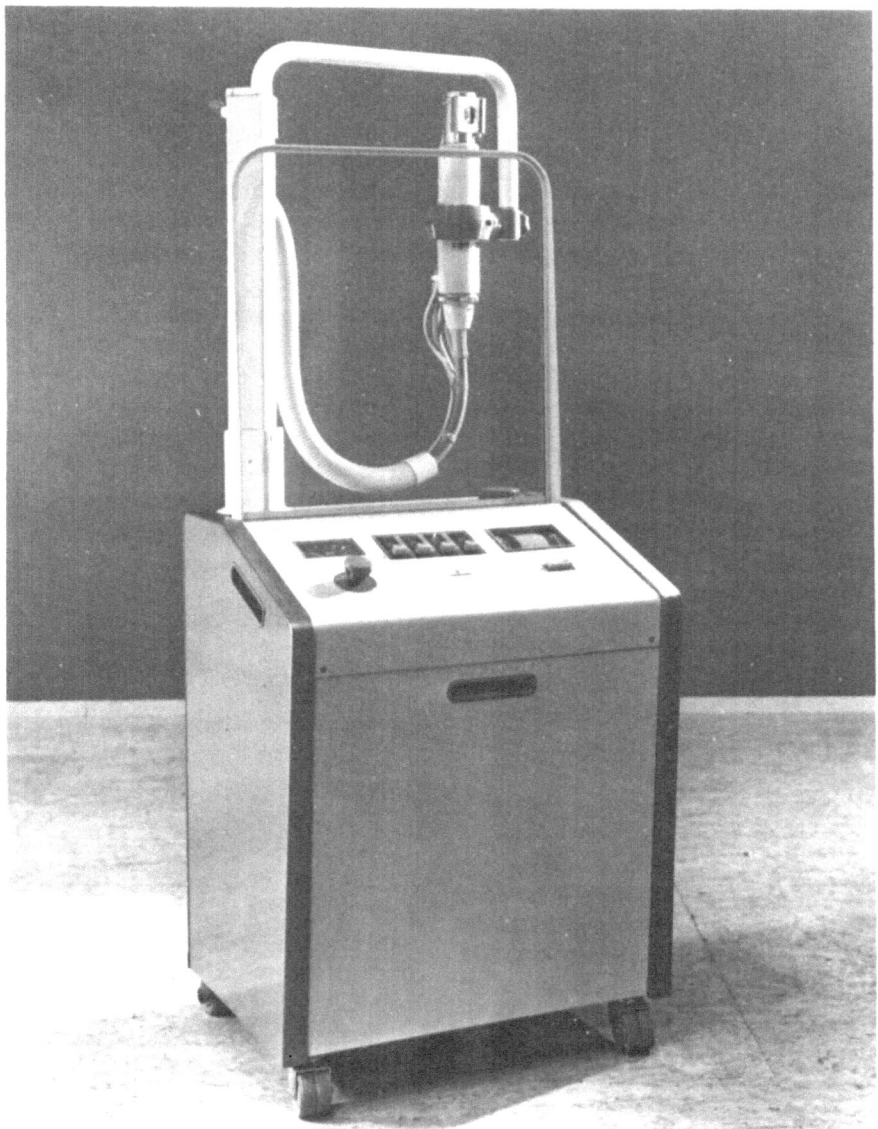

Figure 6-7. Philips RT 100 soft x-ray machine.

Table 6-11 *Model RT 50 Contact X-ray Machine*

Parameter	Specification
Manufacturer	Philips
Address	Philips Medical Systems Inc, 710 Bridgeport Ave.
	PO Box 484, Shelton, Conn 06484
Model	RT 50
Window	Beryllium
mA	2
kV	10–50
HVL range (mm Al)	0.02–0.7
D_{12} range (mm tissue)	0.25–4.5
Safety devices	6 standard kV–filter combinations with automatic control
Cooling method	Air
Remarks	Available in the United States

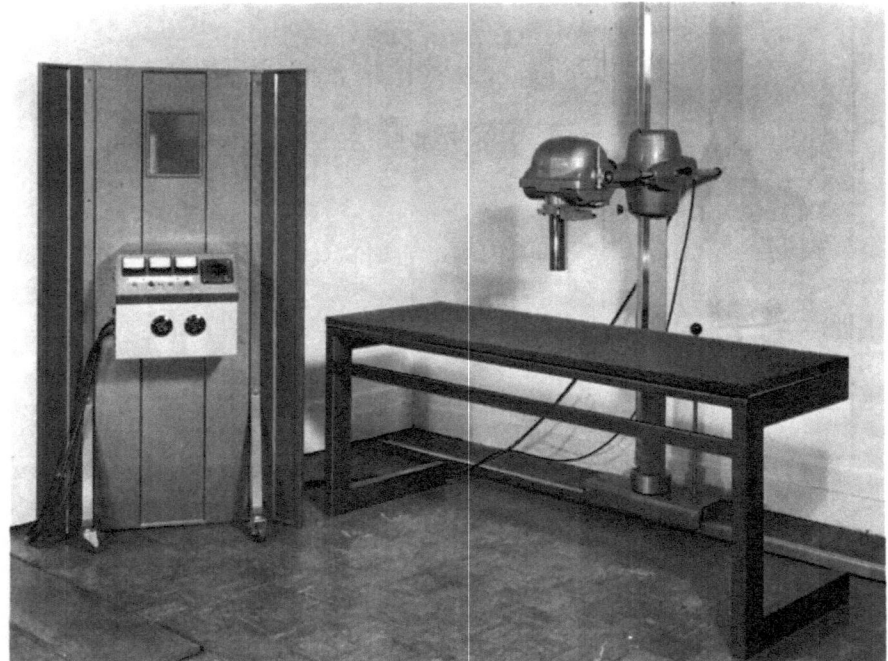

Figure 6-8. Bucky Combination soft x-ray machine.

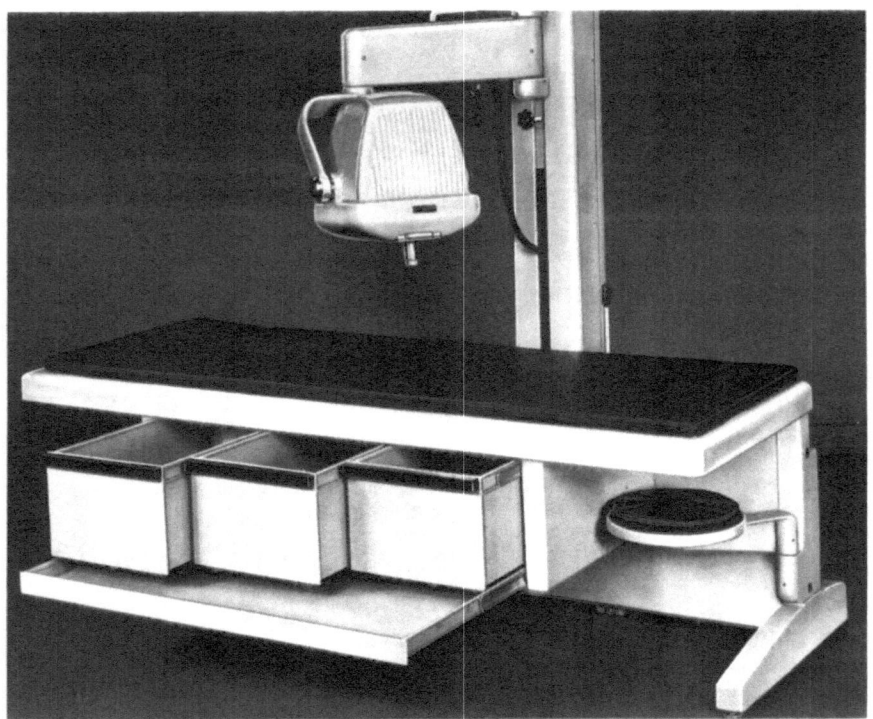

Figure 6-9. General Electric Maximar 100 soft x-ray unit.

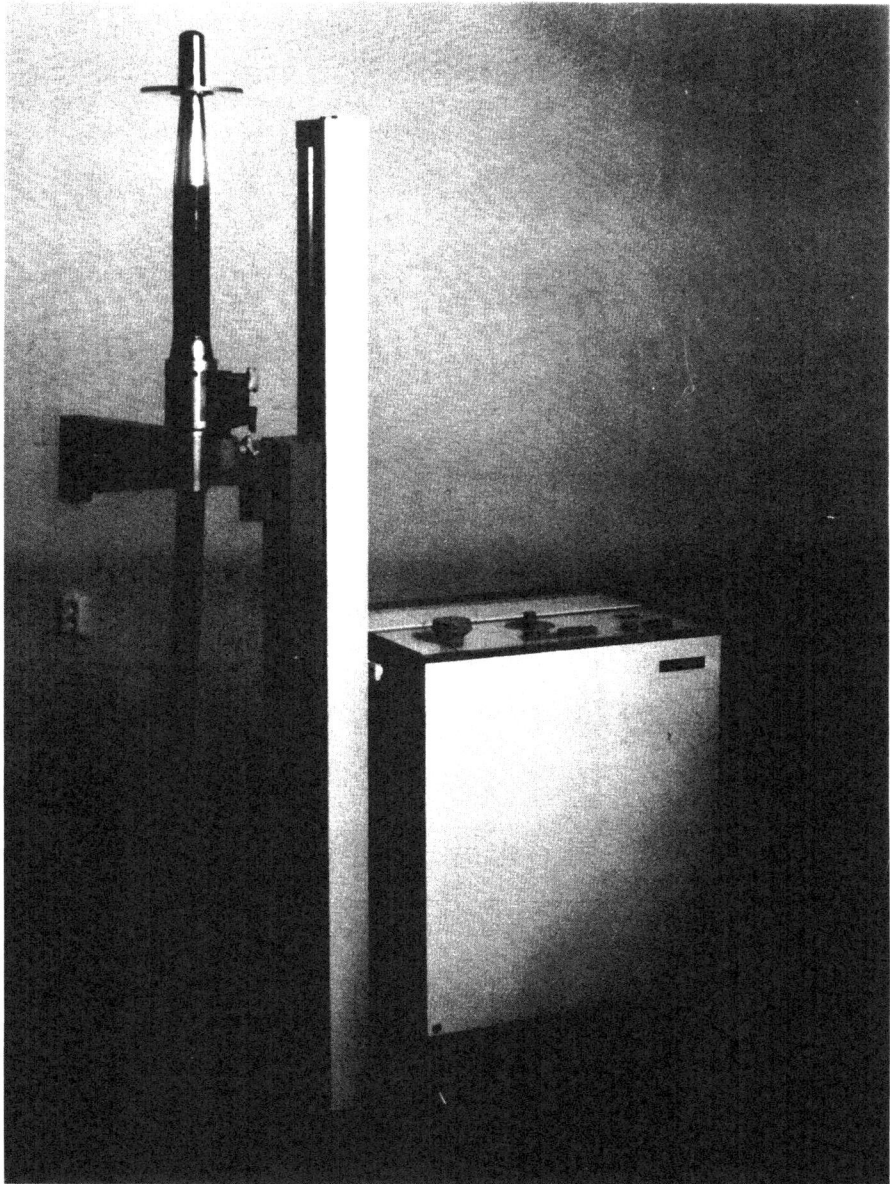

Figure 6-10. Philips RT 50 contact therapy unit.

References

1. Atkinson HR: Skin carcinoma depth and dose homogeneity in dermatological x-ray therapy. Australas J Dermatol 6:208, 1962
2. Braun-Falco O, Lukacs S, Goldschmidt H: Dermatologic Radiotherapy. New York, Springer-Verlag, 1976
3. Bucky G, Combes FD: Grenz Ray Therapy. New York, Springer, 1954
4. Chaoul H, Wachsmann F: Die Nahbestrahlung, 2nd ed. Stuttgart, Thieme, 1953
5. Cipollaro AC, Crossland PM: X Rays and Radium in the Treatment of Diseases of the Skin, 5th ed. Philadelphia, Lea & Febiger, 1967
6. Domonkos AM: Treatment of eyelid carcinoma. Arch Dermatol 91:364, 1965
7. Goldschmidt H: Dermatologic radiation therapy. In Moschella S, Pillsbury DM, Hurley HJ (eds): Dermatology. Philadelphia, Saunders, 1975
8. Goldschmidt H: Ionizing radiation therapy in dermatology. Current use in the United States and Canada. Arch Dermatol 111:1511, 1975

9. Goldschmidt H: Die Roentgentherapie von Dermatosen. In Jadassohn (ed): Handbuch der Haut- und Geschlechtskrankheiten (Suppl), Vol V/2. Berlin, Springer, 1959, pp 486–598

10. Goldschmidt H: Radiotherapy of skin cancer. Cutis 17:253, 1976

11. Goldschmidt H: Dermatologic radiotherapy. Selection of radiation qualities and treatment techniques. Int J Dermatol 15:171, 1976

12. Hollander MB: UltraSoft X Rays. Baltimore, Williams and Wilkins, 1968

13. Jennings WA: Physical aspects of the roentgen radiation from a beryllium tube operated over the range 2–50 K. V. P. for clinical purposes. Acta Radiol (Stockh) 33:435, 1950

14. Jennings WA: Low voltage x-ray therapy with a beryllium window tube. II. The achievement of optimum depth dosage distribution from the physical standpoint. Br J Radiol 24:135, 1951

15. Jennings WA, Gager RM: Physical characteristics of soft roentgen rays. Am J Roentgenol Radium Ther 62:91, 1949

16. Johns HE, Cunningham JR: The Physics of Radiology, 3rd ed. Springfield, Ill, Thomas, 1969

17. Schirren CG: Die Röntgentherapie gutartiger und bösartiger Geschwülste der Haut In Jadassohn J (ed): Handbuch der Haut- und Geschlechtskrankheiten (Suppl) Vol V/2. Berlin, Springer, 1959

18. Selman J: The Basic Physics of Radiation Therapy. Springfield, Ill, Thomas, 1960

19. Tuddenham WJ: Half-value depth and fall-off-radiation as functions of portal area, target–skin distance, and half-value layer. Radiology 69:78, 1957

20. Wachsmann F: In Meyer HJ, Matthes R (eds): Die Strahlentherapie, Physikalische Grundlagen der Röntgentherapie und Dosimetrie. Stuttgart, Thieme, 1949

21. Witten VH: Place of grenz radiation in dermatologic practice. Arch Dermatol 81:110, 1960

22. Zoon JJ, Werz JFC: The quality of x rays in the treatment of skin diseases. Arch Dermatol Syph 75:733, 1957

7

Megavoltage Radiation Therapy

Lawrence W. Davis

In most instances of dermatologic irradiation, the lesions to be treated are quite superficial and the tolerance of normal tissue, with the exception of the skin, for radiation is not a serious consideration in the techniques used. There are some exceptions to this generalization, such as the treatment of a squamous cell carcinoma of the ear which has invaded the underlying cartilage. In this chapter we will review some of the techniques and equipment used in therapeutic radiology and some of the considerations of normal tissue tolerance in planning a course of radiotherapy.

Interactions of Radiation with Matter

Since the manner in which photons (x and γ rays) interact with matter accounts for some of the differences observed between the superficial x-ray units used in dermatology and the larger units used in therapeutic radiology, a brief review of these interactions will be helpful. (For further details see Chapter 1.) A photon may interact by any of the following three processes [5]: (1) photoelectric absorption, (2) Compton absorption, or (3) pair production.

Photoelectric Absorption

Photoelectric absorption involves the inner, bound electrons of atoms and results when a photon displaces one of the electrons in the K,

L, M, or N shells. In this process the energy of the photon is absorbed and an electron is displaced. Photoelectric absorption has the greatest probability of occurring when the energy of the photon is just sufficient to displace the electron; as a result, it accounts for most of the interactions of x rays generated at mean energies of 50 keV or less. In addition, the amount of energy absorbed by an atom is proportional to the fourth power of its atomic number. Thus, when this process is the primary type of absorption, heavy atoms such as calcium absorb much more energy than does the hydrogen or oxygen of soft tissue. With photoelectric absorption, bones and cartilage absorb about 6 times more radiation than does soft tissue; this explains the white appearance of bones on diagnostic radiographs.

Compton Absorption

In Compton absorption, the photon interacts with the outer electrons of the atom. Since very little energy binds the outer electrons to the atom, they are often considered "free" electrons. When a photon collides with a free electron, the electron will recoil, having gained a portion of the photon's energy. The remaining energy will result in a scattered photon. Thus, some of the photon's energy is absorbed and some is scattered. Since this process involves free electrons, it is independent of the atomic number of the atom involved; therefore, absorption per g due to the Compton interaction is nearly identical for all materials. In general, the fraction of energy scattered decreases with increasing photon energy, while the fraction of energy transferred to the electron increased with increasing photon energy. In soft tissue, Compton absorption is the most important process for mean photon energies between 100 keV and 10 MeV. With mean photon energies between 60 and 90 keV, photoelectric and Compton absorption are equally important; while from 200 keV to 2 MeV, Compton absorption alone is present. Since all materials absorb radiation equally per g with Compton absorption, bones appear only vaguely on radiographs made at Compton energy levels; this slight appearance is due to their increased density rather than to the increased absorption of heavy atoms.

Pair Production

As a photon with energy greater than 1.02 MeV passes near the nucleus of an atom, it may be converted to a positive (positron) and negative electron. Since each particle has an equivalent electronic mass of 0.511 MeV, this accounts for the required minimum photon energy of 1.02 MeV. If the photon has more energy than 1.02 MeV, this additional energy is shared by the positron and electron. Since both a positive and negative particle are formed, no electronic charge results. As the positron slows down, it combines with an electron and produces 2 photons of radiation.

In contrast to photoelectric and Compton absorption which decrease as photon energy increases, the likelihood of pair production increases with increasing photon energy above 1.02 MeV. Thus, as a photon increases in energy above 1.02 MeV, it is increasingly less penetrating than is the lower-energy beam.

Absorption by pair production increases with increasing atomic weight and bones will absorb twice as much radiation by this process as will soft tissues. Pair production assumes importance with photon beams of mean energy greater than 5 MeV, and is the most important type of absorption for x rays of mean energy greater than 50 MeV.

Types of Megavoltage Therapy Units

Three common types of high-energy radiation therapy devices are now in use. These include the following: (1) cobalt-60 units; (2) linear accelerators, from 4 to 35 MeV; and (3) betatrons, from 18 to 45 MeV.

Other high-energy devices including cesium-137 units, resonant transformers (1 to 2 MeV), and Van de Graaff generators (2 MeV) are still in use, but these older devices are being replaced with newer units.

Cobalt-60 Units

Cobalt-60 (^{60}Co) units (see Figure 7-1) produce radiation by means of a decaying radioactive cobalt source. Radioactive cobalt has a half-life of 5.2 years; therefore, the radiation dose from such a source decreases 1.1% every month. In the decay of ^{60}Co, 2 photons result with energies of 1.17 and 1.33 MeV. Since[6] ^{0}Co produces photons with only two particular energies rather than a spectrum of energies, as do x-ray machines, ^{60}Co is equivalent in energy to a 2- or 3-MeV x-ray machine.

Since most ^{60}Co sources are 1 to 2 cm in diameter, rather than 1 to 2 mm as is the focal spot of an x-ray unit, the edge of the cobalt beam is less sharp than that of a high-energy x-ray beam. This is due to the geometric penumbra resulting from the large-size source. Devices known as penumbra trimmers are included on cobalt-60 units to reduce the fuzziness of the beam edge.

Linear Accelerators

In a linear accelerator, radiofrequency waves are fed into a wave guide, and electrons are injected onto the crests of these waves. These electrons may either strike a target at the end of the wave guide, producing x rays, or they may be extracted for electron therapy.

Currently available linear accelerators may be grouped according to three energy levels. Low-energy accelerators operate at 4 to 8 MeV and generally do not have options for

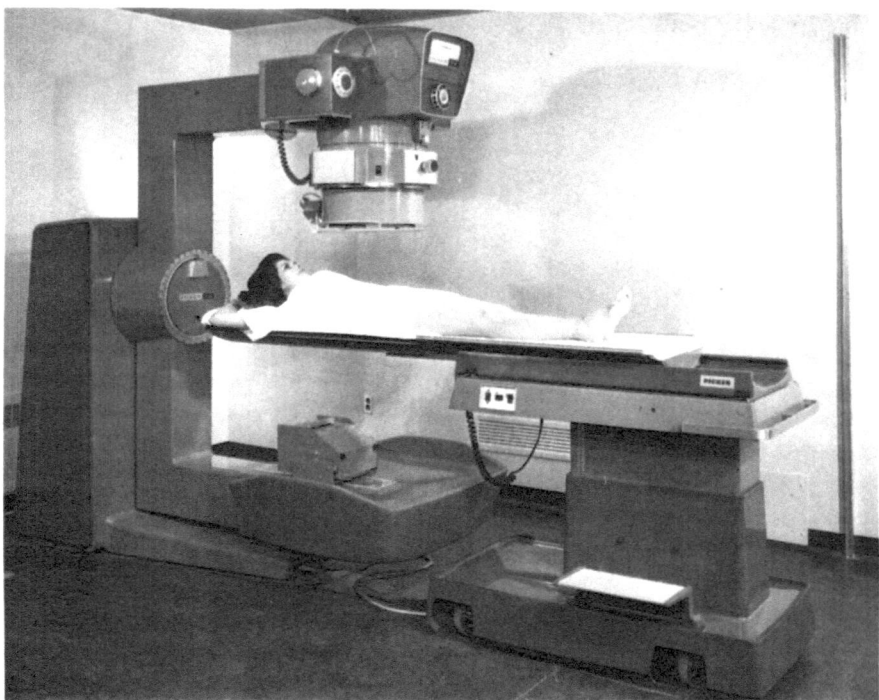

Figure 7-1.   A cobalt-60 unit. Courtesy of Picker Corporation.

electron therapy; medium-energy accelerators operate at 12 to 18 MeV with options for photon or electron therapy; and high-energy accelerators operate at 35 MeV. Most of the medium- and high-energy accelerators have energy options for both photons and electrons, but generally use 8 to 10 MeV photon beams.

Betatrons

Betatrons accelerate electrons. In these devices (see Figure 7-2), electrons are injected into a doughnut-shaped envelope which is situated between two large magnets. The electrons are constantly accelerated and their paths are kept circular by the magnetic field. When the energy of the accelerated electrons is at a particular level the electrons may be directly extracted, or allowed to strike a target producing x rays. The efficiency of the betatron is very high for x-ray production at its maximum energy; however, as the energy of the electrons is decreased, the dose rate of these devices decreases. While the electrons available for therapy can be selected from several MeVs to the

maximum energy of the betatron, the photon energy level is generally near the higher range.

With all high-energy radiation devices, the size of the treatment field must be limited either by a cone-shaped device which attaches to the machine (as with low-energy x-ray units) or more commonly by a collimating device. A collimator consists of a set of metal jaws which can be continually adjusted to produce fields ranging in area from several to 30 × 30 or 40 × 40 cm², depending on the particular therapy machine. Unlike low-energy therapy units which operate at a treatment distance of 15 to 30 cm, cobalt-60 units have treatment distances of 80 cm and other megavoltage units have treatment distances of 100 cm or greater.

Advantages of Megavoltage Therapy Units

There are three main advantages of the megavoltage units used in radiation therapy: (1) skin sparing, (2) increased depth dose, and (3) more uniform absorption [3].

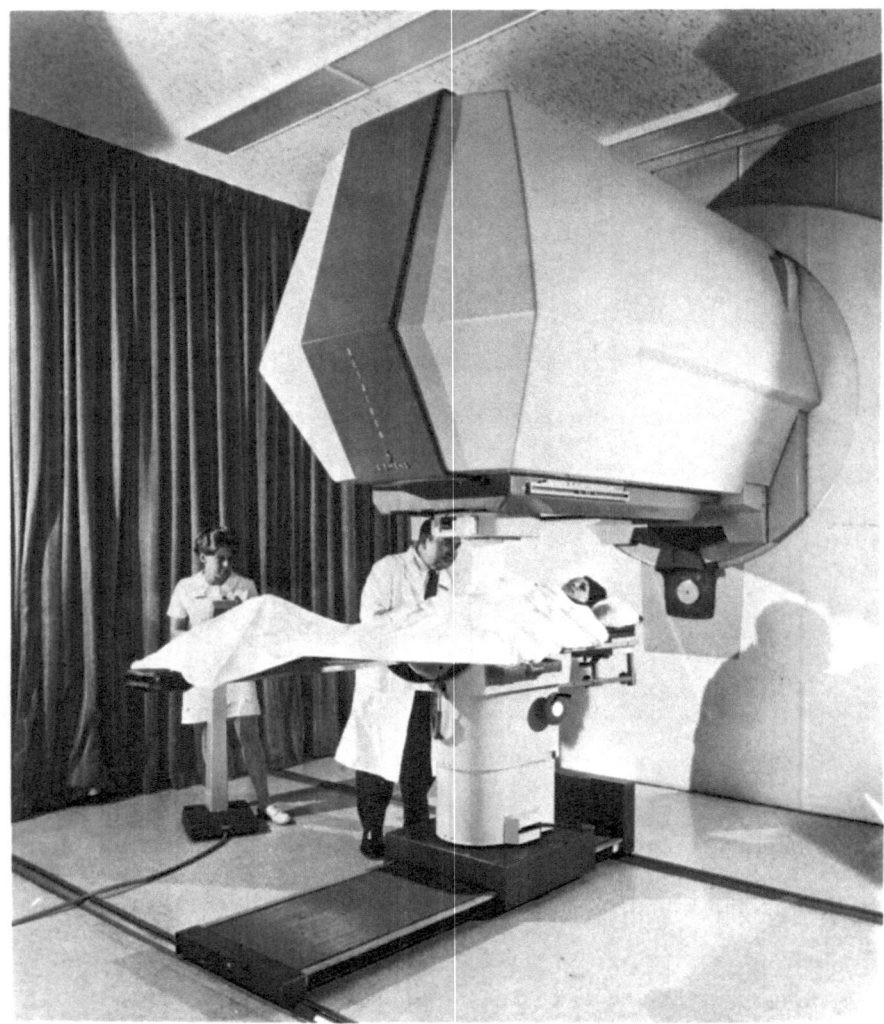

Figure 7-2.   A 42 MeV betatron. Courtesy of Siemens Corporation.

Skin Sparing

Several processes account for the deposition of a photon beam's energy in tissue. The photon undergoes one of the several interactions listed above, producing electrons as a result. These electrons travel in numerous directions and finally come to rest, depositing additional energy. The range of these electrons is related to the energy of the photon that released them, and may be several cm from the site of photon interaction. As the energy of the photon increases, the proportion and range of the electrons traveling in the same direction as the photon increases compared to the number scattered in other directions. Thus, with increasing

photon energy, fewer electrons are scattered backward. As the photon penetrates deeper into tissue the photon beam is absorbed, and a point occurs at which the number of electrons depositing energy is equal to the number being scattered forward. At this juncture, the energy deposition is at its maximum. With low-energy x-ray beams, the maximum dose occurs at the surface, but with megavoltage beams, this maximum dose occurs beneath the skin. With ^{60}Co radiation it occurs at a depth of 0.5 cm, with 6 MeV x rays it occurs at 1.5 cm, and with 31 MeV x rays it occurs at 5 cm. As a result, the maximum dose in the treated field is not at the skin but is in the tissues beneath the skin. Therefore, in these cases, the skin reaction is less than with low-energy radiation—a phenomenon termed skin sparing.

In the early days of radiation therapy, the skin dose was the limiting factor in treating a tumor, and patients were treated until a brisk, moist desquamation of the skin developed. Before techniques of radiation dosimetry were well developed, the amount of treatment was judged by the appearance of the skin. When higher-energy beams were introduced an occasional patient was overtreated, due to the absence of the expected skin reaction from the skin-sparing properties of the higher-energy radiation. As a result of this increased dose to the subcutaneous tissues, late radiation complications are more frequently related to the dose to these deeper structures than to the dose to the skin. Although dry desquamation is common in patients receiving a course of radiotherapy, moist desquamation of the skin is infrequent. Six to 12 months following radiotherapy fibrosis of the subcutaneous tissues frequently results, especially in areas containing a large amount of subcutaneous fat, such as the buttock or supraclavicular area.

Increased Depth Dose

Most of the tumors treated by therapeutic radiologists are located deep in the body, and the intent of treatment is to deliver a large dose of radiation to the tumor with a minimum dose to the surrounding normal tissues. The megavoltage radiation sources aid in accomplishing this purpose, since the radiation is more penetrating than that of the small sources commonly used in dermatology. Table 7-1 compares the percentage depth dose of 100-kV, 6-MeV, and 20-MeV x rays. Two points may be noted in particular. Since the maximum dose with 20-MeV x rays occurs at 4 cm, doses to areas more superficial and deeper than 4 cm are less than that at 4 cm. Since the maximum dose of 6-MeV x rays occurs at 1.5 cm, the doses in the table become progressively smaller with increasing depth [2]. Also, as the energy of the radiation increases, the beam becomes more penetrating, and a larger proportion of the dose occurs at a given depth as compared to the skin.

In addition to the improved penetration of high-energy radiation, the shape of the dose

Table 7-1 *Comparison of Depth Dose for Several X-ray Energies*

Depth (cm)	X-ray Energy		
	100 kV	*6 MeV*	*20 MeV*
2	60%	99%	90%
5	35%	87%	99%
10	5%	67%	82%

pattern at the edge of the treatment field is improved. Isodose curves from a superficial 100-kV unit show a much lower dose at the edge of the field than do those from a 6-MeV linear accelerator, which are relatively flat across the treatment field. Thus, with megavoltage beams, the dose at the edge of the field decreases much less, but beyond the edge of the radiation field the dose falls markedly. Because of the decreased dose at the edge of the field of the 100-kV beam, an adequate margin must be left around a tumor treated with this radiation.

More Uniform Absorption

As the energy of the radiation beam increases and Compton absorption becomes predominant, the absorption of radiation becomes more uniform. As a result, the amount of energy absorbed by bone is less than with lower-energy beams. Because of this more uniform absorption, complications in bone are fewer and tumors adjacent to bone are not shielded. While this is generally not an important consideration in dermatologic applications, there are a few instances where it might be, as in treatment of a carcinoma of the skin invading the cartilage of the ear or nose, or a large carcinoma involving the bone of the skull.

Constitutional Symptoms

Superficial x-ray units primarily cause local symptoms when used for treatment. These include skin erythema and dry and moist desquamation. However, because of the increased penetration of the megavoltage units and the larger volume of tissue treated, systemic symptoms often accompany radiotherapy with these units. These symptoms are probably related to the breakdown of tissue as well as being associated with a particular organ which may be within the irradiated volume. Malaise and increased fatigue are common symptoms. When treatment fields are in the abdominal area, symptoms may include anorexia, nausea, vomiting, and diarrhea [1].

Treatment Planning

Since the intent of treatment with radiation is to deliver a maximum dose to the tumor and a minimum dose to the surrounding normal tissues, the number, size, and angles of the treatment fields to be used must be planned, except in those instances where the tumor is so superficial that a single treatment field may be used [4]. In most cases, a cross section of the patient at the level of the tumor is made and drawn on a sheet of paper. The tumor is drawn within this cross section, using whatever means are available to determine the extent of the tumor, such as physical examination and routine and special radiographic studies. Also within this cross section are placed the normal structures which may be critical in limiting the total radiation dose delivered. On the basis of a prescribed dose to the tumor and normal tissue, the most suitable field arrangement is determined to accomplish the therapy.

Summary

Megavoltage units used in therapeutic radiology produce radiation which is more penetrating and more uniformly absorbed, and which has a smaller skin dose than that of the superficial units commonly used in dermatology. While these units are especially useful for the treatment of deep-seated tumors, they could be used to treat superficial lesions that involve bone or cartilage. The electrons produced by these units are useful in the treatment of extensive, superficial lesions. This will be more completely discussed in Chapter 11.

References

1. Buschke F, Parker RG: Radiation Therapy in Cancer Management. New York, Grune Stratton, 1972
2. Cohen M, Jones DEA, Greene D (eds): Central axis depth dose data for use in radiotherapy. Br J Radiol (Suppl) 11:1, 1972
3. Fletcher GH: Textbook of Radiotherapy. Philadelphia, Lea & Febiger, 1966
4. Hale J, Raventos A: Treatment planning with 2 mV x rays. Radiol Clin North Am 1:245, 1963
5. Johns HE, Cunningham JR: The Physics of Radiology. Springfield, Ill, Thomas, 1969

8

Current Usage of Dermatologic Radiotherapy in the United States and Canada

Herbert Goldschmidt

A comprehensive survey of the Task Force on Ionizing Radiation of the National Program for Dermatology of the American Academy of Dermatology evaluated the usage of ionizing radiation by dermatologists in the fall of 1974 [1]. A detailed questionnaire was mailed to 4560 dermatologists in the United States and Canada; 2444 replies were received and evaluated by computer. Almost one-half (49%) of all replies came from dermatologists in practice only 1 to 10 years (and from residents in training). One-fifth (21%) were from dermatologists who have practiced for more than 20 years. The main findings of this survey can be summarized as follows.

Equipment

Superficial x-ray and/or grenz-ray equipment is available in 55.5% of dermatologic offices (2305 replies). Types of ionizing radiation equipment are listed in Table 8-1.

Usage

Almost half of all respondents use x-ray therapy every week (44.3%; 2316 replies). Almost one-third (29%) use x rays in 1 to 5 patients each week, 10.2% in 6 to 25 patients each week, 3.1% in 26 to 50 patients each week, and 2% in more than 50 patients each week. The frequency of usage was directly proportional to

patient load (number of patients seen each week), number of malignant neoplasms treated each week, and experience and age (number of years in practice).

Value of Dermatologic Radiotherapy

Many respondents (2308) expressed their opinions on the value of x-ray therapy. One-eighth (12.5%) find it indispensable; 67.1%, valuable in selected cases; 16.6%, valuable in rare cases; 2.9%, not valuable; and 0.9%, completely contraindicated.

Indications

The main indications for *superficial x-ray therapy* include the following: basal cell cancers (89.3%), squamous cell cancers (79.8%), mycosis fungoides (78.5%), Kaposi's sarcoma (74.6%), lymphocytoma (55.8%), and keloids (55.5%). (Percentages indicate proportion of over 2000 dermatologists with or without x-ray equipment using or recommending x-ray therapy for these indications.) Detailed data are listed in Table 8-2.

The main indications for *grenz-ray therapy* include eczematous conditions (44.5%), pruritus ani and vulvae (35%), lichen simplex chronicus (30.4%), and psoriasis (30.1%). Detailed data are listed in Table 8-3.

Table 8-1   *Types of Ionizing Radiation Equipment Used in Dermatologic Offices*

		Replies			
		YES		NO	
Equipment	TOTAL	NO.	%	NO.	%
Grenz-ray units (5 to 20 kV)	1361	604	44.4	757	59.6
Beryllium-window units (soft-ray machines, 10 to 50 to 100 kV)	1095	141	12.8	954	87.2
Superficial low-voltage machines (60 to 120 kV)	1589	984	61.9	605	38.1
Contact therapy units	1025	14	1.4	1011	98.6
Other x-ray machines	1008	71	7.0	937	93
Radium	1063	102	9.6	961	90.4
Other radionuclides	933	12	1.3	921	98.7

Residency Training

Practical clinical instruction during residency training was considered good by 37.4%, adequate by 22.2%, and poor by 27.1% of respondents. One-fifth received no practical training (18.3%).

Future Training

The need for future training in residency programs was evaluated by 2352 respondents. One-third (29.5%) want more emphasis in future training programs; 51.3%, the same emphasis; 7.4%, less emphasis; and 11.8% want training discontinued. Increased *practical* instruction was requested by 65.8% of 2273 dermatologists.

Reasons for Nonusage

Many (1250) dermatologists *not* using x rays gave the following major reasons for nonusage (one or more answers given): better treatments available (1039), potential hazards (radiodermatitis) (641), lack of training (520), medicolegal reasons (496), and cost of malpractice insurance (440).

Instruction at American Academy of Dermatology

Almost one-fifth (17.1%) of 2304 dermatologists desire that instruction in ionizing therapy at annual meetings be increased; 66.1%, continued; 6.6%, decreased; and 10.2%, discontinued.

Examination in Radiation Therapy by American Board of Dermatology

Many (2345) dermatologists (including over 200 residents) stated their opinions on the need for special knowledge in the field of dermatologic radiotherapy during examinations for board qualification. Almost one-tenth (9.1%) desire greater emphasis on the field of radiotherapy, 55.3% want the present emphasis continued, 20.4% want questions on radiotherapy deemphasized, and 15.2% wish such questions to be discontinued.

Table 8-2 *Indications for Selective Use of Superficial X-ray Therapy*

Diagnosis	Not Used	Used	Frequency of Use			
			1–5%	*6–20%*	*21–50%*	OVER 50%
Basal cell	226	1880	1087	403	158	232
carcinoma	10.7%	89.3%	51.6%	19.1%	7.5%	11.1%
(2106 replies)						
Squamous cell	417	1648	848	311	172	5
carcinoma	20.2%	79.8%	41.4%	15.1%	8.3%	0.3%
(2064 replies)						
Kaposi sarcoma	470	1278	325	170	230	653
(1848 replies)	25.4%	74.6%	17.6%	9.2%	12.4%	35.4%
Lymphocytoma	848	1030	348	188	180	314
(1878 replies)	45.2%	55.8%	18.5%	10%	9.6%	16.7%
Keloid	937	123	561	245	150	167
(2060 replies)	45.5%	55.5%	27.2%	11.9%	7.3%	8.1%
Acne	1210	869	660	126	46	37
(2079 replies)	58.2%	41.8%	31.7%	6.1%	2.2%	1.8%
Verruca plantaris	1203	861	534	134	90	103
(2064 replies)	58.3%	41.7%	25.9%	6.5%	4.3%	5.0%
Hidradenitis	1291	759	357	183	109	110
suppurativa	63%	37%	17.4%	8.9%	5.3%	5.4%
(2050 replies)						
Eczema	1292	683	431	139	63	50
(1975 replies)	65.4%	34.6%	21.8%	0.7%	3.2%	0.6%
Lichen simplex	1311	690	382	143	79	86
chronicus	65.5%	34.5%	19.1%	7.1%	3.9%	4.4%
(2001 replies)						
Paronychia	1420	633	275	142	110	105
(2053 replies)	69.2%	30.8%	13.4%	6.9%	5.4%	5.1%
Hemangioma	1463	543	408	67	37	31
(2006 replies)	72.9%	27.1%	20.4%	3.4%	1.8%	1.5%
Psoriasis	1503	471	351	83	22	15
(1974 replies)	76.1%	23.9%	17.8%	4.2%	1.1%	0.8%
Verruca vulgaris	1554	488	366	69	31	22
(2042 replies)	76.1%	23.9%	17.9%	3.4%	1.5%	1.1%
Pruritus ani and	1525	473	278	105	41	49
vulvae	76.2%	23.8%	13.9%	5.3%	2.1%	2.5%
(1998 replies)						
Furuncle and	1680	466	202	54	50	60
carbuncle	82.1%	17.9%	9.9%	2.6%	2.4%	2.9%
(2046 replies)						
Granuloma	1654	359	181	79	51	48
annulare	82.8%	17.8%	9.0%	3.9%	2.5%	2.4%
(2013 replies)						
Lentigo maligna	1631	265	146	60	31	28
(1896 replies)	86%	14%	7.7%	3.2%	1.6%	1.5%
Seborrheic	1760	244	146	43	33	22
dermatitis	87.8%	12.2%	7.3%	2.1%	1.6%	1.2%
(2004 replies)						

Table 8-3 *Indications for Selective Use of Grenz-ray Therapy*

Diagnosis	Not Used	Used	Frequency of Use			
			1–5%	6–20%	21–50%	OVER 50%
Eczema	843	677	304	165	95	113
(1520 replies)	55.5%	44.5%	20%	10.9%	6.2%	7.4%
Pruritus ani and	966	521	213	115	77	116
vulvae	65%	35%	14.3%	7.7%	5.2%	7.8%
(1487 replies)						
Lichen simplex	904	487	234	143	92	118
chronicus	60.6%	30.4%	15.7%	9.6%	6.2%	7.9%
(1491 replies)						
Psoriasis	916	588	264	147	86	91
(1504 replies)	60.9%	30.1%	17.5%	9.8%	5.7%	6.1%
Lichen planus	1089	409	159	102	64	84
(1498 replies)	72.7%	27.3%	10.6%	6.8%	4.3%	5.6%
Seborrheic	1166	318	122	65	55	76
dermatitis	78.6%	21.4%	8.3%	4.3%	3.7%	5.1%
(1484 replies)						
Basal cell	1175	158	101	18	13	16
carcinoma	88.8%	11.2%	7.6%	1.4%	0.9%	1.3%
(1323 replies)						
Granuloma	1271	154	77	30	25	22
annulare	89.2%	10.8%	5.4%	2.1%	1.8%	1.5%
(1425 replies)						
Paronychia	1267	154	74	37	19	24
(1421 replies)	89.2%	10.8%	5.2%	2.6%	1.3%	1.7%
Lymphocytoma	1143	136	67	32	19	18
(1279 replies)	89.4%	10.6%	5.2%	2.5%	1.5%	1.4%
Kaposi sarcoma	1089	120	46	19	19	36
(1209 replies)	90.1%	9.9%	3.8%	1.6%	1.6%	2.9%
Lentigo maligna	1269	105	47	13	16	29
(1374 replies)	92.4%	7.6%	3.4%	0.9%	1.2%	2.1%
Acne	1325	102	58	24	12	8
(1427 replies)	92.9%	7.1%	4.1%	1.7%	0.7%	0.6%
Hemangioma	1327	96	53	19	11	13
(1423 replies)	93.3%	6.7%	3.7%	1.3%	0.8%	0.9%
Keloid	1280	76	46	16	6	8
(1356 replies)	94.4%	5.6%	3.4%	1.3%	0.4%	0.5%
Squamous cell	1276	66	41	15	5	5
carcinoma	95.1%	4.9%	3.2%	1.1%	0.3%	0.3%
1342 replies)						
Verruca vulgaris	1363	63	42	12	6	3
(1426 replies)	95.7%	4.3%	2.9%	0.8%	0.4%	0.2%
Verruca plantaris	1354	57	40	6	8	3
(1411 replies)	96%	4%	2.8%	0.4%	0.6%	0.2%
Hidradenitis	1348	51	36	4	5	6
suppurativa	96.4%	3.6%	2.6%	0.3%	0.3%	0.4%
(1399 replies)						
Furuncle and	1383	28	18	4	2	4
carbuncle	98%	2%	1.3%	0.3%	0.1%	0.3%
(1411 replies)						

Reference

1. Goldschmidt H: Ionizing radiation therapy in dermatology. Current use in the United States and Canada. Arch Dermatol 111:1511, 1975

9

Radiotherapy of Cutaneous Malignancies

Arthur H. Gladstein, Alfred W. Kopf, and Robert S. Bart

Most of the uncertainties and pitfalls encountered in the early years of x-ray therapy have been eliminated with modern equipment and techniques. Despite this, the use of radiation by dermatologists has declined since the close of World War II. The major decline has been in its use for the management of benign dermatoses, for which other excellent treatments are now available. X-radiation is still extensively used in the treatment of cutaneous malignancies, especially basal and squamous cell carcinomas, Kaposi's sarcoma, and mycosis fungoides. For these malignant neoplasms x-ray therapy is an effective modality and, indeed, is the treatment of choice in certain circumstances. If appropriate principles are followed and precautions taken, x-radiation is a safe and effective method of therapy.

To treat a particular cutaneous malignancy, the dermatologist has available scalpel surgery, curettage–electrodesiccation, Mohs' surgery, chemotherapy, and cryosurgery, as well as radiation. Thus, experienced dermatologists have a multidisciplinary approach that permits selection of the most appropriate modality for each tumor.

X-ray Therapy of Basal Cell Carcinomas

X-ray therapy is effective for the treatment of many basal cell carcinomas. The 5-year cure rate in our published series of 500 histologically proved basal cell carcinomas was 93% [4]. Al-

though there are occasional exceptions, we prefer not to irradiate patients who are less than 40 to 45 years of age or lesions below the head and neck.

Advantages

Based on our experience in treating a very large number of basal cell carcinomas, we consider the following as advantages of x-ray therapy:

1. Elderly patients, some of whom fear and refuse surgery, will frequently consent to having their cancers treated with x-radiation.
2. For patients on anticoagulant therapy, radiation therapy avoids the risk of excessive bleeding associated with surgical procedures.
3. Since little emotional or physical stress is produced by radiation therapy, it can be used safely for patients in poor mental or medical condition.
4. During the course of treatment the patient usually can pursue his routine activities. Toward the end of a course of x-ray therapy there may be some soreness and discomfort, but this is of short duration and is rarely of great concern to the patient. Since hospitalization is rarely necessary, costs are minimized.
5. Unlike surgery, x-ray therapy preserves the contours of the normal tissues surrounding the tumor; this is a great advantage. Adequate cancer therapy requires that the lesion

and a margin of normal-appearing skin be treated. This usually poses no problem for the radiotherapist since he can easily adjust the field size to the required area of treatment: tumor margins may be made as generous as necessary without sacrifice of normal tissue and the port may be easily designed for treatment of lesions with very irregular borders. In those areas where tissue cannot be readily sacrificed because of its cosmetic or functional importance, radiation is therefore often the method of choice. The nose, canthal areas, and eyelids are good examples of such areas. The difficult reconstructions after surgery are often avoided with x-ray therapy. Ectropion of the eyelid and retraction of the lip are less common following irradiation than after surgical procedures.

6. Radiation therapy may be preferred to surgery for patients and locations prone to keloid formation. Many superficial basal cell carcinomas occur on the chest, shoulders, and back—areas tending to keloid formation. Furthermore, these lesions may be quite extensive in surface area. Radiation in the grenz-ray range (see below) is effective for this type of basal cell carcinoma. It is, however, frequently more convenient to use another modality, especially for the smaller lesions.

7. Postoperative radiation therapy can be successfully used for basal cell carcinomas known or thought to have been inadequately removed surgically. In such instances careful evaluation must be given to insure proper margins.

8. Recurrences after any modality except radiation can be treated with x rays. Unfortunately, the re-recurrence rate after radiation may be high, and was 27% in our study [15]. However, in that study [15], the re-recurrence rates after excision and especially after curettage–electrodesiccation were higher still (40 and 59%, respectively). Mohs' surgery, with a cure rate of over 90% for recurrent basal cell carcinomas, is more effective [16].

Disadvantages

As with any modality, there are also some disadvantages to radiotherapy for basal cell carcinomas. These include the following:

1. Although it is possible to cure a basal cell carcinoma with a single x-ray treatment, this one-exposure method is mentioned only to be condemned, except for the most unusual circumstance where it would be impossible for the patient to return and surgical approaches are strictly contraindicated. Good radiation therapy employing the principles of protraction and fractionation requires multiple visits, usually more than do surgical approaches, and this is a relative disadvantage for the patient. This is especially true for the elderly patient who may find travel difficult.

2. Cosmetic results tend to worsen with time after radiation therapy. The published New York University Skin and Cancer Unit experience can be summarized as follows (Table 9-1): Excellent or good cosmetic results were observed in 74% of the lesions within the first year after treatment, in 68% in the third to fifth year after treatment, and in 49% in the ninth to twelfth year. Although uncommon, patients treated with radiation sometimes find the cosmetic result unacceptable subsequently, and surgical revision may be necessary.

3. Cosmetic results following conventional x-ray therapy of lesions on the trunk and extremities are frequently poor and healing is slow. Thus, lesions below the neck are generally best treated by surgical modalities.

4. X-ray therapy for basal cell carcinomas always produces permanent alopecia. Patients must be warned about this effect when the treatment fields involve the eyebrows, eyelashes, bearded area, or scalp. Resulting cosmetic deficits can often be minimized with eye makeup, false hair pieces, and long hair styles. Hair transplantation can be used in scalp and eyebrows [15a].

Table 9-1 *Cosmetic Results after X-ray Therapy of 500 Basal Cell Carcinomas*

Cosmetic Result	Years After Treatment	% Patients
Excellent to Good	0–1	74
	3–5	68
	9–12	49
Fair to Poor	0–1	26
	3–5	32
	9–12	51

After Bart et al [4].

5. Careful shielding around and below lesions of the eyelids and canthi is imperative to prevent damage to the ocular lens. No radiation cataracts have been encountered at the Skin and Cancer Unit over the many years during which hundreds of cancers of the eyelids and canthi have been treated using the shielding techniques described below. Radiation cataracts are clinically distinct from ordinary cataracts, and had any occurred, they would have been readily identified. Furthermore, studies in our department using thermoluminescence dosimeters indicate that the lens receives less than 50 R with our method of treating eyelid and canthal basal cell carcinomas [14]. The minimum cataractogenic dose reported in the literature is about 200 rads [6].

6. Some failures and recurrences occur with all forms of therapy; they are sometimes retreated with the modality originally used. This is usually inadvisable with radiation because of potential serious sequelae. Although the schedule for basal cell carcinomas at the Skin and Cancer Unit is characterized by low total dose and relatively low x-ray energies (Table 9-5, on p. 119), we very rarely retreat with any type of radiation, and then only under extraordinary circumstances.

Technique

The first step in treating a basal cell carcinoma with x rays is to outline the visible and/or palpable border of the lesion with a skin marker. Ordinarily this presents no difficulty since most basal cell carcinomas have fairly well-defined clinical margins. If the lesion is poorly defined, the physician may either estimate its extent or, preferably, do multiple biopsies to determine its dimensions.

Many basal cell carcinomas extend laterally beyond what can be readily seen or felt and, therefore, a margin of normal-appearing skin is always included in the area treated. At the Skin and Cancer Unit, 5 mm is the margin used if the clinical borders are reasonably distinct. If the margins are indistinct, as they may be with morphea-type basal cell carcinomas (which we find are often curable with x radiation [3]), a wider margin, up to 10 mm, is used. Thus, if the maximum tumor diameter of a well-defined lesion is 20 mm, the minimum diameter of the port used is 30 mm. A field diameter less than 20 mm is not used with our radiation schedule regardless of the smallness of the lesion.

The outline of the radiation port, which is usually 5 mm beyond the clinical perimeter of the lesion, is next marked on the skin. The port is cut in lead sheeting of appropriate thickness (p 98) to conform accurately to the outline around the "normal" margin. The edges of the port are then serrated (p 98); this prevents a sharply defined postradiation outline which may compromise the cosmetic result. The shield is then taped in position on the patient (Fig. 9-1a–e).

Special Shielding Techniques

The subject of shielding is discussed in chapter 4. Additional shielding techniques are necessary in the treatment of basal-cell carcinomas of eyelids and canthi, nose, lips, and ears.

Eye

Nowhere is protection from unwanted radiation more important than in the region of eye. External eye shields must be used whenever radiation is applied to the head and neck, and internal eye shields used in the treatment of palpebral and canthal lesions, in order to adequately protect the lens. Radiation cataracts are preventable with proper shielding techniques. Permanent alopecia of eyelashes always occurs when lids or canthi are treated with cancericidal doses of x rays and the patient should be so advised.

Figure 9-2 shows the materials used in treating eyelid and canthal lesions. The location of the tumor determines the type of internal eye shield required (Fig. 9-3). Should the lesion be located on the upper eyelid (Fig. 9-3a), a lead shield in the shape of a tongue-blade is applied over the lower lid and under the upper lid. Only the upper eyelid will be exposed to radiation and the lens is protected. A lesion on the lower eyelid requires that the tongue-blade–shaped shield be inserted in the lower cul-de-sac covering the upper lid and lens during exposure. Originally these shields consisted of lead sheeting 0.92 mm in thickness. After observing several instances of benign conjunctival leukoplakia following x-ray therapy, the shield was modified in an attempt to reduce or eliminate this complication by de-

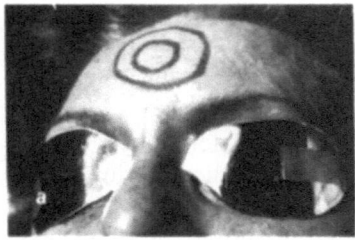

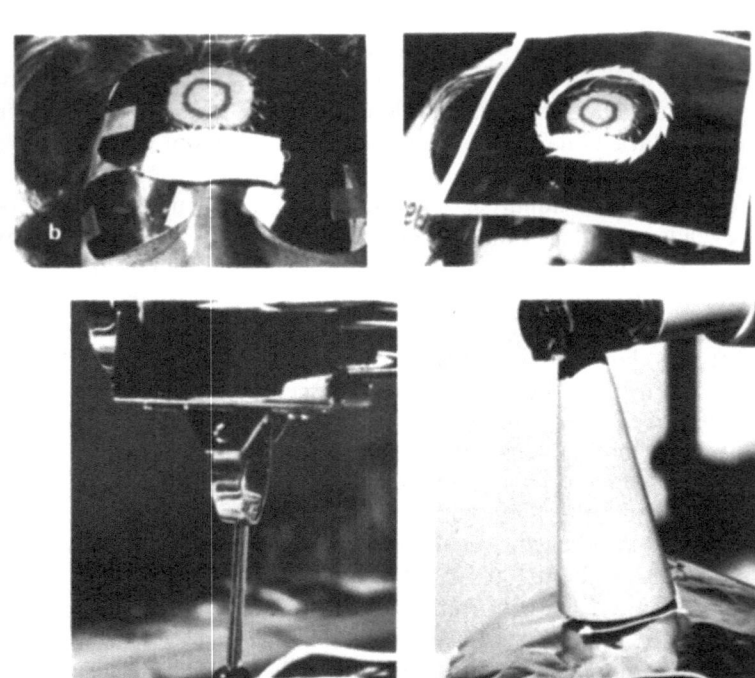

Figure 9-1. Method of shielding for treatment of cutaneous malignancies with x rays. a. Outline of lesion with 5-mm border of normal-appearing skin. b. Serrated lead shield taped in position; eyes are protected by lead shields. c. Overlay shield in place. d. Open field (no cone) method. Only to be used in rare instances where cones not suitable. e. Cone applied to port—preferred method.

creasing backscatter [14]. This new shield (Fig. 9-4) consists of a lead core 0.92 mm in thickness, electroplated with 0.25 mm of copper and covered with 0.0075 mm of cadmium. Finally, the shield is coated with a layer of paraffin to ensure a smooth surface, eliminating the dan-

ger of corneal abrasion. Backscatter is decreased by the new eyelid shields, so that the amount of x radiation received by the palpebral conjunctiva is reduced by approximately 20%.

Lesions located at the canthi (Fig. 9-3c and d) require that portions of both lids be exposed during therapy. For this situation two types of cup-shaped shields are available. The Gougelman shield (Fig. 9-5) is made of silver-plated lead; the other (Fig. 9-6) is made of brass. Both of these shields have been modified

Figure 9-2. Shielding materials used in the treatment of periocular lesions. Upper row, left to right: mineral oil for lubricating shields, Butyn Sulfate (local anesthetic), Liquifilm (artificial tears) for dry eyes. Pontocaine (local anesthetic). Lower row, left to right: brass eye shield with suction cup, Gougelman eye shield, "tongue" (tongue-blade shaped) eye shield, topical antibiotic, eye pad.

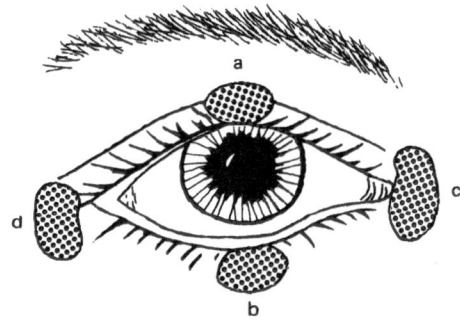

Figure 9-3. Classification of periocular lesions into canthal (requiring exposure of both lids) and lid (requiring exposure of one lid only).

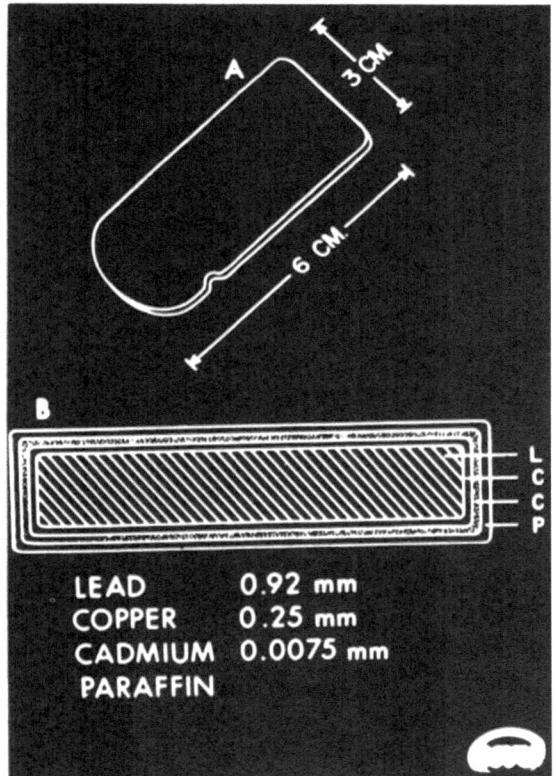

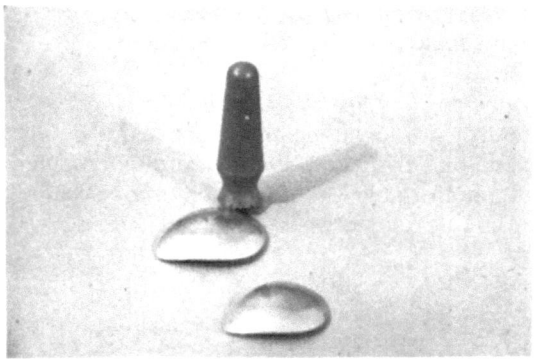

Figure 9-6. Brass eye shield with suction cup.

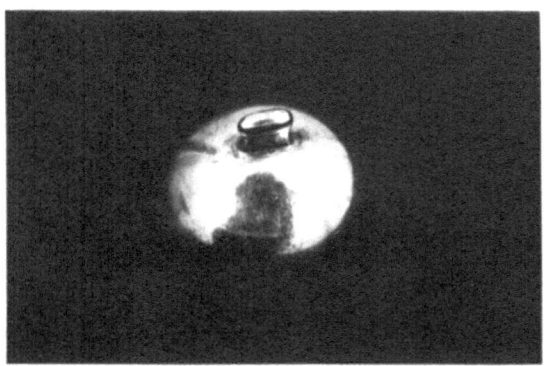

Figure 9-4. "Tongue" eye shield.

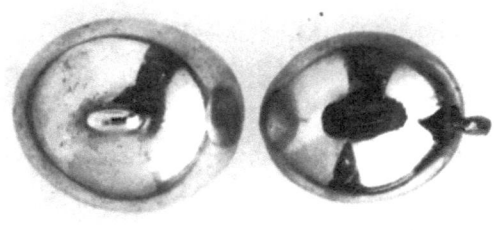

Figure 9-7. Modified Gougelman eye shield. Handle has been moved to one end.

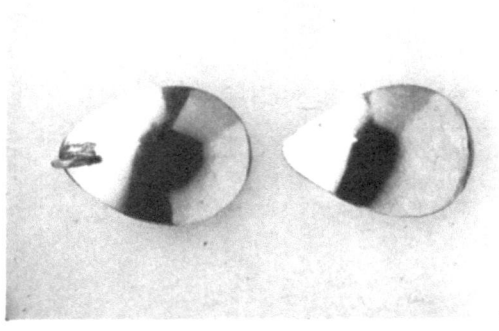

Figure 9-5. Gougelman eye shield.

Figure 9-8. Modified brass eye shield. A handle has been affixed to the narrow end.

for easy manipulation (Figs. 9-7 and 9-8) by placing handles at the end of the shields [10].

Procedure for Insertion of Eyelid Shield A few drops of local anesthetic are instilled. The tongue-blade–shaped shield is carefully molded to fit comfortably into the upper or lower palpebral cul-de-sac. It is then coated with heated paraffin and allowed to cool. After it is inserted, the shield is taped in position so that it is firmly secured and will not move during therapy. Overlay shielding is then applied. After each x-ray treatment the shields are removed, an ophthalmic antibiotic ointment is instilled into the conjunctival cul-de-sac, and an eye patch applied for about 2 hr (Fig. 9-9).

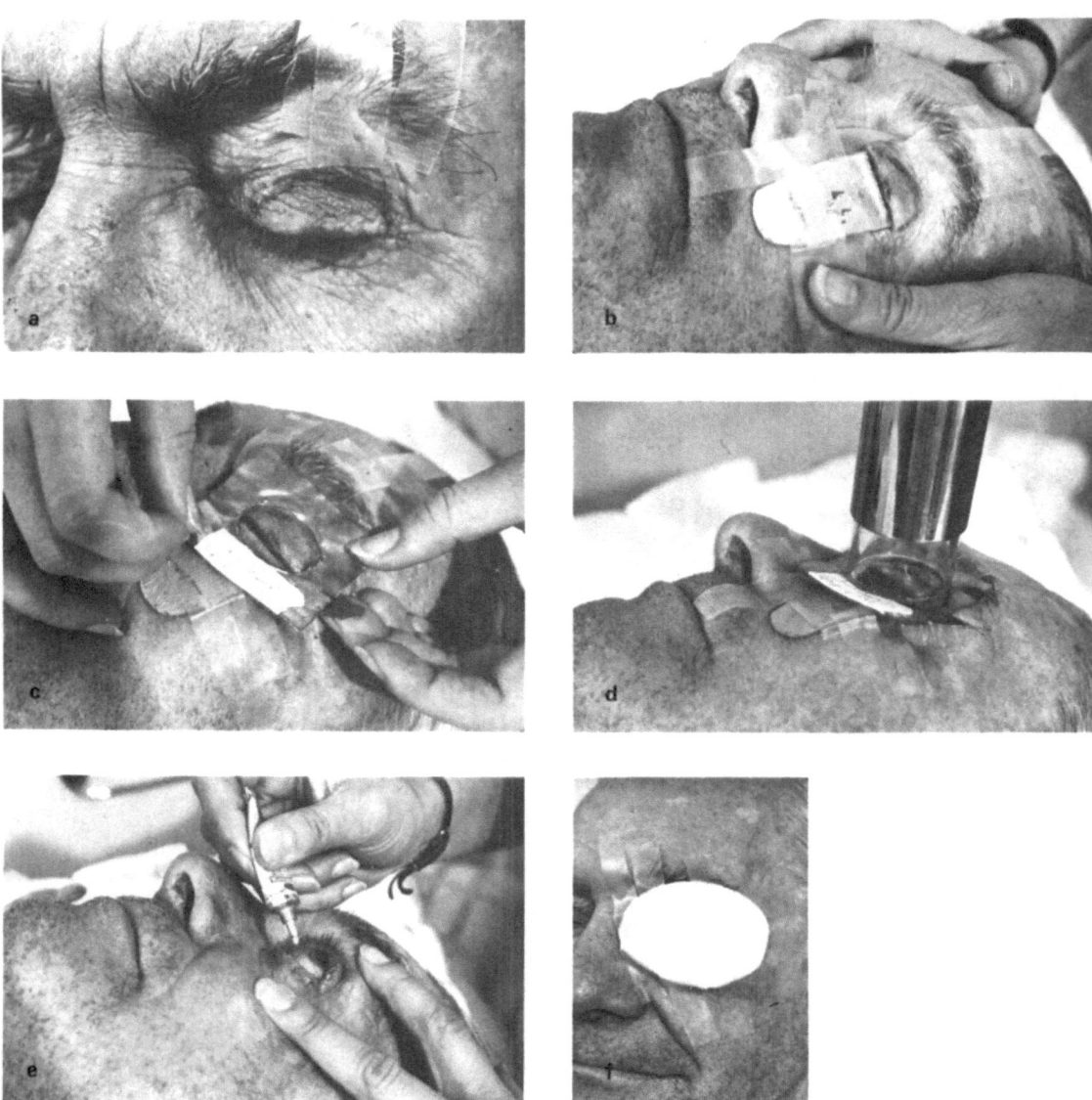

Figure 9-9. Method of shielding eye when treating upper lid with x rays. a. Outline of area to be treated. b. "Tongue" eye shield has been inserted into the palpebral conjunctival cul de sac, molded to fit contour of patient's face, and taped in place. c. Outer shield is placed into position. d. Cone is positioned over port. e. Ophthalmic antibiotic ointment is applied after completion of therapy and removal of shield. f. Eye patch is applied; it can be removed 2 hours later.

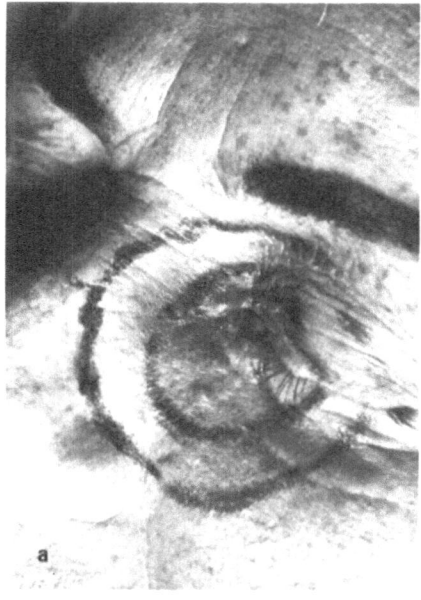

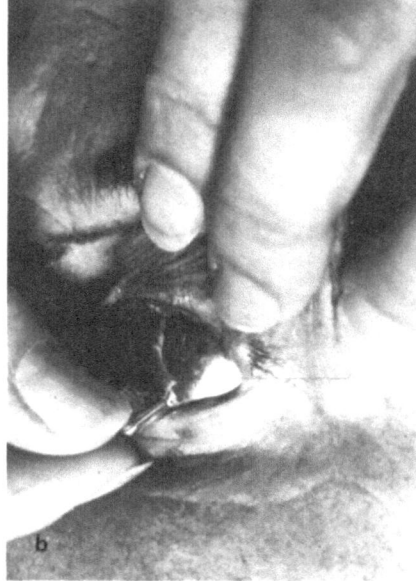

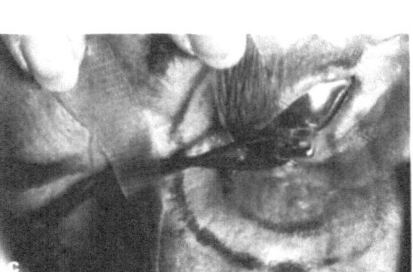

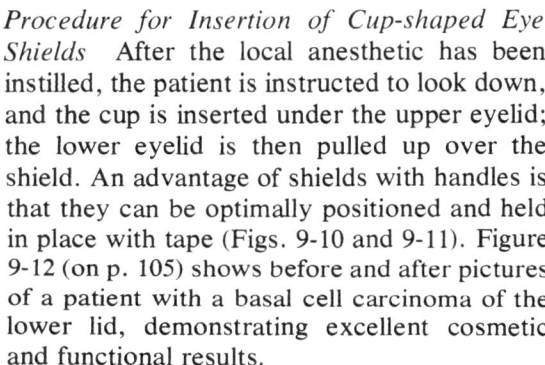

Figure 9-10. Method of shielding eye when treating inner canthus with x rays. a. Outline of lesion with 5-mm border or normal-appearing skin. b. Insertion of Gougelman eye shield. c. Suture material looped through hole in handle facilitates removal. d. Outer shield placed in position just prior to exposure.

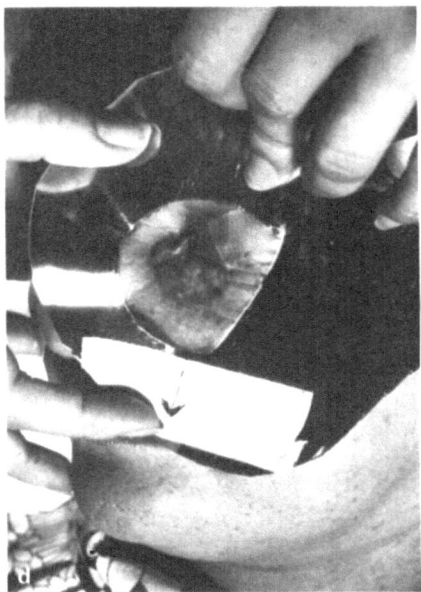

Procedure for Insertion of Cup-shaped Eye Shields After the local anesthetic has been instilled, the patient is instructed to look down, and the cup is inserted under the upper eyelid; the lower eyelid is then pulled up over the shield. An advantage of shields with handles is that they can be optimally positioned and held in place with tape (Figs. 9-10 and 9-11). Figure 9-12 (on p. 105) shows before and after pictures of a patient with a basal cell carcinoma of the lower lid, demonstrating excellent cosmetic and functional results.

Nose

When the skin of the nose is treated by x rays, the eyes must always be shielded and the nasal septum should be protected if possible. Eyes should always be covered by external lead sheeting (Fig. 9-13). To protect the septum from exit dose, lead sheeting is molded to fit easily, covered by a finger cot (usually lubricated with mineral oil), and inserted either into one or both nostrils, depending upon the area to be treated. These shields are most useful when the sides and tip of the nose are treated.

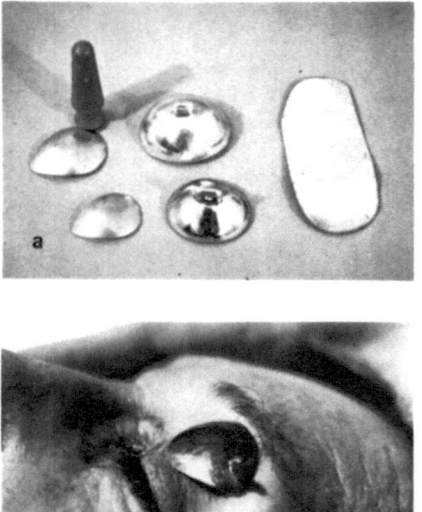
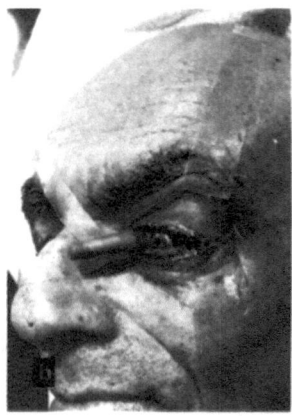

Figure 9-11.   Use of brass eye shield. a. From left to right: brass eye shield with suction cup, Gougelman eye shield, multilayered tongue-blade–shaped eye shield. b. Insertion of brass eye shield with suction cup. c. Handle on brass shield is always placed opposite to the area of pathology.

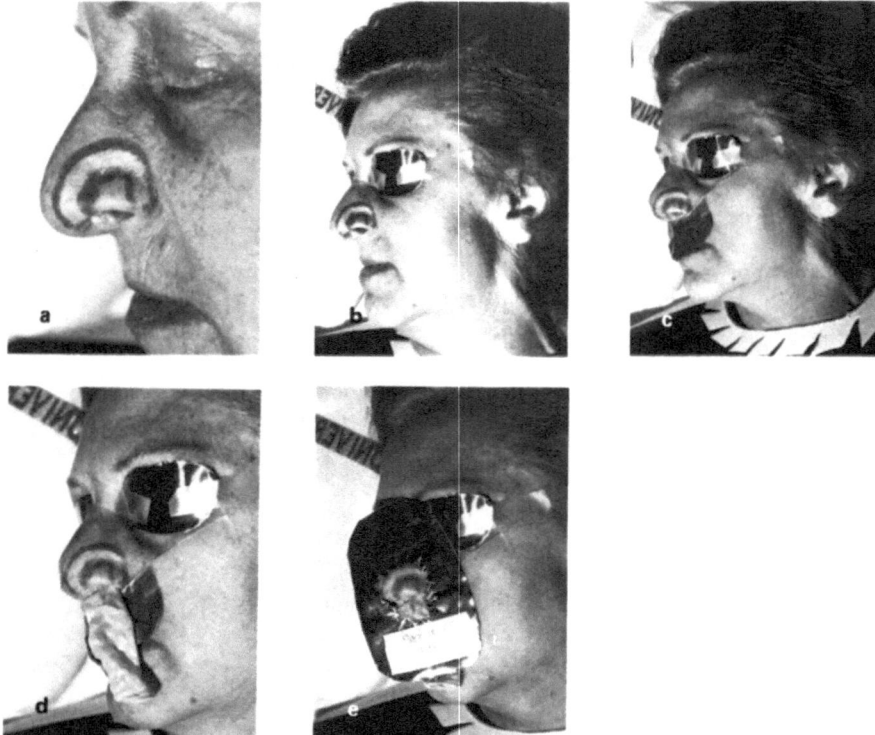

Figure 9-13.   Method of shielding for lesions on one side of nose. a. Outline of lesion with 5-mm border of normal-appearing skin. b. Eye and thyroid protected with lead shielding. c. Lead shielding to protect upper lip. d. Lead covered with finger cot in nostril to protect septum. e. Outer serrated lead shield defining port.

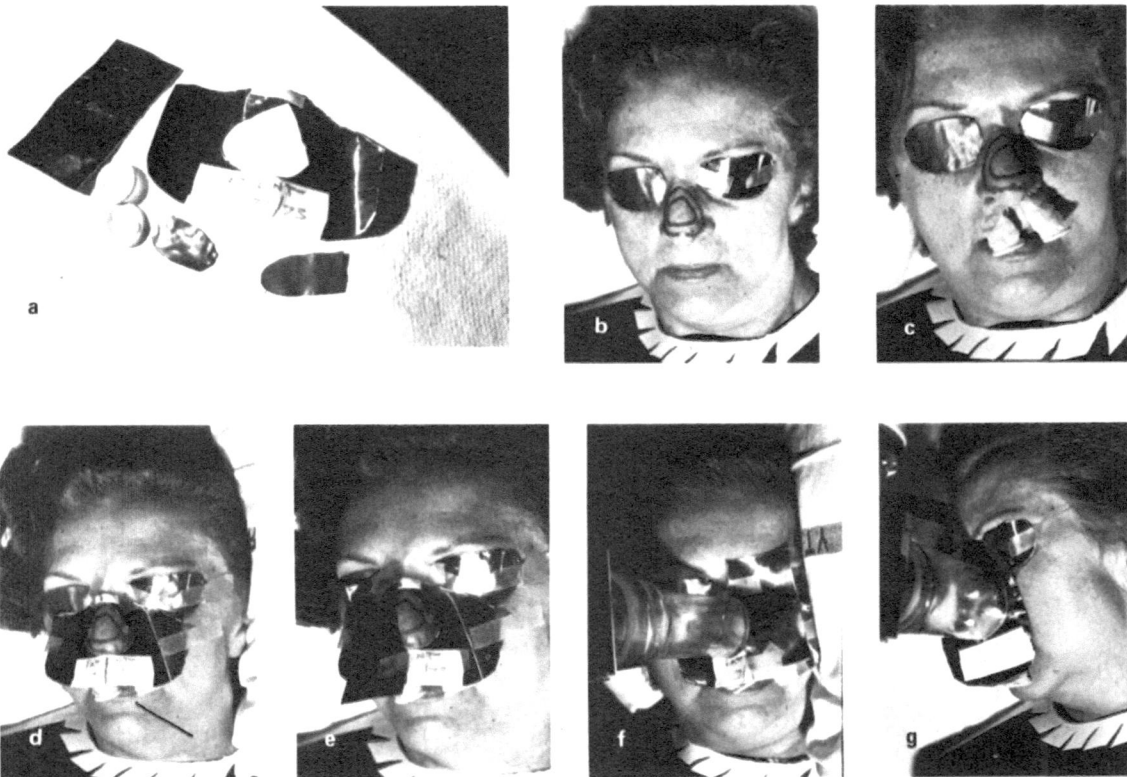

Figure 9-14. Method of shielding for x-ray treatment of lesions on both sides of nose. a. Lead shielding, from left to right: shield for upper lip, external shield with x-ray port, and two pieces of lead to be covered with finger cots for insertion into nostrils. b. Outline of lesion with 5-mm border of normal-appearing skin. c. Eyes and thyroid protected with lead shielding; lead shielding in nostrils. d. Outline of port with vertical line drawn through upper and lower poles. e. Supplementary lead shielding positioned to fit on the two vertical lines. One side of nose will be treated; after first exposure, supplementary lead shield will be positioned to permit treatment of the other side of nose. f. Right side of nose receiving treatment. g. Left side of nose receiving treatment.

It is helpful to instruct the patient to breathe through his mouth when internal nasal shields are inserted, because an uncomfortable patient will find it difficult to remain motionless. External shielding is, of course, also used when treating malignancies of the nose.

When the lesion extends to both sides of the nose, special shielding is required (Fig. 9-14). First, a shield is prepared as in Fig. 9-14a. This should encompass the extent of the area to be irradiated. Vertical lines are drawn across the shield from top to bottom. The shield is then shaped and taped securely in position. A supplementary lead shield is fashioned so that it may be positioned to fit on the two vertical lines. This will permit exposure of part of the lesion. After exposure, the supplementary

shield is rotated—again positioning it along the vertical axis, so that it covers the irradiated side. The previously shielded area is now irradiated. The area of the nose to be treated should be made to lie as flat as possible by the judicious use of adhesive tape. Figure 9-15 (on p. 105) shows before and after pictures of a patient with a very large basal cell carcinoma with excellent functional result.

Ear

Tumors of the pinna may occur on the anterior surface, on the posterior surface, or may be "wrap-around" lesions involving both surfaces of the helix or lobule. To clarify the discussion of shielding, the various possibilities will be considered separately. As for all x-ray treatments to the face and neck, external eye shields must be applied.

Anterior Surface of Ear   To protect the retroauricular skin and the scalp from exit dose, lead should be placed between the posterior surface of the ear and the head whenever possible. A crescent-shaped lead shield is often ap-

propriate. The anterior surface is protected in the usual way with lead sheeting with an appropriate port cut in it (Fig. 9-16).

Posterior Surface of Ear   To properly expose the posterior surface, the ear is bent forward. Lead shielding must be applied to the two surfaces of the ear. The pinna is firmly fixed with

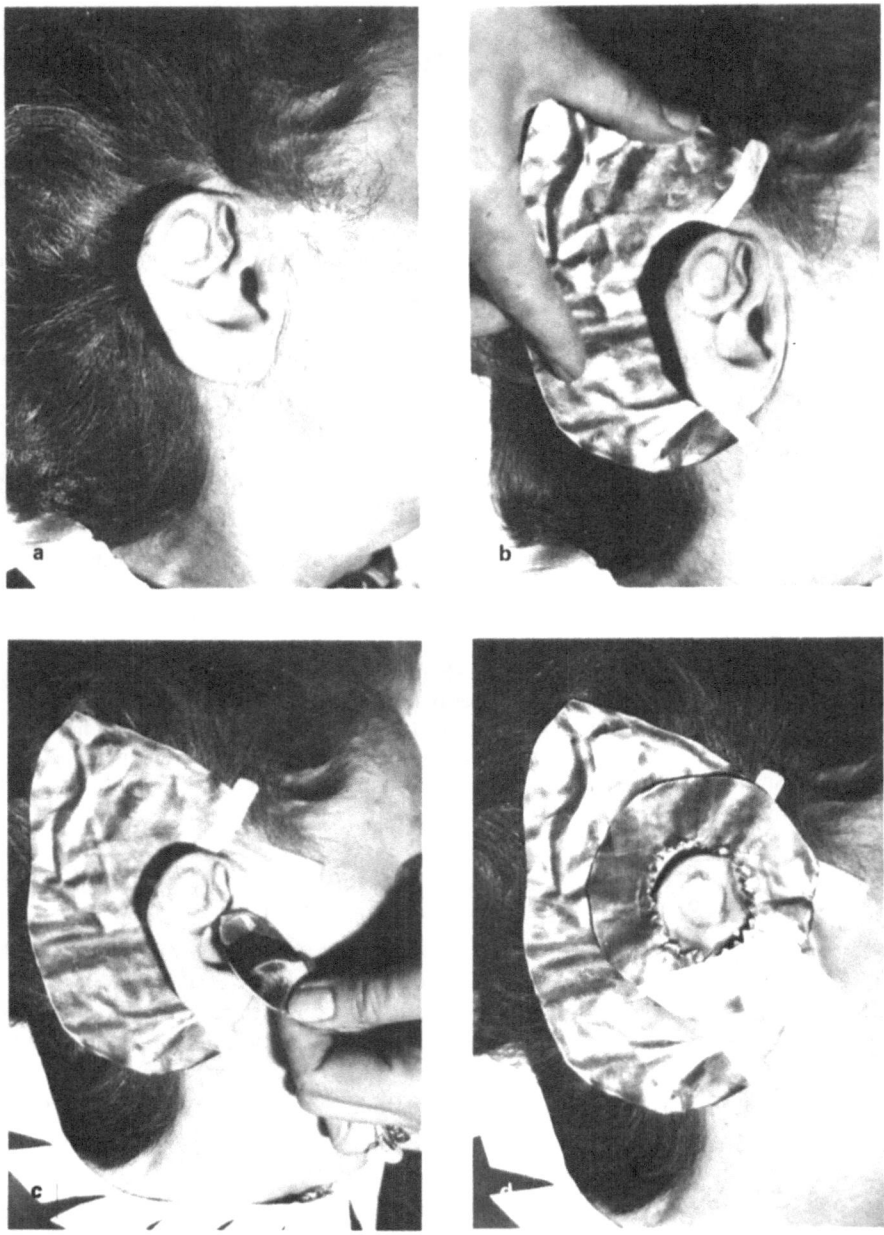

Figure 9-16.   Method of treating anterior surface of ear with x rays. a. Outline of lesion with 5-mm border of normal-appearing skin. b. Lead sheeting cut to fit behind ear to absorb exit dose. c. Lead inserted under antihelix to absorb exit dose. d. Outer serrated shield in place.

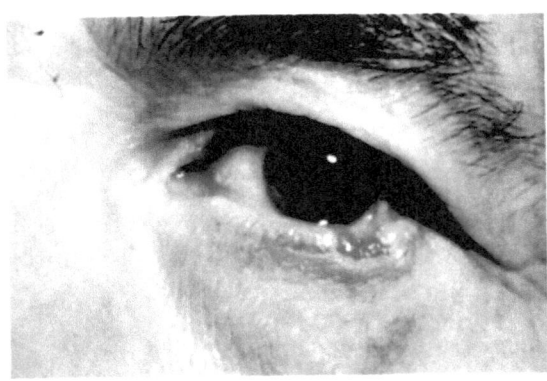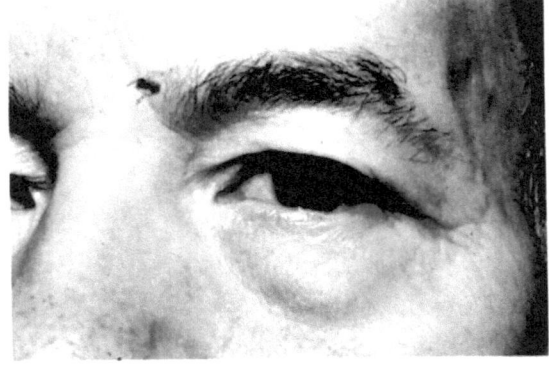

Figure 9-12. Before (a) and after (b) pictures of a patient with basal cell carcinoma.

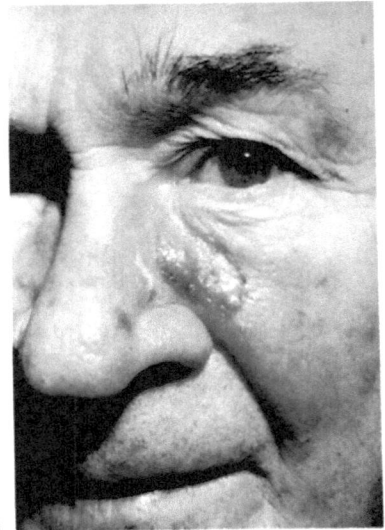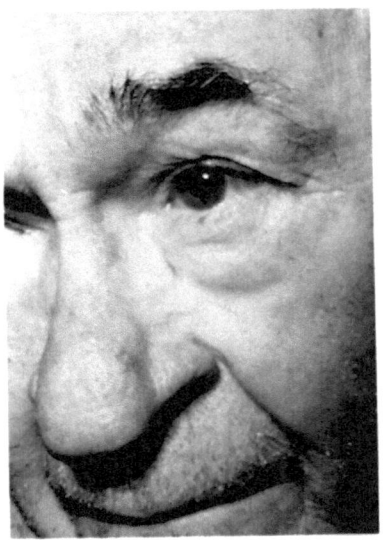

Figure 9-15. Before (a) and after (b) pictures of patient with basal cell carcinoma.

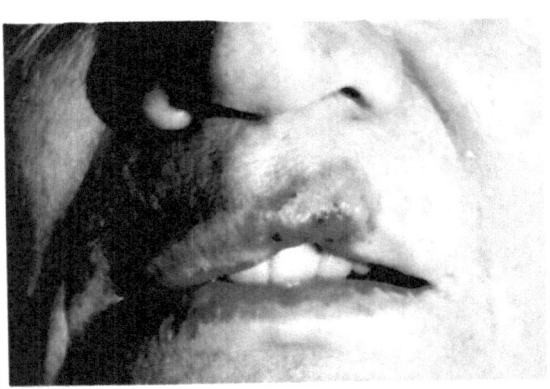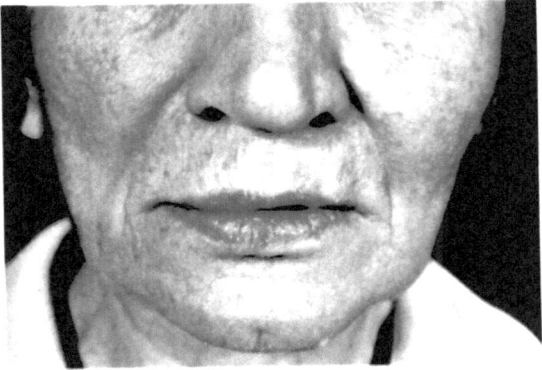

Figure 9-22. Before (a) and after (b) pictures of patient with basal cell carcinoma.

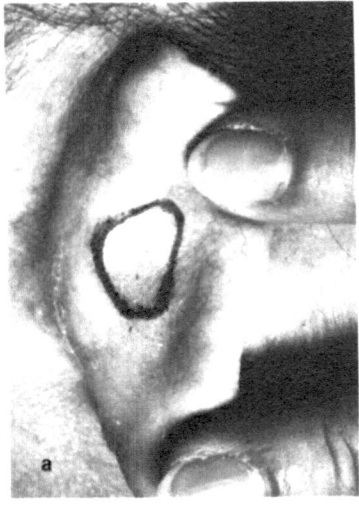
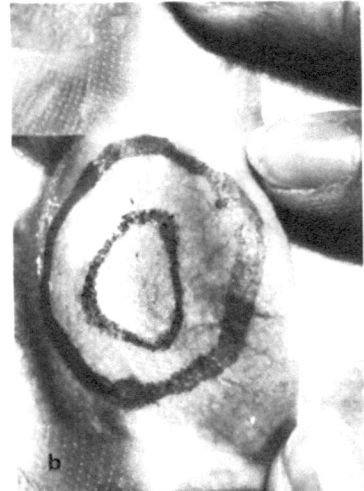
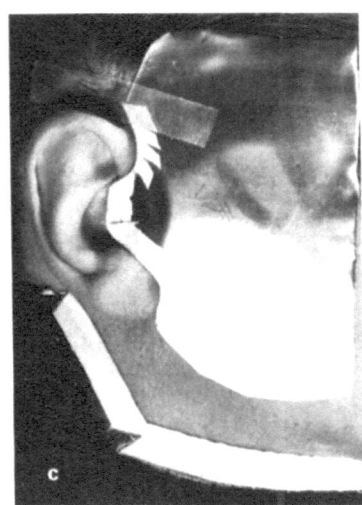

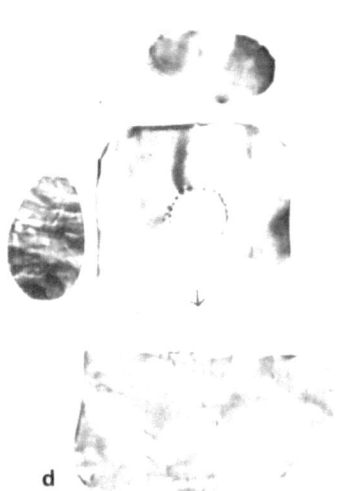
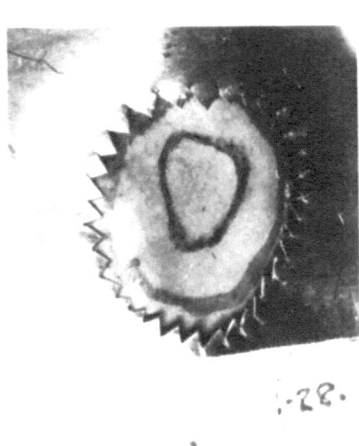

Figure 9-17. Method of treating the posterior surface of the ear with x rays. a and b. Outline of lesion with 5-mm border of normal-appearing skin. c. Lead shielding inserted to absorb exit dose. d. External lead shielding. e. Close-up of port.

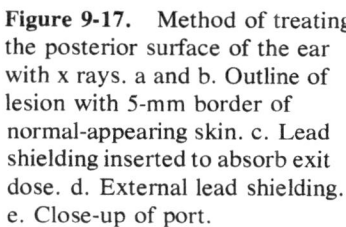

tape to assure as flat a surface as possible after the lead is placed between the preauricular skin and the anterior auricular surface (Fig. 9-17).

Lesions of Helix and Lobule Lesions of the helix and lobule can be handled by one of several methods. The part can be positioned, firmly fixed, and shielded; the area to be treated is then exposed in the usual way. This may result in a considerable difference in dosage received between the center and edges of the lesion because the surfaces will not be flat. The inverse square rule can be used; increasing the target–skin distance increases the relative amount of radiation reaching that part of the lesion furthest from the target of the tube.

Another approach, when possible, is to treat the lesion with both anterior and posterior exposures. The amount of exit radiation must be considered in determining the dose of each exposure. This method can also be used for lesions involving both sides or the full thickness of part of the ear. Another means of managing lesions that involve both sides of the ear is to have the exit dose equal one-half the surface dose; eg, if the ear lobe is thought to be filled with tumor and is 10 mm in thickness, half the surface dose can be made to reach the other side when one surface is irradiated (see below).

Preauricular Lesions Preauricular lesions are shielded as in Fig. 9-18.

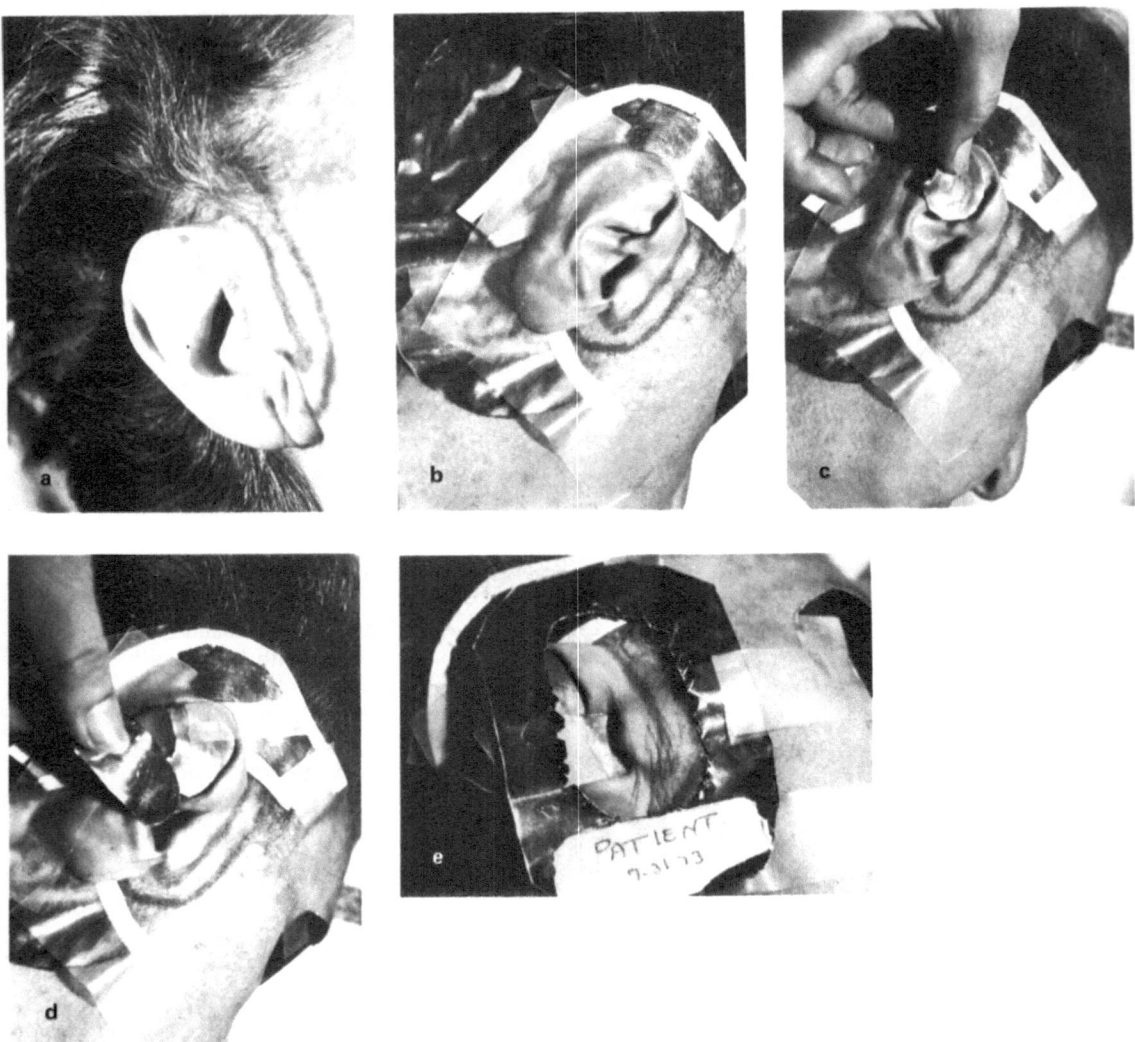

Figure 9-18. Method of treating preauricular area with x-rays. a. Outline of lesion with 5-mm border of normal-appearing skin. b. Lead sheeting cut to fit behind ear to absorb exit dose. c. Lead shielding to protect ear. d. Lead shielding to protect posterior aspect of ear canal. e. Close-up of port.

External Auditory Canal   Lesions that extend into the external auditory canal are usually not suitable for superficial x-ray therapy, but can be managed by other radiation techniques such as radium molds.

Lip

The problems involved in treating malignancies of the lip are similar in many respects to those of the eye and ear. In an analogous situation to that of the eyelids, the pathology may either be localized to the upper or lower lip or it may involve the commissures.

As in all head and neck x-ray therapy, the eyes must be protected by external eye shields (p 98). The patient should be warned that permanent alopecia will occur in the moustache and bearded areas if they are to be irradiated.

Upper or Lower Lip Only   A lead shield covered with a rubber finger cot is inserted behind the lip to protect the gums and teeth from the exit dose (Fig. 9-19). It is firmly taped to the skin. Some therapists use gauze to cover the shield. Frequently, mucositis develops during the course of therapy and the gauze has a tendency to stick; rubber is therefore preferable.

If the pathology is confined to the inner or outer surface only, the lip is taped appropriately, the overlay shield is applied, and therapy is administered. Should the tumor extend to both inner and outer surfaces, treatment can be given as for ear lesions: alternate exposures are applied to each surface, or the $D_{1/2}$ concept may be used (see below).

If the pathology is mainly on one surface and extends only slightly to the other, eversion of the lip using adhesive tape and cotton dental pledgets or rolls may be necessary (Fig. 9-20). The target–skin distance is increased in this instance to ensure proper depth dose, since this lessens the fall-off of radiation due to curvature.

Both Lips Commissural lesions present no special difficulty in shielding. Internal shields are easily made to protect teeth and gums. Again, the internal shield is covered with a finger cot to provide a smooth and comfortable

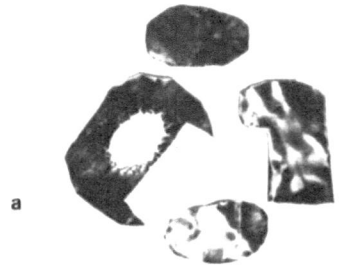

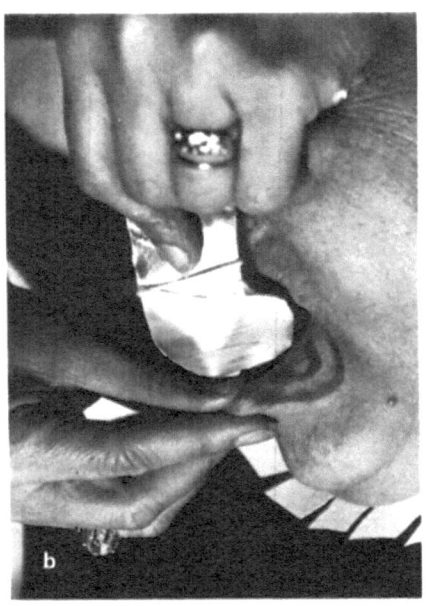

Figure 9-19. Method for treating lower lip with x rays. a. Lead shielding: top and bottom, eye shields; left, serrated outer shielding; right, "hockey stick" shield to protect gums and teeth from exit dose. b. "Hockey stick" shield covered with finger cot inserted behind lower lip. c. Outer serrated shield taped in position. d. "Hockey stick" shield taped in position.

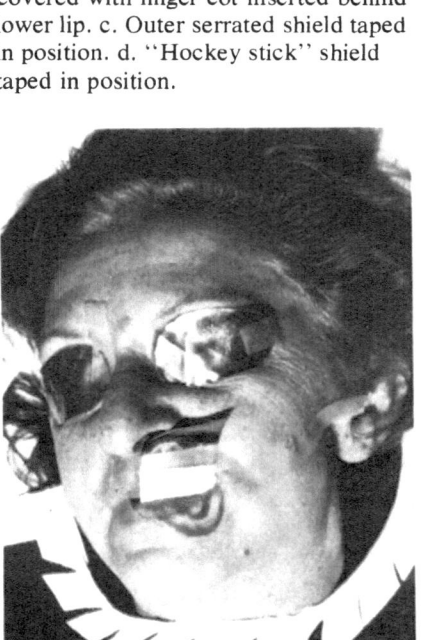

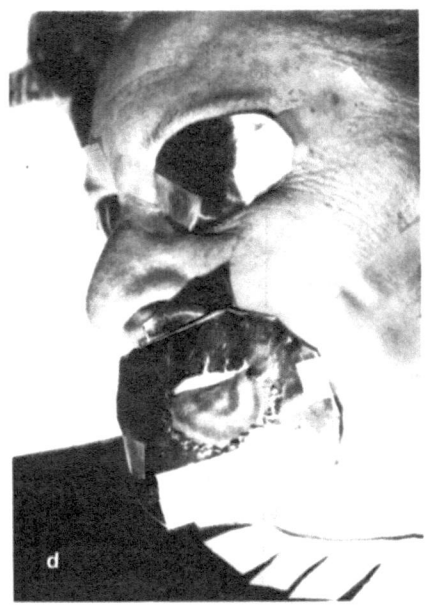

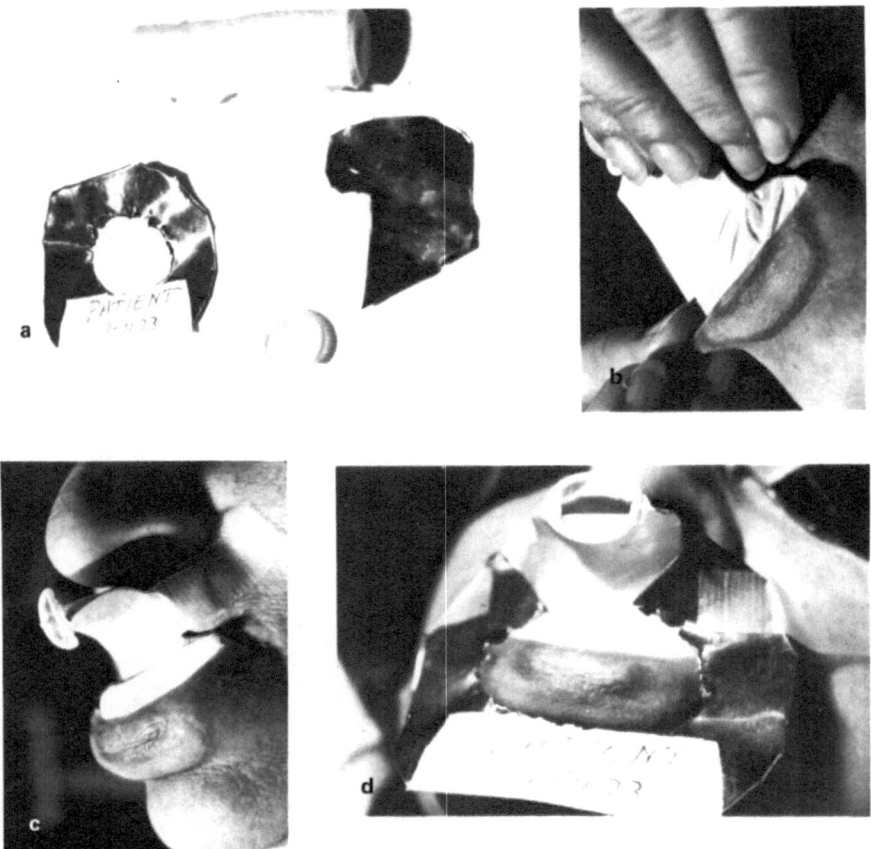

Figure 9-20.   Method of treating vermilion surface of lip with x rays. a. Top, cotton roll; right, "hockey stick" shield to absorb exit dose; left, outer serrated shield. b. Insertion of shield covered with finger cot. c. Cotton roll everts lip, exposing entire pathology. d. Outer serrated shield taped in position.

surface (Fig. 9-21). During the course of therapy the lips may swell, ooze, and become acutely tender. The patient should be advised, before therapy, that mucositis is commonly encountered. Figure 9-22 (on page 105) shows before and after pictures of a patient with basal cell carcinoma of the upper lip. After x-ray therapy there is usually little defect with excellent functional result.

Radiation Factors

Table 9-2 outlines the schedule used for treating basal cell carcinomas at the Skin and Cancer Unit from about 1950 to 1970. All of the long-term follow-up data on cutaneous malignancy cited in this section are based on this schedule. After the installation of Siemens Der-

mopan II equipment in 1971, some of the factors were modified (see below). By examining the schedule in Table 9-2, one sees that added filtration was not used. Tumors that infiltrated very deeply or invaded bone were not treated by this method. Superficial basal cell carcinomas and Bowen's disease were also not treated with this quality of radiation because it is considered too penetrating for such superficial pathology (see below for a discussion of grenz-ray treatment of these conditions).

Radiation Reactions

Immediate

After completion of 1 or 2 exposures, there is generally no visible radiation reaction. Erythema is the first manifestation, usually ap-

Table 9-2 *Radiation Therapy Schedules for Basal and Squamous Cell Carcinomas (Using Picker 120 X-ray Unit)*

Factor	Basal Cell Carcinoma	Squamous Cell Carcinoma
HVL (mm Al)	0.9	0.9
Voltage (kV, peak)	100	100
Added filtration	None	None
TSD (cm)	20 cm	20 cm
Current (mA)	5–10	5–10
Dose per treatment (R, air dose)	680	680
Total dose (R, air dose)	3400	5440
Number of treatments	5	8
Interval (days)	2–3	2–3
Time span (days)	9–12	17–20
Minimum port diameter (cm)	2	2

Abbreviations: HVL, Half-value layer; kV, kilovoltage; TSD, Target–skin distance; mA, Milliamperes.

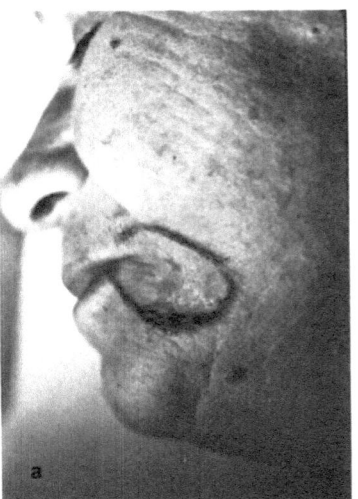
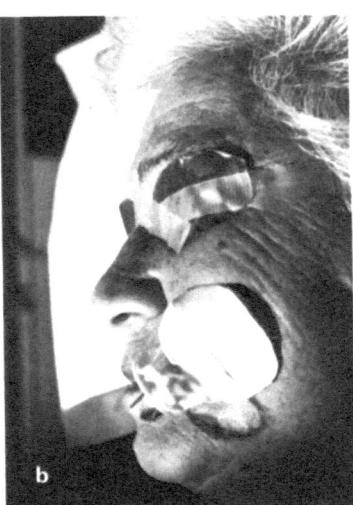
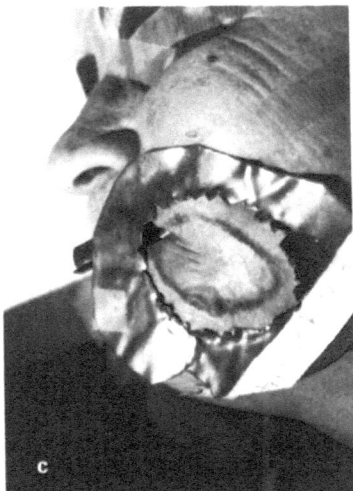
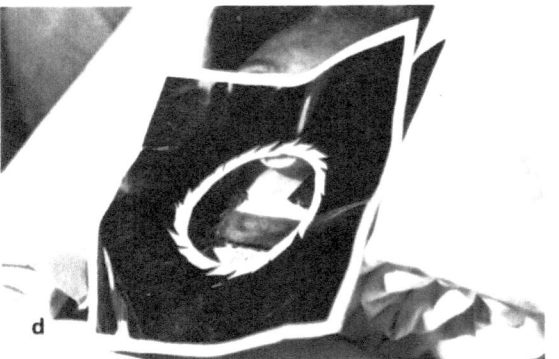
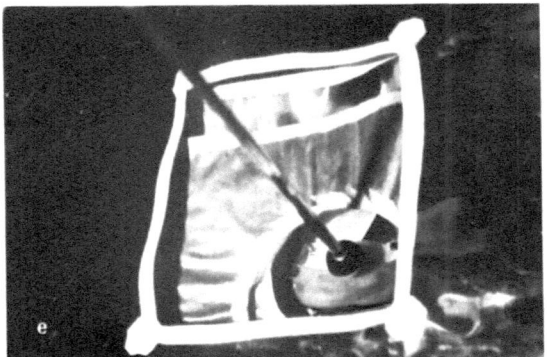

Figure 9-21. Method of treating both lips. a. Outline of the lesion. b. Lead shielding to prevent exit dose. c. Close-up of port. d. Lead shield laid across rolled sheet. e. Distance indicator measures target–skin distance.

pearing at the time of the fourth or fifth treatment. Once it appears, erythema increases in intensity as the therapy progresses and may increase further after treatments are completed. It usually lasts from 2 to 4 weeks after the last treatment. Erythema is the hallmark of successful therapy with our schedule. Should it not appear within 1 week after the last treatment, which is rare, another dose is administered. If it does not appear after a second additional exposure (making a total of seven treatments or 4760 R), some explanation must be sought, such as a defect in the x-ray apparatus.

Oozing and crusting may later accompany the erythema. Some patients complain of burning or itching and, occasionally, that something is "crawling" in or on the skin. The crust may alarm the patient. It may be thick, and its presence seemingly duplicates the circumstances that brought the patient to the physician in the first place. The patient can be confidently assured that this time it has no sinister significance.

Underlying the crust is the ulceration caused by necrosis of the tumor. The volume of the cancer (depth and width) determines the size and duration of the ulcer. Healing of the ulcer may take considerable time ranging from weeks to several months, depending on the site and the volume of tumor irradiated.

Treatment of nose and lip lesions presents special problems. A mucositis frequently develops on the underside of the irradiated area, often accompanied by serosanguineous oozing. Although generally of short duration, the oozing may cause concern to the patient unless he is forewarned. The lip may also swell during therapy. This, plus the pain from the mucositis, may cause some temporary difficulty in eating. All of the above signs and symptoms are generally mild and subside within 2 weeks without therapy.

Three Months Later

The swelling, oozing, crusting, and mucositis have all run their course and disappeared. In most instances, little or nothing can be seen on the treated site, or there may be some hyperpigmentation.

One Year Later

Often very little is seen at the treated site, and it may be difficult to find. There may be mild dyschromia (hyper- and/or hypopigmentation), telangiectasia, and/or mild atrophy.

Three Years Later

Atrophy and fine telangiectasic vessels will generally be evident within the portal area. There may be hyper- and/or hypopigmentation. This aspect will be discussed in some detail below.

Results of X-ray Therapy of Basal Cell Carcinomas

The most complete report of the experience of the Skin and Cancer Unit in the treatment of basal cell carcinomas is that of Bart et al [4]. Much of the following discussion is based on that report.

Clinical Material

Over a 10-year period 500 biopsy-proved basal cell carcinomas in 459 patients were treated as outlined in Table 9-2, using the shielding methods described above. All lesions were located on the head and neck except for 4 on the trunk and extremities. No lesions invaded bone and none had received previous radiation.

Recurrence Rate

Of the 33 recurrences in this series of 500 lesions, 21 appeared within 2 years after treatment and only 2 after 5 years. Twenty two recurrences were at the periphery of the irradiated field, 9 were in the center, and in 2 instances locations were not recorded.

Tumors treated varied in size from 2 to 111 mm diameter with a median of 10 mm. If they were divided into 4 almost equal groups according to size, differences in recurrence rates among the groups were not statistically significant. Tumors of the scalp, nose, paranasal area, and neck showed a higher recurrence rate than did those of the forehead, ear, face, eyelids, and canthi. For the 500 basal cell carcinomas treated, the 5-year recurrence rate was 7%.

Is it possible to improve these results? One should note that 22 recurrences were at the periphery of the treated fields, indicating geographic misses. Should there be any question about the size of a lesion, a border larger than 5 mm is recommended. Some therapists routinely employ 10-mm margins. With our technique, failures due to inadequate borders were more likely than failures due to the quality of radiation.

We have had success in the management of morphea type basal cell carcinomas; for this condition margins larger than 5 mm are frequently employed [3].

Cosmetic Results

A cosmetic evaluation is done each time the patient returns for follow-up. The results are classified as excellent, good, fair, or poor. If the site displays gross scarring, atrophy, multiple telangiectasias, and pigmentary changes (hyper- and/or hypopigmentation) the results are considered poor; if the site is difficult to find and blends in well with the surrounding skin, it is judged excellent.

Based on 803 observations over a period of 1 to 12 years, the cosmetic results were as follows: excellent to good results were noted in 74% of treatment sites within the first year after therapy, in 68% in the third to fifth year after therapy, and in 49% in the ninth to twelfth year; fair to poor cosmetic results were seen in 26, 32, and 51%, respectively (Table 9-1).

Although the cosmetic results tend to worsen with time, this does not present a serious contraindication for radiotherapy since, in the great majority of instances, the cosmetic results are acceptable. However, in a small series of morphea-type basal cell carcinomas treated with x radiation, we found the cosmetic results generally inferior [3].

Sequelae of Radiation Therapy

"Pseudorecidives" Ordinarily, a few weeks after therapy has been completed, no evidence of the treated cancer is discernible clinically. Occasionally, in the area treated a new tumor appears [1]. Such growths usually do not resemble the original tumors. They may be single or multiple, and of varied colors and sizes. The first thought is that they represent recurrences, but they disappear without treatment. Such lesions are called "pseudorecidives." Among the entities which have been recognized as pseudorecidives are keratoacanthomas, cutaneous horns, and lesions simulating verrucae or seborrheic keratoses. Microscopically, the pathology in these lesions includes marked epidermal acanthosis, sometimes appearing pseudoepitheliomatous.

Delayed Tumor Regression In contrast to the above, sometimes an event occurs in which the tumor has not disappeared several weeks after completion of therapy. The concern here is that the cancer is radioresistant. At this time, biopsy may still be positive for basal-cell carcinoma. However, conclusions concerning the future biologic potential of the lesion cannot be drawn from this finding. Sufficient radiation may have been absorbed to render it incapable of further growth. If the tumor is not clinically enlarging or if it is slowly shrinking, the area should be observed monthly for up to 6 months after completion of therapy. Should the tumor still be present after this time, it must be considered radioresistant, excised, and the specimen examined microscopically. Alternatively, Mohs' surgery may be used.

Delayed Ulceration Delayed radiation ulcers appear in the healed site in approximately 1% of basal cell carcinomas of ears and nose treated with the radiation technique outlined. Typically, the patient returns months to years after the lesion site has healed completely. The presenting complaint is that of an ulceration of short duration. It may have been precipitated by some mild mechanical injury, exposure to cold, or excessive sun exposure. Biopsy of such an ulcer shows no recurrence of the cancer. These delayed radiation ulcers usually heal spontaneously, although complete healing may require several months.

Eye Sequelae Permanent alopecia will always develop if the eyebrows or eyelashes are included in the port.

Conjunctival leukoplakic plaques developed on the eyelids in 5 of 50 lesions in our series treated with the radiation technique outlined. These plaques represent benign, radiation-induced keratoses [13]. They usually disappear slowly, and are generally asymptomatic. The new eye shield previously described was designed to reduce backscatter to the conjunctiva in the hope of reducing the incidence of this complication [14].

Squamous Cell Carcinomas The most significant complication is the development of squamous cell carcinomas after x-ray therapy for basal cell carcinomas. This was found after therapy in 3 of the 500 basal cell carcinomas in our published series [4].

It has been known for many years that chronic radiodermatitis can lead to malignancy (basal and squamous cell carcinomas). However, this kind of radiodermatitis is usually that which follows treatment for benign conditions: repeated exposures to low doses of radiation can produce this kind of "carcinoma-prone" radiodermatitis. After the appearance of chronic radiodermatitis, a long latent period (from 1 to 40 or more years) ensues before the radiation-induced tumor emerges. Only rarely does the radiodermatitis following x-ray therapy for skin cancers have such an outcome [5].

Squamous Cell Carcinoma

Squamous cell carcinomas may develop in skin, semimucous membranes, or mucous membranes. Unlike basal cell carcinomas, they have the potential for metastases. It is our policy to limit x-ray therapy to squamous cell carcinomas having the following characteristics: maximum diameter of 6 cm; location on head or neck; no evidence of lymph node or distant metastases; absence of bony involvement; and origin from skin or semimucous membranes but not from mucous membranes. Excluded from dermatologic x-ray therapy are those lesions that: are not located on head or neck; are over 6 cm in diameter; occur intraorally; invade bone; extend from upper lip into a nostril; or are secondary to radiodermatitis, osteomyelitis, chronic ulcers, and burn scars. Basically, then, the following schedule will be concerned with the x-ray therapy of relatively small, uncomplicated squamous cell carcinomas located on the lip and on the skin of the head and neck. Lesions at the angle of the mouth are easily irradiated and heal well, whereas surgical reconstruction of the commissure is often difficult. In addition, those lesions that are reported as basal–squamous cell or metatypical carcinomas are considered as squamous cell carcinomas when planning therapy.

Technique

Dosage
Squamous cell carcinomas have a tendency to infiltrate more deeply than do basal cell carcinomas. To assure an adequate depth dose, 8 treatments of 680 R are given 2 to 3 times per week for a total dose of 5440 R. Radiation factors used for both types of carcinomas are summarized in Table 9-2.

Shielding
Shielding techniques are the same as those employed for basal cell carcinomas.

Keratoacanthoma

Keratoacanthoma is a benign pseudocarcinoma usually located on the light-exposed areas of the body. Typically, it is a lesion which has a rolled border and a keratin-filled central crater; it is skin colored or pink, grows rapidly over several weeks or a few months, and disappears spontaneously [5]. The differentiation clinically and histologically from squamous cell carcinoma is often difficult and sometimes impossible.

X rays are effective in eradicating keratoacanthomas. The technique we have employed is that used for squamous cell carcinoma (ie, 680 R per treatment for 8 treatments over a 3-week period, through a port including a 5-mm border of normal-appearing skin surrounding the perimeter of the lesion).

Bowen's Disease and Superficial Basal Cell Carcinoma

These two neoplasms often mimic each other clinically since both are usually erythematous, scaly, and sometimes crusted plaques. A biopsy may be the only way to distinguish between them. Both respond satisfactorily to radiation in the grenz-ray range (15 kV; HVL, 0.035 mm Al; $D_{1/2}$, 0.9 mm tissue).

The following discussion applies to both lesions since they are irradiated by us in an identical manner. Bowen's disease of true mucous membranes, such as that of the rectum or vagina, is usually treated surgically in our medical center. It is not treated by dermatologic radiation techniques. (For a more detailed discussion of radiotherapy of Bowen's disease see [17].)

Technique

A 5-mm border of normal-appearing skin is included in the port. For lesions over 10 cm in diameter, as may occur in superficial basal cell carcinomas, wider borders are recommended.

External shielding with lead sheeting is used. Grenz-ray doses of 500 R are usually given 3 times a week [17]. Ten such treatments, for a total dose of 5000 R, are given. This schedule was arrived at by striving to achieve high cure rates and acceptable cosmetic results.

Reactions following completion of therapy are similar to those seen after conventional x-ray therapy. However, they are usually not as severe and the eventual atrophy is less apparent.

Whereas malignant cutaneous lesions have been rarely reported after multiple grenz-ray treatments for benign dermatoses [7], they have not been observed after therapy for malignant disease using the schedule outlined above.

Radiation therapy for Bowen's disease and superficial basal cell carcinoma finds its greatest application in those patients who either refuse surgery or in whom the lesions are extensive and where surgery might lead to severe scarring, mutilation, and/or keloid formation [17]. Lesions on the fingers respond admirably.

Grenz-ray therapy is superior to conventional radiotherapy in the treatment of both Bowen's disease and superficial basal cell carcinoma because the pathology of these diseases is quite superficial. For very extensive lesions, the lack of significant backscatter with grenz-ray therapy makes this modality quite safe to use. It should be stressed that grenz-ray therapy as outlined above is *not* recommended for Bowen's disease or superficial basal cell carci-use. It should be stressed that grenz-ray therapy as outlined above is *not* recommended for Bowen's disease or superficial basal cell carcinomas in which the thickness of the disease process exceeds the $D_{1/2}$ of the x-ray beam.

Mycosis Fungoides

Clinically, mycosis fungoides is divided into three stages: I. premycotic; II. infiltrative or plaque; III. tumorous. Marked pruritus is the hallmark of this malignant lymphoma and may be an important clue in its diagnosis. The duration of the disease is extremely variable, ranging from months to many years. Patients have been known to suffer from this illness for 40 years or more. In a series of 165 patients with mycosis fungoides, the mean duration was 8.1 years in 106 deceased patients and 12.5 years in 59 living patients [8].

Radiation may be beneficial for both the symptoms and lesions of mycosis fungoides. Because of its great effectiveness, x-ray therapy often plays a key role in the management of this condition. Before using x-ray therapy, the diagnosis should be firmly established and the stage of the disease ascertained.

X-ray Treatment of Stage I

If the condition is relatively localized, grenz rays (15 kV (peak); HVL, 0.035 mm Al; $D_{1/2}$, 0.9 mm) are used in doses of 200 to 300 R generally administered once or twice per week. For widespread pathology (including universal involvement), teleroentgen therapy (50 kV; HVL, 0.2 mm Al; $D_{1/2}$, 2 mm) is used (Chapter 12). There are two reasons for using such a "soft" x-ray beam. In Stage I, the pathology is relatively superficial; also, mycosis fungoides has a tendency to recur repeatedly over many years. Soft radiation can be given repeatedly as needed with much less tendency to produce severe radiodermatitis. Of course, superficial x rays (100 kV (peak); HVL, 0.9 mm Al; $D_{1/2}$, 12 mm) can also be used in stage I. However, there are several disadvantages. It cannot be used over wide areas without causing severe side effects including radiation sickness and leukopenia. With repeated administration, all the serious sequelae of radiation dermatitis are likely to occur. It should not be inferred that grenz rays and teleroentgen therapy, as defined above, are harmless and without side effects. Radiodermatitis may occur with both if the dosages given are sufficiently high. However, atrophy is less marked than with harder radiations.

X-ray Treatment of Stage II

The treatment of stage II mycosis fungoides requires careful estimation of the depth of the lymphomatous process. For lesions with appreciable infiltration, grenz rays are ineffective as insufficient energy reaches the depth of the process. Widely disseminated, relatively superficial lesions can be treated with teleroentgen therapy. Localized, increasingly infiltrated lesions are treated with superficial x-rays (100 kV (peak); HVL, 0.9 mm Al; $D_{1/2}$, 12 mm). Low dosages are employed because of the high degree of radiosensitivity of the tumor and the sparing effect on the skin in terms of chronic radiodermatitis. Doses of 85 R to 170 R are administered once or twice weekly for about 4 to 6 treatments. Such small doses are generally sufficient both to determine the radiosensitivity of the lesions and to cause their clinical involution when they are radiosensitive.

X-ray Treatment of Stage III

Stage III mycosis fungoides is characterized by the presence of tumors in various phases of development. They may be single or multiple, small or large, smooth or ulcerated, clean or infected, localized or generalized. Patients may have severe burning and pain. This stage is treated with superficial x rays (100 kV (peak); HVL, 0.9 mm Al; $D_{1/2}$, 12 mm), except in those instances where the tumors are considered deeper than 1.5 cm. For such deeper lesions, filtration is added to harden the beam. Employing a 1- or 2-mm aluminum filter changes the HVL to about 2 or 3 mm, respectively. Dosage used is 170 R once or twice per week. A 5- to 10-mm border of normal-appearing skin beyond the perimeter of the tumor is always included in the port. Since these patients are in the advanced phases of the lymphoma, treatment is continued as long as there is satisfactory response. A cumulative dose to an area may reach several thousand roentgens.

Table 9-3 summarizes the technical specifications of the x-ray equipment used at the Skin and Cancer Unit in the treatment of mycosis fungoides.

Teleroentgen therapy as used in derma-

tology may be a new concept for the reader. The target is 2 meters from the patient, giving a maximum field diameter of 2 meters. The patient lies on a table and first the entire front and then the entire back of the body are irradiated. (Fig. 9-23). On the following day each side (right and left) is exposed to assure reasonably even distribution of the radiation. The factors associated with this treatment are shown in Table 9-4.

A course of therapy consists of 10 treatments given on 10 consecutive weekdays (excluding Saturdays and Sundays). The course may be repeated as needed (see below). Because of its superficial absorption, this technique is not suitable for the tumor stage of mycosis fungoides. There is a more thorough discussion of teleroentgen therapy in Chapter 12.

Most cases of mycosis fungoides, whatever the stage, respond to radiation, often dramatically. The lesions involute and the itching and burning usually abate promptly. X-ray therapy has many advantages over other forms of treatment. It can usually be given on an ambulatory basis. The patient may be treated without any loss of time from work. Often the results are extremely gratifying. Foul-smelling, ulcerated tumors may heal in a matter of 2 to 3 weeks. Not only is the therapy easy to administer and painless, but there are usually no apparent side effects. Unlike systemic chemotherapy, no significant bone marrow suppression results from irradiation given as outlined here.

As with all modalities of treatment, x-ray

Table 9-3 *Radiation Factors in Treatment of Mycosis Fungoides*

Stage of Disease	Radiation	kVp	HVL (mm Al)	Added Filter (mm Al)
I. Premycotic				
Localized	Grenz	15	0.03	0
Generalized	Teleroentgen	50	0.2	0
II. Infiltrative				
Localized	Superficial	100	0.9	0
Generalized	Teleroentgen (Whole body if necessary)	50	0.2	0
III. Tumor				
Relatively deep	Superficial	100	0.9	0
Deep (1.5–2 cm)	Superficial	100	2.0	1
Very deep (2–3 cm)	Superficial	100	3.0	2

Abbreviations: HVL, Half-value layer; kVp, Kilovoltage (peak).

The term "cure" appears in the literature for Hodgkins' disease after treatment with radiation [12]. This new concept of utilizing very large doses to completely eliminate all neoplastic cells has now also been applied to mycosis fungoides. Modifying the Stanford Medical Linear Accelerator to permit total skin irradiation with the electron beam, Bagshaw and Eltringham [2] use much more aggressive dosage schedules than employed previously. Fuks and Bagshaw [9] have raised the total dose of electrons to between 3000 and 4000 rads in order to attempt total destruction of all the neoplastic cells. With this method they have reported long-term cures in 8 patients who had early disease.

Kaposi's Sarcoma

Kaposi's sarcoma is generally regarded as a malignancy presenting as reddish–purplish plaques, nodules, and tumors principally on the skin of the lower and upper extremities. They may, however, occur anywhere on the body. Internal involvement with Kaposi's sarcoma or associated malignant lymphoma is not uncommon, and may be the cause of death.

While surgery may be used for the removal of solitary plaques and nodules, radiation is the mainstay of treatment because the lesions are usually radiosensitive, often numerous, and exhibit a great tendency to recur. The lesions most frequently requiring treatment are tumors of various sizes and depths. The mere presence of a Kaposi's sarcoma lesion is not

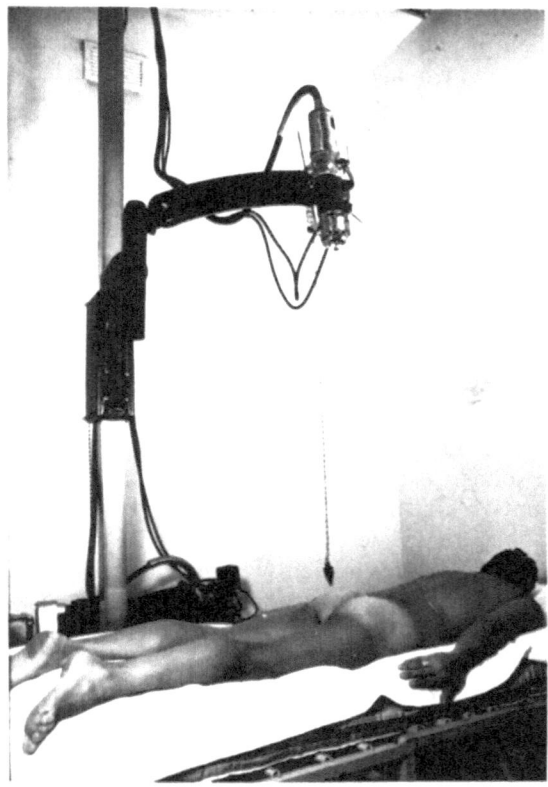

Figure 9-23. Teleroentgen therapy.

therapy of mycosis fungoides is not suited for all lesions or all stages of the disease. Some lesions may not respond, even to high doses of radiation. Many lesions will respond initially only to become radioresistant subsequently. The opposite is also true. Some lesions may not respond at first only to become radiosensitive later. The reasons for such radiobiologic changes are not known. Many patients may be clear of lesions for years and subsequently relapse. Up to the present, the result of x-ray therapy has been palliation, not cure.

A new dimension was added to the radiation therapy of mycosis fungoides in 1953 by Trump et al [18] when they introduced electron-beam therapy for the treatment of this disorder. Employing a Van de Graaff generator, they treated patients who had previously received all known modalities including x rays and chemotherapy. They reported a satisfactory to excellent treatment response to the first course of electrons in well over 90% of the patients. While life might be prolonged and symptoms relieved, this also did not prove to be a cure. Again, only palliation was achieved.

Table 9-4 *Teleroentgen Specifications for Whole Body Irradiation in Mycosis Fungoides*

kVp	50
HVL (mm Al)	0.2
$D_{1/2}$ (mm tissue), H-DD	2.0
TSD (meters)	2
Areas treated on days 1, 3, 5, 9, 11	Front and back
Areas treated on days 2, 4, 8, 10, 12	Right and left sides
Number of R per treatment	50
Total number of R per course of treatment	250
Apparatus	Picker 60, beryllium-window Machlett tube (OEG)

Abbreviations: HVL, Half-value layer; kVp, Kilovoltage (peak); TSD, Target–skin distance; H-DD, (D½), Half-dose depth (half-value depth).

sufficient reason for irradiation, since it may remain stationary for years without therapy. If the tumor is ulcerated, painful, infected, or cosmetically disfiguring, x-ray therapy should be considered. Radiation should be applied judiciously as patients may live as long as 10 to 40 years with this condition; if at all possible, radiodermatitis should be avoided.

Grenz rays (15 kVp; HVL, 0.035 mm Al; $D_{1/2}$, 0.5 mm) and teleroentgen techniques (50 kVp; HVL, 0.2 mm Al; $D_{1/2}$, 2 mm) are used infrequently in this disorder as their effects are too superficial. Harder beams are usually employed in doses of 85 to 170 R once or twice per week until flattening of the lesions occurs. The x-ray treatment of a tumor of Kaposi's sarcoma is identical to that of a tumor of mycosis fungoides.

Half-dose Depth ($D_{1/2}$) Concept

In the past, most dermatologists considered cutaneous malignancies, e.g., basal cell carcinomas, as either "ordinary" or "deep." For the former, "superficial" (e.g., about 100 kVp) radiation was employed; for the latter, added filters or higher kilovoltages were used to increase penetration. Indeed, much of the work cited in this chapter was done at the Skin and Cancer Unit using a Picker 120 x-ray machine operating at 100 kV with a HVL of 0.9 mm Al. No really precise effort had been made to correlate the hardness or penetrability of the beam with the depth of the lesion. This system has been modified relatively recently at our unit; it has been altered based on the concept of half-value depth ($D_{1/2}$) as recommended by Jennings [11], although we prefer the term half-dose depth (H-DD). Only a brief summary of these concepts will be given here since there is a thorough discussion elsewhere in this book.

To provide proper treatment, the hardness or penetrability of the x-ray beam must be known. Originally, x-ray beams were identified solely by the voltages used to generate them. The half-value layer (HVL) replaced voltage as a means of classification because of its greater accuracy in characterizing the actual quality of

radiation. The HVL is that thickness of material, usually aluminum (Al) in dermatologic therapy, which reduces the intensity of the incident beam by 50%. The greater the HVL, the harder the beam, and the more penetrating its effects. While accurate and useful, the concept of HVL seems less appropriate than that of the H-DD. Skin, instead of aluminum, is the index of the hardness of the radiation (special waxes are actually used for the measurements). If the H-DD of an x-ray beam is said to be 3 mm, it means that 50% of the dose applied at the surface will reach 3 mm into the skin. The depth of the lesion is estimated by careful scrutiny of its clinical features or by findings on histologic examination of a biopsy specimen. Suppose that a dose of 1700 R at the base of the tumor is considered sufficient for its eradication. If one uses a beam whose H-DD matches the estimated depth of the lesion, then 3400 R applied to the surface of the lesion will result in 1700 R reaching its base.

Our new Dermopan equipment, installed in 1971, allows utilization of the H-DD concept in which we select that quality of radiation of which will be 50% absorbed within the lesion. For example, to treat a basal cell carcinoma we still use 680 R for each of 5 treatments (3400 R total dose) over 9 to 12 days, but select the Dermopan "step" according to the depth of the cancer. Tables 9-5 to 9-9 list the factors we now use in treating basal cell carcinomas, squamous cell carcinomas, keratoacanthomas, mycosis fungoides, and Kaposi's sarcoma. It should be emphasized that such a wide range of factors is also possible with other soft x-ray beryllium-window machines besides the Dermopan equipment, i.e., Philips RT-100 x-Ray (Table 9-8).

Acknowledgments

The calibration of Appendix #2 was done by Mr. Edgar N. Grisewood. The authors wish to thank Miss Sylvia Buchanan, Mrs. Nettie Alderman, and Miss Herta Samson, radiation technicians, New York University Skin and Cancer Unit, for their cooperation.

Table 9-5 *Present Schedule for Treating Basal Cell Carcinomas at NYU Skin and Cancer Unit*

Thickness of Lesion (mm)	HVL (mm Al)	kVp	Added Filtration (mm Al)	H-DD or $D_{1/2}$ (mm tissue)	TSD (cm)	mA	Dose per Treatment	Total Dose	No. of Treatments	Interval (days)	Time Span (days)	MPD (cm)
2–3	0.1	29	0.3	2–3	15–30	25	680	3400	5	2–3	9–12	2
6–7	0.35	43	0.6	6–7	15–30	25	680	3400	5	2–3	9–12	2
10–12	0.85	50	1.0	10–12	15–30	25	680	3400	5	2–3	9–12	2
13–17	1.3	50	2.0	13–17	15–30	25	680	3400	5	2–3	9–12	2

Abbreviations: HVL, Half-value layer; kVp, kilovoltage (peak); TSD, Target–skin distance; MPD, Minimum port diameter; H-DD, ($D_{1/2}$) Half-dose depth (half-value depth); mA, Milliamperes.

Table 9-6 *Present Schedule for Treating Squamous Cell Carcinomas and Selected Keratoacanthomas at NYU Skin and Cancer Unit*

Thickness of Lesion (mm)	HVL (mm Al)	kVp	Added Filtration (mm Al)	H-DD or $D_{1/2}$ (mm tissue)	TSD (cm)	mA	Dose per Treatment	Total Dose	No. of Treatments	Interval (days)	Time Span (days)	MPD (cm)
2–3	0.1	29	0.3	2–3	15–30	25	680	5440	8	2–3	17–20	2
6–7	0.35	43	0.6	6–7	15–30	25	680	5440	8	2–3	17–20	2
10–12	0.85	50	1.0	10–12	15–30	25	680	5440	8	2–3	17–20	2
13–17	1.3	50	2.0	13–17	15–30	25	680	5440	8	2–3	17–20	2

Abbreviations: HVL, Half-value layer; kVp, kilovoltage, TSD, Target–skin distance; MPD, Minimum port diameter; H-DD, ($D_{1/2}$). Half-dose depth (half-value depth); mA, Milliamperes.

Table 9-7 *Calibration for Siemens Dermopan 2*

	kVp	mA	Filter	HVL (mm Al)	H-DD or $D_{1/2}$ (mm tissue)	TSD (cm)	R/min in Air	85 R MIN	85 R SEC	100 R MIN	100 R SEC	340 R MIN	340 R SEC
Step 1	14	25	none	0.025	0.5	15	2360				2.5		
				0.032	.9	30	350				17		
Step 2	29	25	0.3	0.1	2	15	430			12	14		48
					3	30	104			49	58	3	17
Step 3	43	25	0.6	0.35	6	15	448			11	13		46
					7	30	109			47	55	3	7
Step 4	50	25	1.0	0.85	10	15	408			13	15		50
					12	30	100			51		1	3	24
Step 5	50	25	2.0	1.3	13	15	195			26	31	1	45
					17	30	48.0	1	46	2	5	7	5
Teleroentgen:													
Step 4	50	25	none	0.08	1.5	100	158		32		38	2	9
				0.17	2.0	200	20.5	3	55	4	52	16	40

Abbreviations: HVL, Half-value layer; kVp, Kilovoltage (peak); TSD, Target–skin distance; H-DD, ($D_{1/2}$), Half-dose depth (half-value depth); mA, Milliamperes.

Table 9-8   *Calibration for Philips RT-100 X-Ray Tube #46485 NR*

kVp	mA	Added Filter	HVL (mm Al)	H-DD or D₁/₂ (mm tissue)	TSD (cm)	R/min in air	85 R MIN	85 R SEC	100 R MIN	100 R SEC	200 R MIN	200 R SEC	170 R MIN	170 R SEC
15	7	none*	0.025	0.4	10	1025		5		6		12		
			.029	.6	20	225		23		27		53		
			.032	.8	30	70	11	13	1	26	2	52		
20	8	0.15	0.12	2	10	910		5½		6½		13		11
				3	20	210		24		28		57		49
				4	30	90.0		57	1	7	2	14	1	53
30	8	0.30	0.20	3	10	850		6		7				12
				4	20	205		25		29				50
				5	30	90.0		57	1	7			1	54
37	8	0.40	0.35	5	10	890		5½		6½				11
				6	20	210		25		30				51
				7	30	92.0		56	1	6			1	51
45	10	0.55	0.60	7	10	960		5½		6½				11
				8	20	240		21		25				43
				9	30	99.0		51	1	1			1	43
55	10	0.78	0.85	9	10	960		5½		6½				11
				10	20	240		21		25				43
				11	30	99.5		51	1	—			1	42
70	10	1.25	1.1	12	10	1025		5		6				10
				13	20	256		20		23				40
				14	30	100		51	1	—			1	42
100	8	1.70	2.0	18	10	837		6		7				12
				20	20	209		24		29				49
				22	30	93.0		55	1	5			1	50
55	10	none*	0.09	3	100	72.0	1	11	1	23			2	22
				4	200	9.3	9	10	10	48				

Abbreviations: HVL, Half-value layer; kVp, kilovoltage (peak); TSD, Target–skin distance; H-DD, (D½), Half-dose depth (half-value depth).

*Inherent filtration is 1 mm Be.

Table 9-9   *Present Factors for Treating Mycosis Fungoides and Selected Cases of Kaposi's Sarcoma at NYU Skin and Cancer Unit*

	Radiation	kVp	HVL (mm Al)	H-DD or D₁/₂ (mm tissue)	TSD (cm)	Added Filter (mm Al)
Stage of Disease						
I. Premycotic						
Localized	Grenz	14	0.025–0.032	0.5–0.9	15–30	0
Generalized	Teleroentgen (whole body)	50	0.08–0.17	1.5–2.0	100–200	0
II. Infiltrative						
Localized	Superficial	29–50	0.1–0.85	2.0–12.0	15–30	0.3–1.0
Generalized	Teleroentgen (whole body)	50	0.17	2.0	200	0
III. Tumor						
Relatively deep (1.0 cm)	Superficial	50	0.85	10.0–12.0	15–30	1.0
Deep (1.5 cm)	Superficial	50	1.3	13.0–17.0	15–30	2.0

Abbreviations: HVL, Half-value layer; kVp, kilovoltage (peak); TSD, Target–skin distance; H-DD, (D½), Half-dose depth (half-value depth).

*Inherent filtration is 1 mm Be.

References

1. Baer RL, Kopf AW: Complications of therapy of basal cell epitheliomas (based on 1000 histologically verified cases). In 1964–1965 Series of Year Book of Dermatology. Year Book Medical, 1965, pp 7–26

2. Bagshaw MA, Eltingham JR: Observations on the electron beam therapy of mycosis fungoides. Front Radiat Ther Oncol 2:163, 1968

3. Bart RS, Kopf AW, Gladstein AH: Treatment of morphea-type basal cell carcinomas with x-rays. Arch Dermatol 113, 783–786, 1977

4. Bart RS, Kopf AW, Petratos MA: X-ray therapy of skin cancer. Evaluation of a "standardized" method for treating basal-cell epitheliomas. In Proceedings of the Sixth National Cancer Conference. Lippincott, 1970

5. Belisario JC: Cancer of the Skin. London, Butterworth, 1959

6. Blatz H: Introduction to Radiological Health. New York, McGraw-Hill, 1964, p 109

7. Braun-Falco O, Lukacs S, Goldschmidt H: Dermatologic Radiotherapy. New York, Springer-Verlag, 1976, p 54

8. Cyr, DP, Geokas MC, Worsley GH: Mycosis fungoides. Hematological findings and terminal course. Arch Dermatol 94:558, 1966

9. Fuks Z, Bagshaw MA: Total-skin electron treatment of mycosis fungoides. Radiology 100:145, 1971

10. Gladstein AH: Modifications of eye shields for use in x-ray therapy of eyelid cancers. Arch Dermatol 114:793, 1974

11. Jennings WA: Physical aspects of the roentgen radiation from a beryllium tube operated over the range 2–50 K.V.P for clinical purposes I and II. Acta Radiol 33:435, 1950

12. Kaplan HS: Radiotherapy of advanced Hodgkin's disease with curative intent. JAMA, Jan 1, 1973, Vol 223, No 1

13. Kopf AW, Allyn B, Andrade R, et al: Leukoplakia of the conjunctiva. A complication of x-ray therapy for carcinoma of the eyelid. Arch Dermatol 94:552, 1966

14. Kopf, AW, Grisewood EN, Bart RS, et al: X-irradiation of ocular tissues measured by thermoluminescence dosimetry. J Invest Dermatol 49:512, 1967

15. Menn H, Robins P, Kopf AW, et al: The recurrent basal-cell epithelioma. Arch Dermatol 103:628, 1971

15a. Orentreich N: Personal communication, 1977

16. Robins P, Albom MJ: Mohs' surgery. Fresh tissue technique. J Dermatol Surg 1:49, 1975

17. Stevens DM, Kopf AW, Gladstein A, et al: Treatment of Bowen's disease with grenz rays. Int J Dermatol June 1977, Vol 16, No. 5

18. Trump JG, Wright KA, Evans WW, et al: High energy electrons for the treatment of extensive superficial malignant lesions. Am J Roentgenol 69:623, 1953

10

Radiotherapy of Lentigo Maligna and Bowen's Disease

Helga Hauss, Albin Proppe, and Herbert Goldschmidt

Lentigo Maligna

Lentigo maligna (melanotic freckle) is a relatively rare premalignant disorder occurring predominantly in sun-exposed areas of elderly patients. It can be effectively treated either by surgical methods or by radiotherapy. The selection of the appropriate method of treatment depends on several factors, particularly the age of the patient, his general health, the location of the lesion, and its size. Dermatologists should be trained in all therapeutic methods in order to determine which modality is best for each case.

This report is based on our experience with 56 patients with lentigo maligna treated by irradiation. Our main indications are large lesions where surgical therapy may leave disfiguring scars, and lesions in anatomic regions where unfavorable postoperative cosmetic or functional results can be expected, such as in the canthi of the eye. In many other instances, radiation therapy may also yield better cosmetic results than will surgery. Treatment with curettage and electrodesiccation is often unsatisfactory and frequently followed by recurrences.

Technical Data

Miescher [12] was the first to use ultrasoft x rays (grenz rays) in the treatment of lentigo maligna. The "Miescher technique" utilizes ra-

diation generated by a beryllium-window tube at 12 kV with an additional 1.0-mm thick filter of tissue-equivalent material (Cellon); the half-value depth ($D_{1/2}$) varies from 0.68 to 0.74 mm (as measured in Cellon) and the half-value layer (HVL) is 0.052 mm Al. Miescher recommended fractions of 1000 to 2000 R once or twice weekly up to a total dose of 6000 to 14,000 R, usually 5 × 2000 R. Cellon is a clear plastic material; since its absorption characteristics are not always consistent, the definition of the radiation quality in mm Cellon is not necessarily accurate nor reproducible in all cases.

The most important American publication in this field is by Petratos et al [13], who originally used a beryllium-window machine at 12 kV with additional filtration of 1.0 mm Cellon at 20 cm target–skin distance (TSD) and 12 mA. The HVL was approximately 0.052 mm Al and the $D_{1/2}$ was 1.3 mm of skin. Since Cellon is not readily available in the United States, they replaced it with a 0.6-mm thick cellulose acetate filter (ordinary x-ray film cleared of its emulsion). At 15 kV, 7mA, and 20 cm TSD, the HVL was 0.052 mm Al and the $D_{1/2}$ was 0.7 mm of skin.

Our own technique differs from the original Miescher technique only by a minor variation in the radiation quality. We use a beryllium-window machine at 10 kV at 30 cm TSD and use no additional filtration. The HVL is approximately 0.022 mm Al. The radiation quality in the grenz-ray range depends on the distance in air; at a longer distance, more soft x rays will be absorbed, resulting in a slightly more penetrating radiation. Originally we used a target–skin distance of 10 cm. This short TSD resulted in a very soft radiation with increased postradiation pigmentation; the HVL was only 0.015 mm Al. Thirty-two of our patients were treated with a TSD of 10 cm; the remaining 24 patients, with a TSD of 30 cm. The difference in radiation quality is explained by the differing absorptions in air. The absorption in air also affects the effective dose rate at the skin surface. Care should be taken not to compute the dose rates at different target–skin distances by using the inverse square law.

The biologic term half-value depth has been used to determine the absorption in different depths of tissue. Unfortunately, however, there is no universally accepted skin-equivalent material. Most skin models are based only on the effective atomic number. The tissue density, however, is also important in describing equivalent radiation absorption. For this reason our half-value depths were determined in 3 M wax, according to Markus [10]. The unfiltered 10 kV beryllium-window radiation at 30 cm TSD has a $D_{1/2}$ of 0.3 mm as measured in 3 M wax.

Our variations in kilovoltage and target–skin distance are minimal compared to the original Miescher technique; the main factors remain the same, particularly the use of individual doses of 1500 to 2000 R once or twice weekly up to a total dose of 8000 to 10,000 R.

Clinical Considerations

The therapeutic effect of the Miescher technique in lentigo maligna has been doubted in view of the anatomic depth of some lesions. Microscopic examination often shows involvement along the root sheaths in skin depths that are not reached by significant doses of grenz rays. These theoretical objections are overruled by the actual results of radiation therapy. It is possible that the effects of soft x rays are not directly related to the actual penetration. The potential role of other unknown therapeutic factors is also emphasized by the unusual length of time needed for resolution of the involved areas. Arma-Szlachcic et al [1] and

Braun-Falco et al [2] have also emphasized the very slow rate at which pigment disappears. Pigmentation in small lesions may take 6 months to dissipate; larger lesions may not disappear completely until almost 2 years have passed.

Thirty-two cases were selected to determine the average length of time between treatment and disappearance of pigmentation. Figure 10-1 summarizes the rate of disappearance of lentigo maligna, based on our limited number of observations.

It is important to check patients at regular intervals after treatment. In some cases pigmentation may not change for a lengthy period. Should the pigmented area enlarge, however, one must consider the possibility that the original lesion did not represent lentigo maligna, but rather the initial stage of lentigo maligna melanoma.

Immediate surgical excision would be indicated in this rare circumstance; which should not be interpreted as a radiation-induced transformation of a lentigo maligna into a melanoma, but rather as a subclinical melanoma which was already present before radiotherapy was started.

Kopf et al [8] recently reported 3 cases of metastatic malignant melanoma in a series of 16 patients with melanotic freckle treated with the Miescher technique. We have not encountered any such cases in our group of patients. It should be remembered in this context that the clinical features of these processes are not always characteristic and that malignant degeneration cannot be excluded in all cases, even when incisional biopsies have been taken. The differential diagnosis between lentigo maligna, junction nevus, and superficial spreading melanoma cannot always be decided with certainty. Incisional biopsies of small portions of a melanotic freckle may miss foci of incipient degeneration into a lentigo maligna melanoma. (On the other hand, we have seen lesions which we would currently interpret as superficial spreading melanomas disappear under treatment with soft x rays.) We agree with most authors who prefer excisional biopsies. When they are inadvisable because of the size or location of the lesion, incisional biopsies have been suggested. In Europe, most dermatologists are reluctant to take incisional biopsies of any lesion in which they suspect melanoma or premelanoma. Many

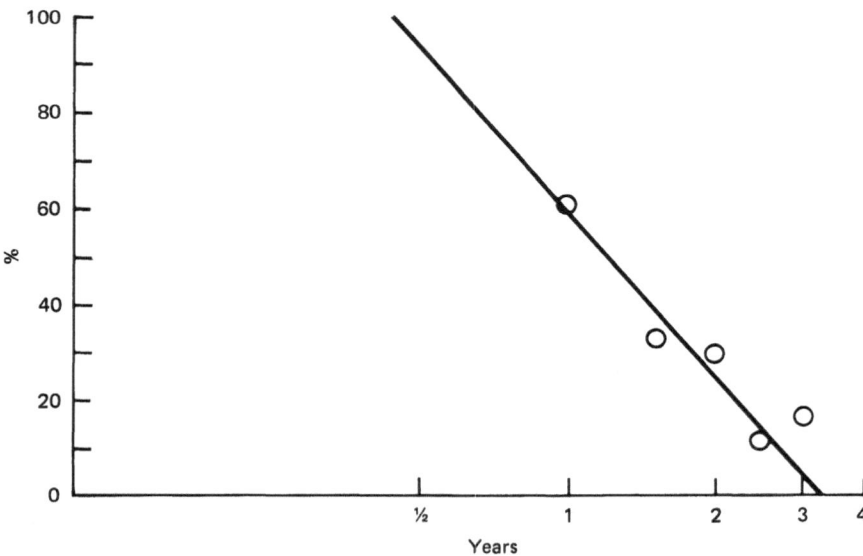

Figure 10-1. Course of lentigo maligna following treatment with the Miescher technique until complete resolution of disease.

leading schools (including Miescher's own department in Zurich; see [1]) maintain that incisional biopsies of melanomas are contraindicated. Arguments in favor of incisional biopsies in all suspected cases of lentigo maligna have not been completely convincing to many European dermatologists.

Even though biopsies were not taken for these reasons in all of our cases, we still consider our statistical data valid. Arma-Szlachcic et al [1] state that other tumors such as pigmented nevi, seborrheic keratoses, and pigmented basal cell cancers "can be ruled out on clinical grounds with a high degree of certainty by an experienced dermatologist"; only 34% of their cases were examined histologically.

The evaluation of therapeutic results is also affected by the former uncertainty concerning the classification of melanomas. Lentigo maligna had been separated from malignant melanoma many decades ago (Hutchinson: senile freckles [1892], lentigo melanosis [1894], now usually classified as Hutchinson's melanotic freckle; Dubreuilh: melanose circonscripte précancéreuse [1912]). Another type of melanoma, ie, the superficial spreading melanoma, has been differentiated only since 1967 [3,4,11,16]. The differentiation of these various types of melanoma is extremely important in view of their differing prognoses, particularly in the evaluation of therapeutic modalities.

In clinical practice it is not always possible to classify individual cases into the 3 groups described by Clark and Mihm [4], ie, into lentigo maligna melanoma, superficial spreading melanoma, and nodular melanoma [9,11]. In our opinion, the distinct differences in sex distribution have been neglected in the biologic assessment of melanomas [6,7]. A personal discussion with Clark and Mihm in December 1971 prompted us to review all cases that were originally classified and treated as lentigo maligna. We found (as did many other clinicians) that our original series included some cases of superficial spreading melanoma. Following reclassification, our series now includes 56 patients with lentigo maligna treated with the Miescher technique (8 of these were treated between 1950 and 1960). The normal mortality rate also complicates the statistical evaluation of long-term therapeutic results regarding potentially malignant skin diseases in older age groups [14]. For this reason we are also presenting the age distribution of our patients (Fig. 10-2). The arithmetic mean age of 60 men (63.7 years) was not markedly different from the arithmetic mean age of 40 women (58.5 years). For this reason the age distribution of patients of both sexes at the onset of therapy is pre-

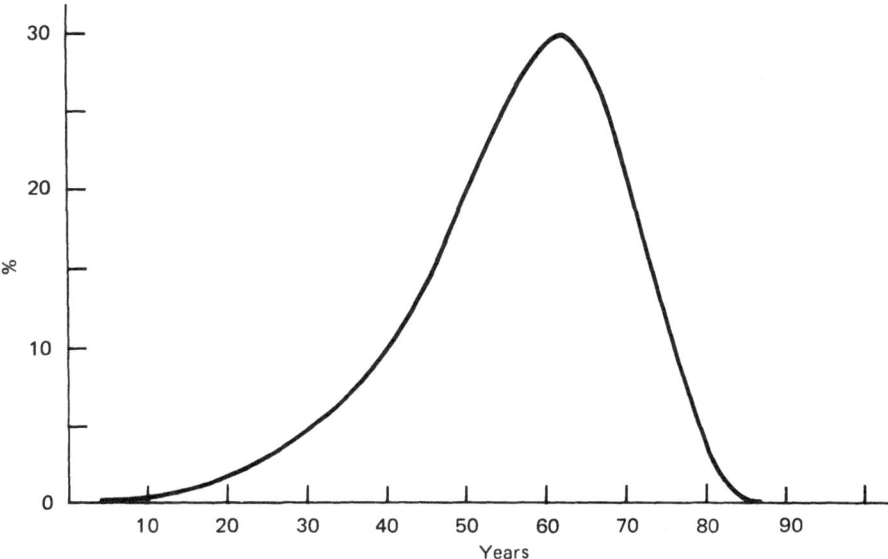

Figure 10-2. Age distribution of patients with lentigo maligna (at onset of radiation therapy).

sented in only one figure. Figure 10-2 shows the percentage frequency in each age group based on the frequency analyses of Daeves and Beckel [5].

Five patients in our series of 56 patients were not included in this analysis because they did not return for follow-up examinations. Sixteen patients were treated only during the past 12 months. These cases were also excluded even though there was no evidence of any unsatisfactory therapeutic results. Follow-up intervals of the remaining 35 patients are presented in Table 10-1. In all of these patients the lesions of lentigo maligna have disappeared completely without any trace of residual pigmentation.

Case Reports

The following cases have been selected to demonstrate therapeutic results. In each case radiation was given with a beryllium-window machine at 10 kV without filtration (Siemens Dermopan 2). The only variable factor was the target–skin distance, which is given for each of the discussed cases.

Case 1: 74-year-old female. Macular brownish pigmentation on left cheek of "many years" duration, growing slowly during the past few months. Figure 10-3 shows this condi-

tion before radiotherapy with 4 × 2000 R (total dose, 8000 R) at a 10 cm TSD. Figure 10-4 shows complete disappearance of lesion 10 months after treatment.

Case 2: 74-year-old male. Hyperpigmented macular lesion in left retroauricular area of 3 years' duration. Clinical and histologic diagnosis: lentigo maligna. Figure 10-5 shows lentigo maligna before radiation therapy. Treatment with 4 × 1500 R at a 30 cm TSD. Figure 10-6 shows complete disappearance of lesion 10 months after treatment.

Case 3: 60-year-old female. The lesion in the lateral corner of the right eye developed

Table 10-1 *Follow-up of Patients with Lentigo Maligna Treated with X Rays*

Years Following Irradiation	No. of Cases
2	9
3	12
4	1
5	1
6	3
7	3
8	4
9	—
10	—
11	1
12	1
Total	35

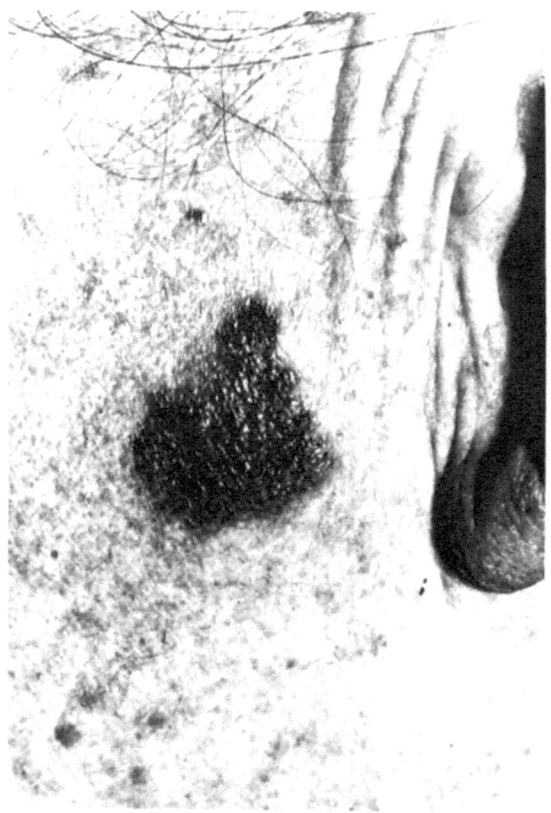

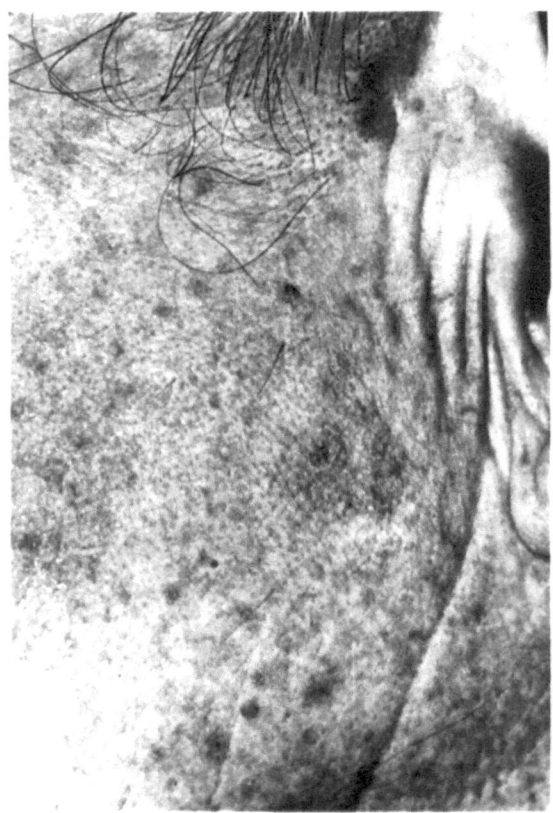

Figure 10-3.   Lentigo maligna of left cheek in 74-year-old female.

Figure 10-4.   Same patient as in Fig. 10-3 10 months following radiation therapy.

approximately 11 years prior to treatment. Figures 10-7 and 10-8 show the lesion before irradiation. Figures 10-9 and 10-10 were taken 11 months after treatment with 4 × 2000 R (TSD, 10 cm). A small residual pigmented area was noted in the right lateral canthus (Figs. 10-9 and 10-10). Figures 10-11 and 10-12 were taken 21 months following irradiation. Lesion disappeared completely without any further treatment.

Case 4: 63-year-old female. A macular area developed on the right temple during the past 8 to 10 years. Figure 10-13 shows the lesion prior to radiation therapy at a TSD of 10 cm with 4 × 2000 R. Nine months later the lesion had disappeared completely with a very satisfactory cosmetic result. Figure 10-14 was taken 18 months after irradiation. Patient has been followed for 7 years post-treatment. Cosmetic result remains excellent.

Case 5: 62-year-old female. Brownish hyperpigmentation in the right zygomatic area of

25 years' duration. Lesion started growing during the past 2 years. Figure 10-15 depicts the lesion before treatment with 3 × 2000 R at a TSD of 10 cm. Figure 10-16 was taken 8 months after radiation therapy; lesion completely disappeared.

Case 6: 67-year-old female. Tan-colored pigmented area on right cheek of 10 years' duration. Following consultation patient was observed for 33 months without any treatment. During this interval the lesion increased 1.3 times in area, from 7.4 to 9.6 cm². Figure 10-17 shows the lesion before treatment with 4 × 2000 R at a TSD of 10 cm. Figure 10-18 was taken 16 months following radiation therapy. Lesion healed completely.

Case 7: 39-year-old male. Patient noted a "mole" on his right upper arm during the past 15 years. Figure 10-19 shows the 14 × 18 mm² lesion before treatment with 6 × 1500 R at a TSD of 30 cm. Figure 10-20 depicts complete clearing of lesion 3 years after treatment.

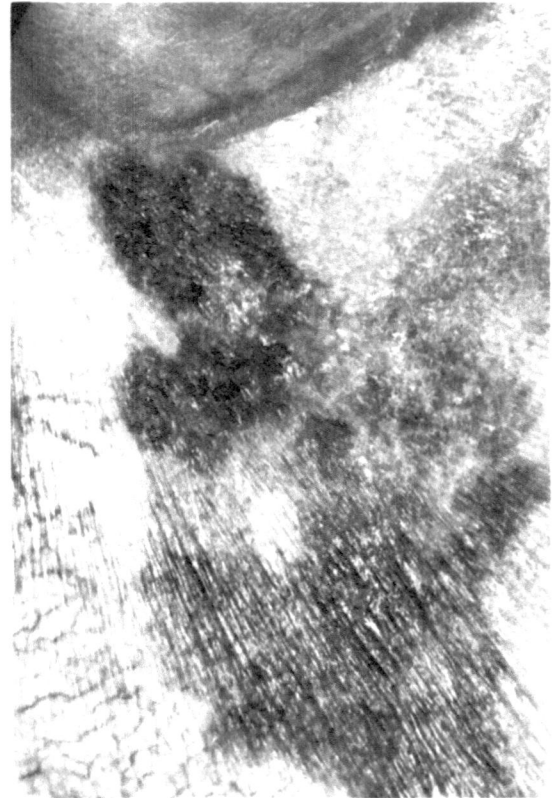

Figure 10-5. Lentigo maligna in left retroauricular area in 74-year-old male.

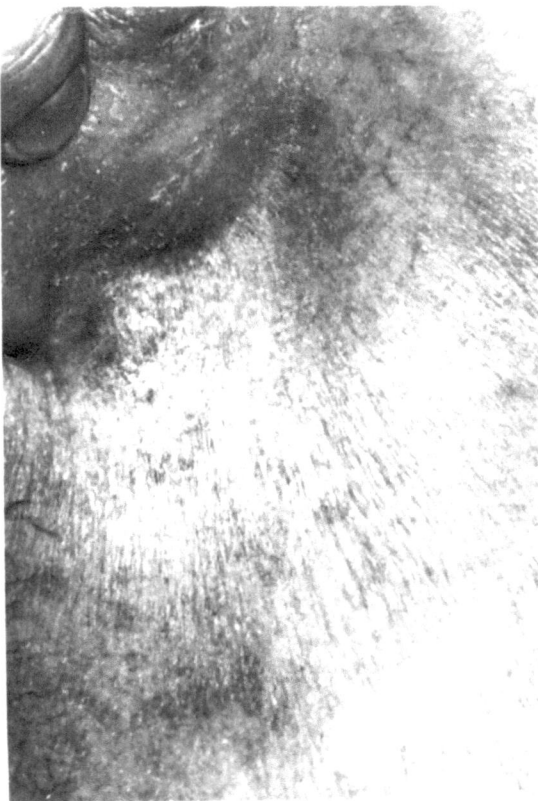

Figure 10-6. Same patient as in Fig. 10-5 10 months following radiation therapy.

Case 8: 68-year-old female. Patient noted a brown lesion on her left cheek 30 years ago. The lesion had been treated twice by electro-desiccation without improvement. The patient was concerned about slow growth during the past 4 weeks. Figure 10-21 shows the 22 × 28 mm² lesion before treatment with 4 × 2000 R at

a TSD of 10 cm. Figure 10-22 shows the excellent therapeutic result 8 months after treatment.

Case 9: 54-year-old female. Slowly growing black-to-brown pigmented area on bridge of nose. Figure 10-23 depicts the 13 × 24 mm² lesion before treatment with 6 × 1500 R at a

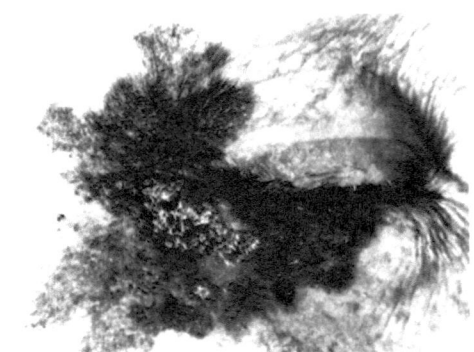

Figure 10-7. Lentigo maligna involving the right lateral canthus and lower lid in 60-year-old female.

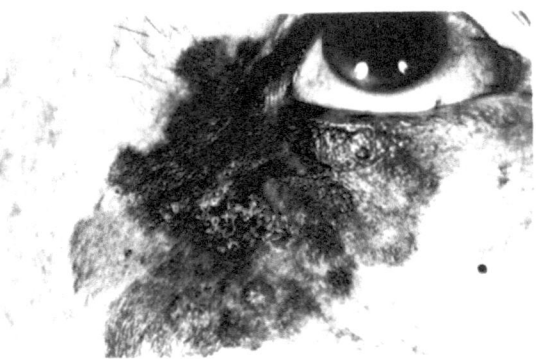

Figure 10-8. Same patient as in Fig. 10-7 with eye opened; note pigmentation of lower lid.

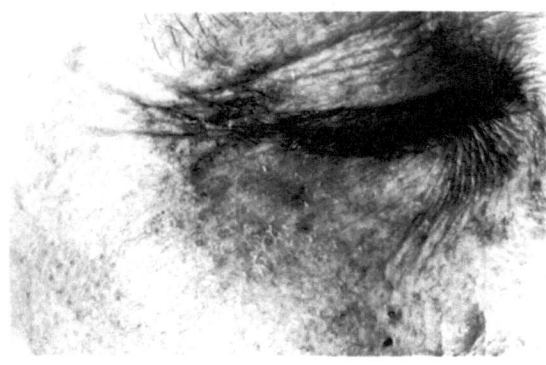

Figure 10-9. Same patient as in Fig. 10-7 11 months following radiation therapy with residual pigmented area.

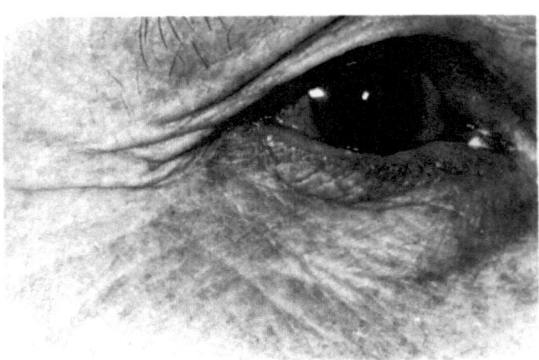

Figure 10-12. Same patient as in Fig. 10-7 with eye opened.

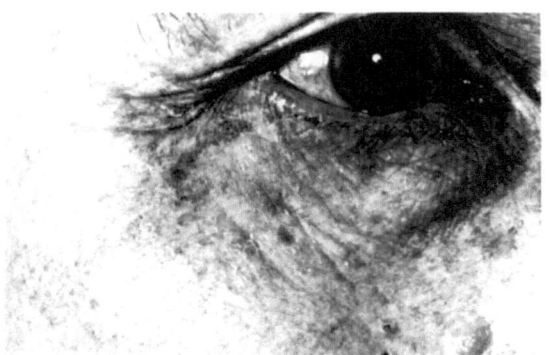

Figure 10-10. Same patient as in Fig. 10-7 with eye opened.

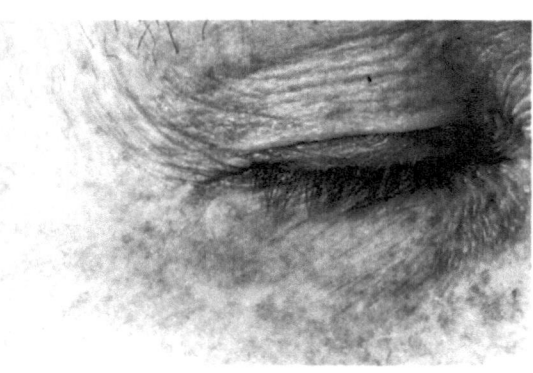

Figure 10-11. Same patient as in Fig. 10-7 19 months following radiation therapy.

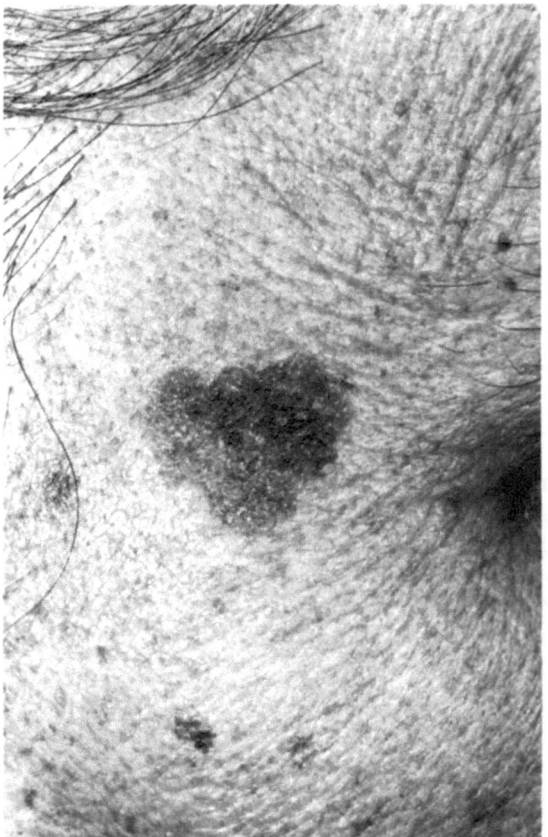

Figure 10-13. Lentigo maligna on right temple of 63-year-old female.

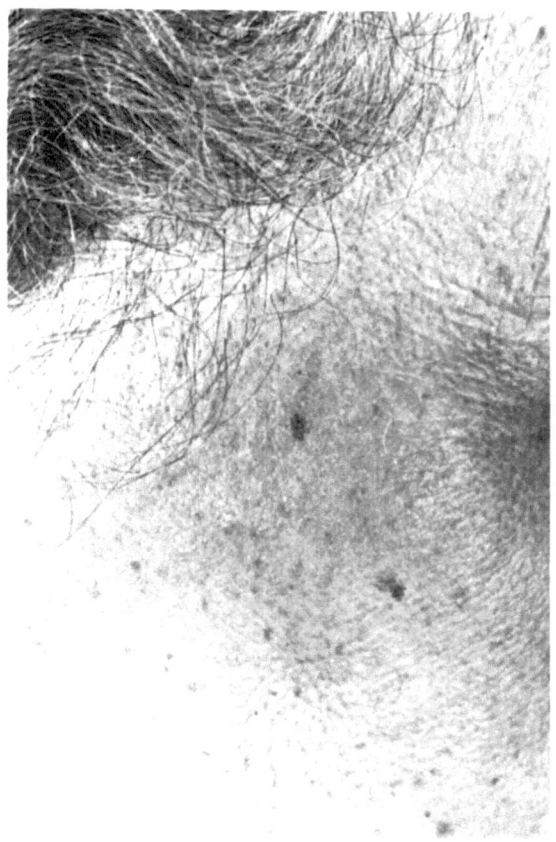

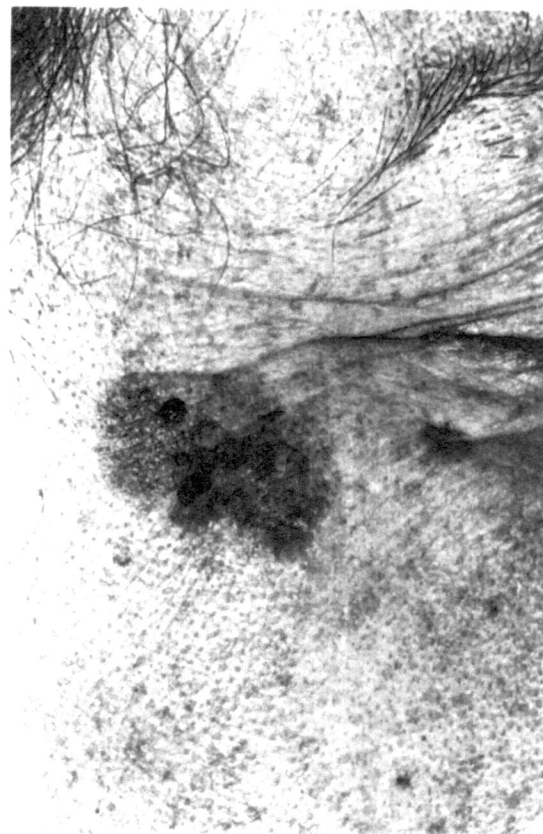

Figure 10-14. Same patient as in Fig. 10-13 1.5 years following radiation therapy.

Figure 10-15. Lentigo maligna in right zygomatic area of 62-year-old female.

TSD of 30 cm. Figure 10-24 shows the therapeutic result 3.5 years following irradiation.

Bowen's Disease

Most cases of Bowen's disease can be treated surgically. Most lesions are relatively small and can be excised completely when the biopsy is taken. Indications for radiation therapy are limited to exceptional cases where neither surgery nor topical chemosurgery with 5-fluorouracil is likely to be effective. Among these rare exceptions are lesions in unusual anatomic areas or extremely large lesions. In contrast to treatment of lentigo maligna, more penetrating x rays are required and radiation is usually given in small fractional doses, as in the radiotherapy of skin cancers. In most patients highly satisfactory cosmetic results can be expected.

Technical Data

This report is based on our experience with 30 patients (14 men, 16 women) with Bowen's disease. In 26 patients a soft radiation with a HVL of only 0.15 mm Al and a $D_{1/2}$ of 2.5 mm of skin was administered. The physical factors correspond to step 2 of the Siemens Dermopan 2 x-ray unit (29 kV, 0.3 mm added filtration, 30 cm TSD).

Case Reports

Case 10: 29-year-old male with a slowly growing tumor on his left thumb of 2 years' duration (Fig. 10-25). The diagnosis of Bowen's disease was confirmed microscopically. Radiotherapy consisted of Dermopan step 2 in 20 individual doses of 300 R each. Figure 10-26 shows a completely healed lesion 2.5 months later.

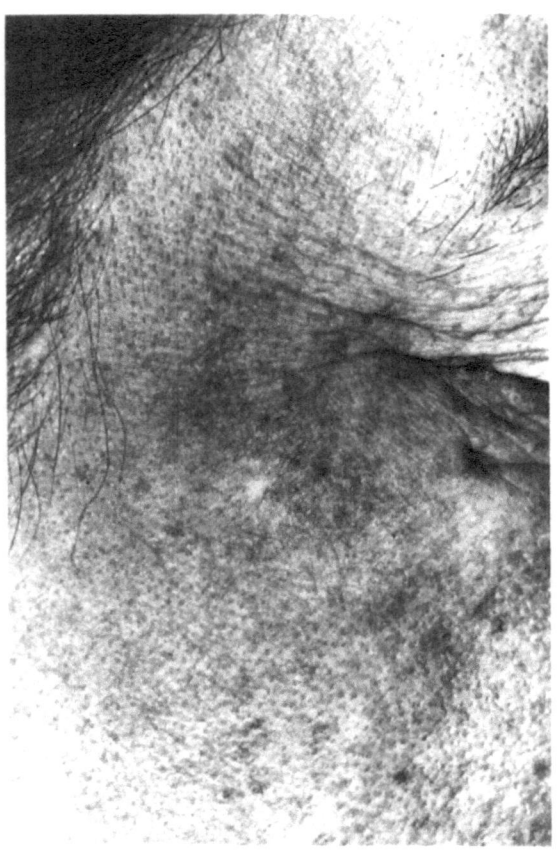

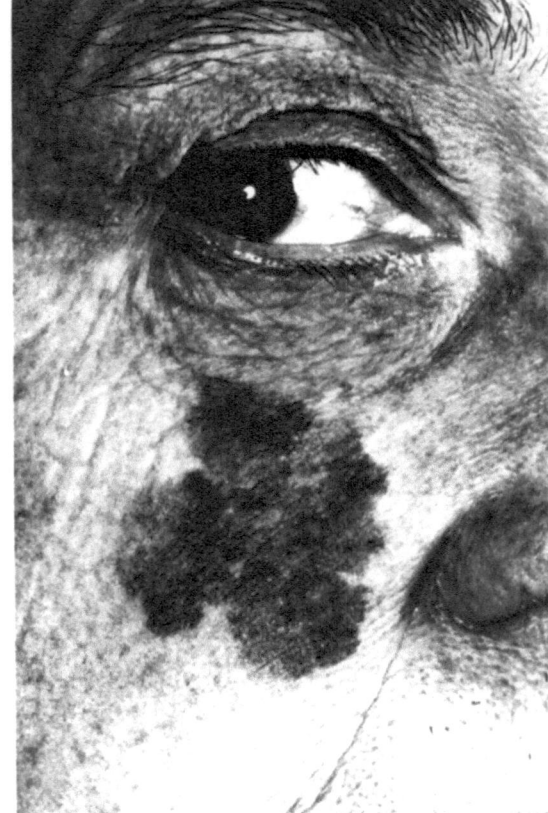

Figure 10-16.   Same patient as in Fig. 10-15 8 months following radiation therapy.

Figure 10-17.   Lentigo maligna on right cheek of 67-year-old female.

Case 11: 72-year-old male noted a slowly increasing growth on his left index finger that showed microscopic changes of Bowen's disease. Radiation therapy consisted of Dermopan step 2 using 14 individual doses of 400 R each.

Case 12: 57-year-old male. Two years ago patient noticed a growth on the shaft of his penis which was originally treated as condyloma acuminatum. Microscopic examination revealed Bowen's disease (Fig. 10-27). Treatment consisted of Dermopan step 2 using 18 doses of 300 R each. Three months after treatment all lesions had healed completely.

Case 13: 64-year-old male who noted well-demarcated, dusky-red, velvety changes on the glans of his penis approximately 3 months ago. The clinical diagnosis was erythroplasia of Queyrat (Fig. 10-28); microscopic examination revealed changes compatible with Bowen's disease. Radiotherapy was started

with Dermopan step 2 in 19 doses of 300 R each. Examination 2.5 years later showed mild scarring with some telangiectasia.

Case 14: 72-year-old female who noted a slowly growing tumor on her upper eyelid for the past 5 years (Fig. 10-29). Microscopic examination revealed Bowen's disease. Since surgical excision of the area would have been mutilating, radiation therapy was started using Dermopan step 2. Following insertion of lead shields into the conjunctival sac, 19 fractions of 300 R each were given at successive intervals. Eight months later a small residual growth was noted at the medial corner of the upper lid which was not adequately treated during the first course. This residual area was retreated using (as an exception) slightly more penetrating radiation with Dermopan step 3 (43 kV; 0.7 mm Al added filter; HVL, 0.39 mm Al; $D_{1/2}$, 6.2 mm as measured in 3 M wax). Nineteen doses

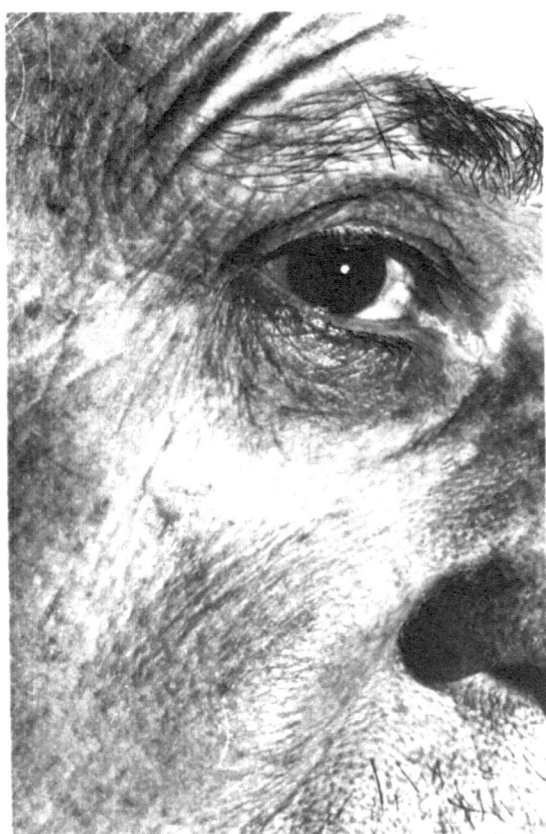

Figure 10-18.   Same patient as in Fig. 10-17 15 months following radiation therapy.

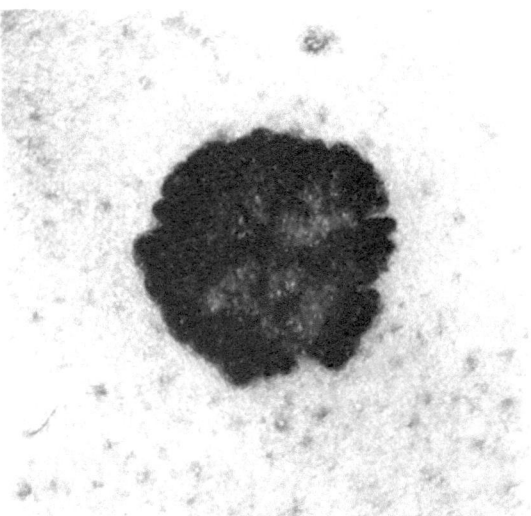

Figure 10-19.   Lentigo maligna on right upper arm of 39-year-old male.

of 300 R each were given with a satisfactory cosmetic result (Fig. 10-30) and without subsequent recurrence.

Whenever possible, the tumor should be treated in a flat plane and the central beam should be perpendicular to the tumor. In the preceding case this could not be achieved due to the extent of the tumor. Similar problems prevail in the genital region. Some authors find irradiation of curved surfaces in this area particularly difficult. The next case will demonstrate that good results are entirely possible when imaginative techniques are used [15].

Case 15: 74-year-old female with a history of oophorectomy and radium treatment for cervical cancer. The skin changes of the external genitalia started 10 years ago and were treated as "eczema" of the vulva with various ointments. During the initial examination the skin showed verrucous changes extending from

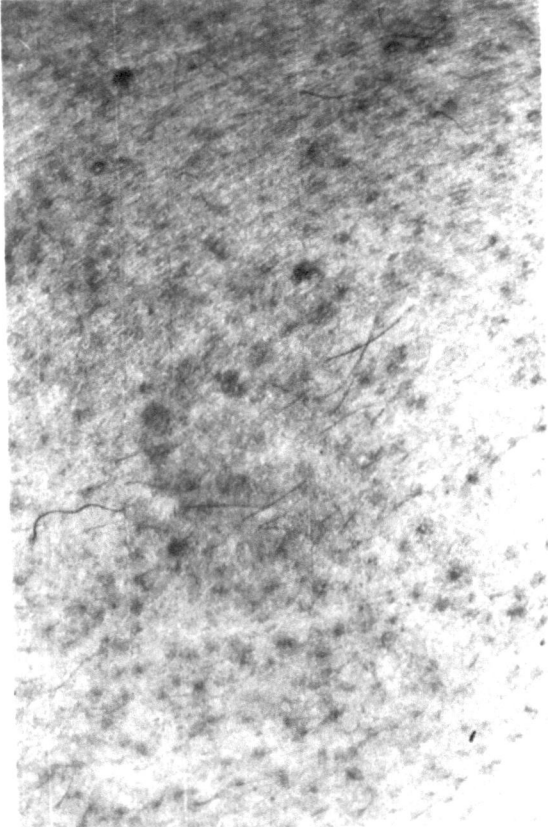

Figure 10-20.   Same patient as in Fig. 10-19 3 years following radiation therapy.

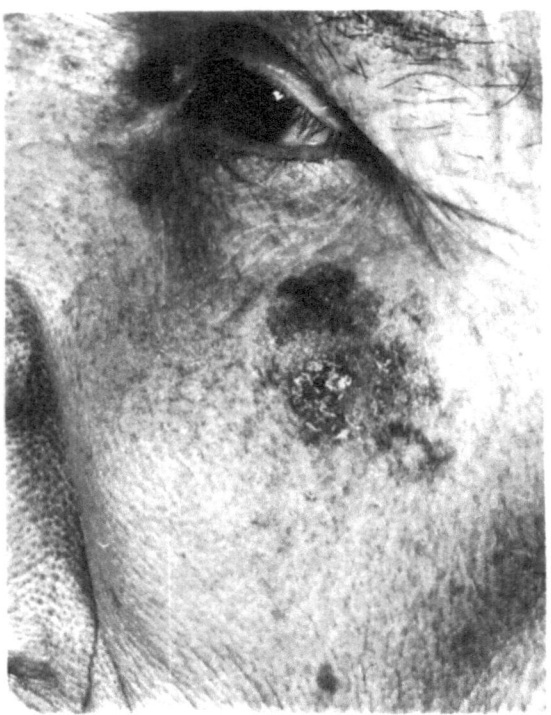

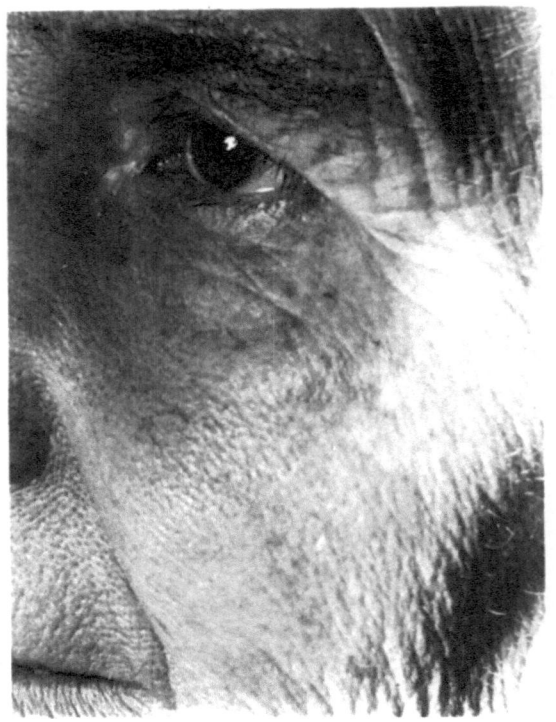

Figure 10-21.   Lentigo maligna on left cheek of 68-year-old female.

Figure 10-22.   Same patient as in Fig. 10-21 8 months following radiation therapy.

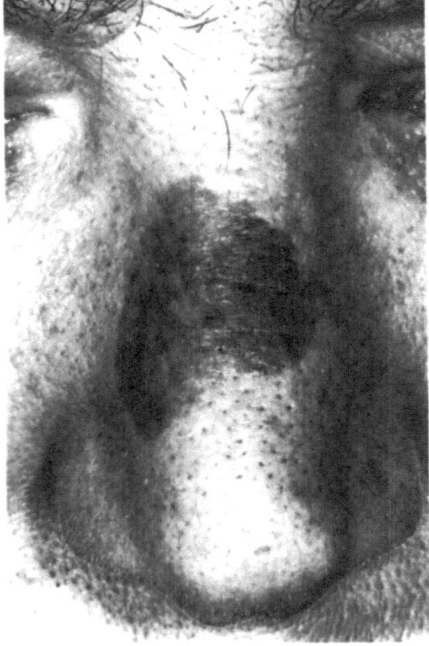

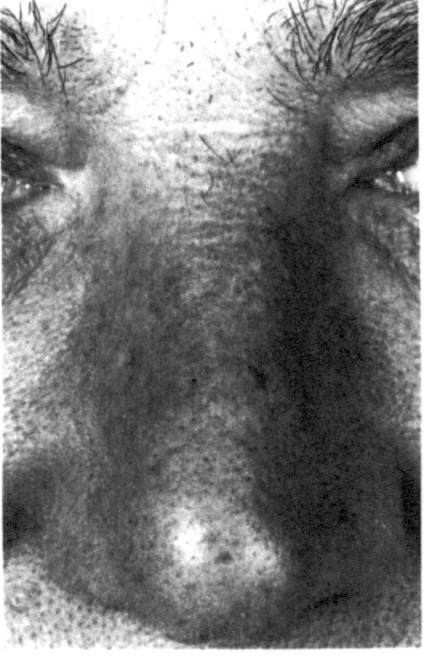

Figure 10-23.   Lentigo maligna over the dorsum of the nose in a 64-year-old female.

Figure 10-24.   Same patient as in Fig. 10-23 3.5 years following radiation therapy.

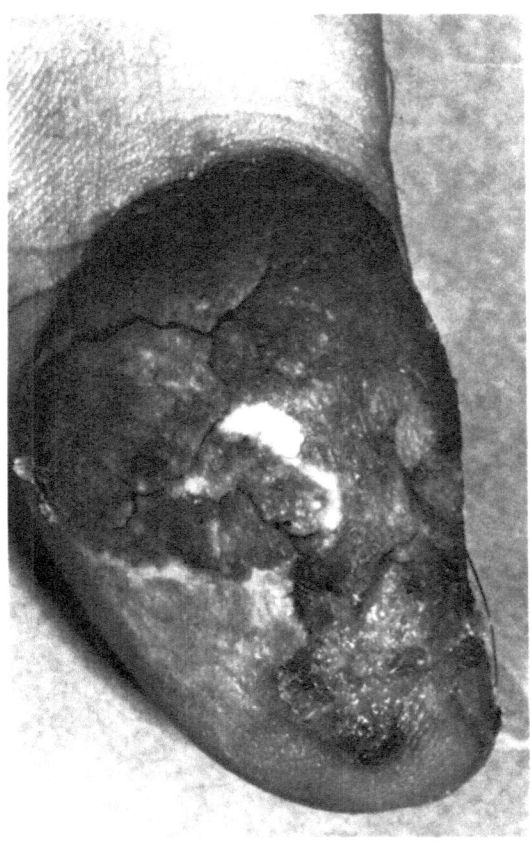

Figure 10-25. Bowen's disease on left thumb of 29-year-old male.

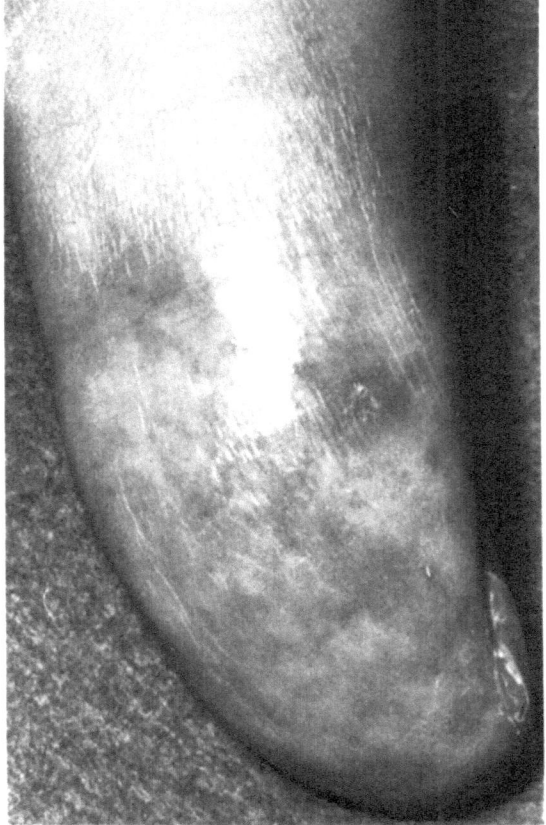

Figure 10-26. Same patient as in Fig. 10-25 2.5 months following radiation therapy.

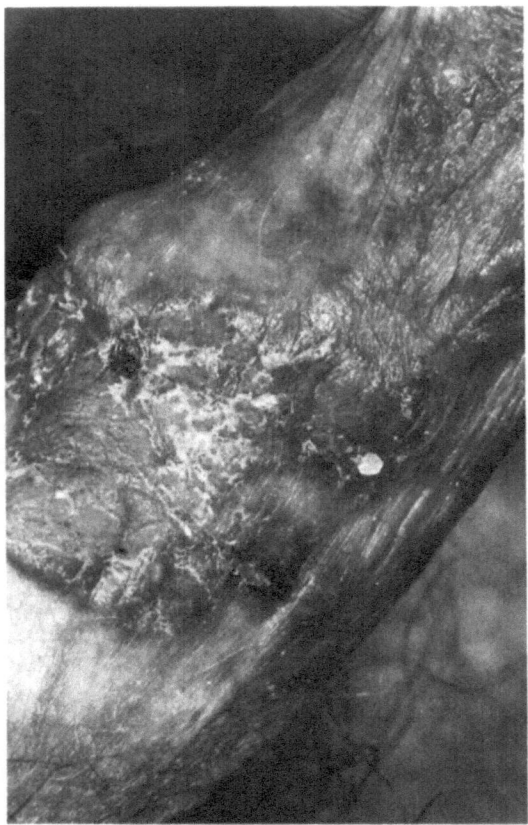

Figure 10-27.   Bowen's disease on shaft of penis in 57-year-old male.

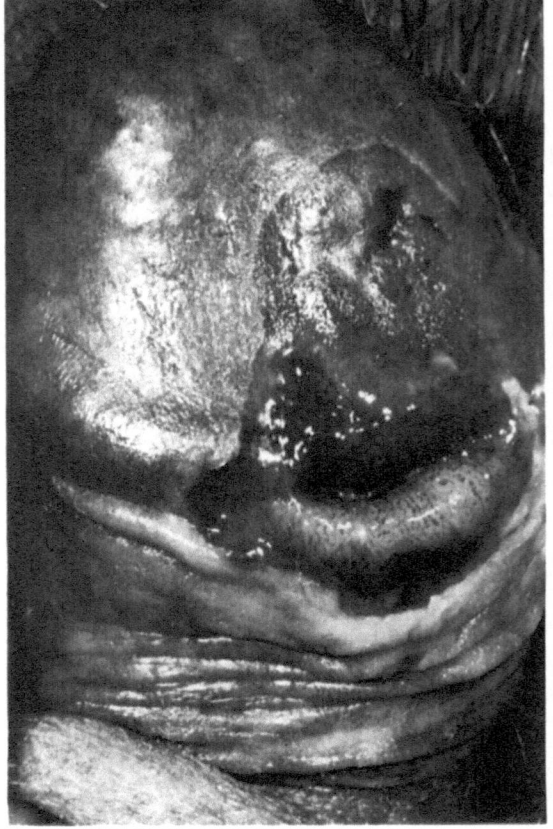

Figure 10-28.   Erythroplasia of Queyrat on glans penis of 64-year-old male.

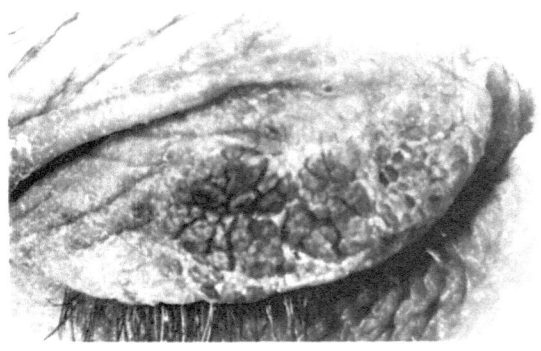

Figure 10-29. Bowen's disease on upper lid of 72-year-old female.

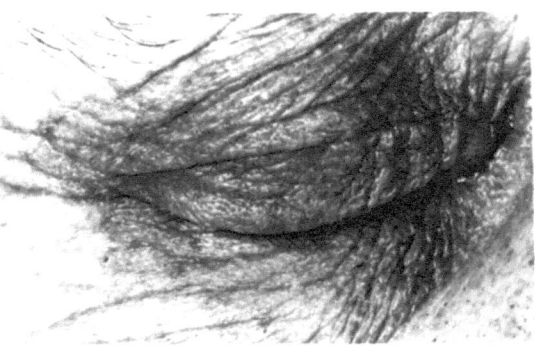

Figure 10-30. Same patient as in Fig. 10-29 7 months following radiation therapy.

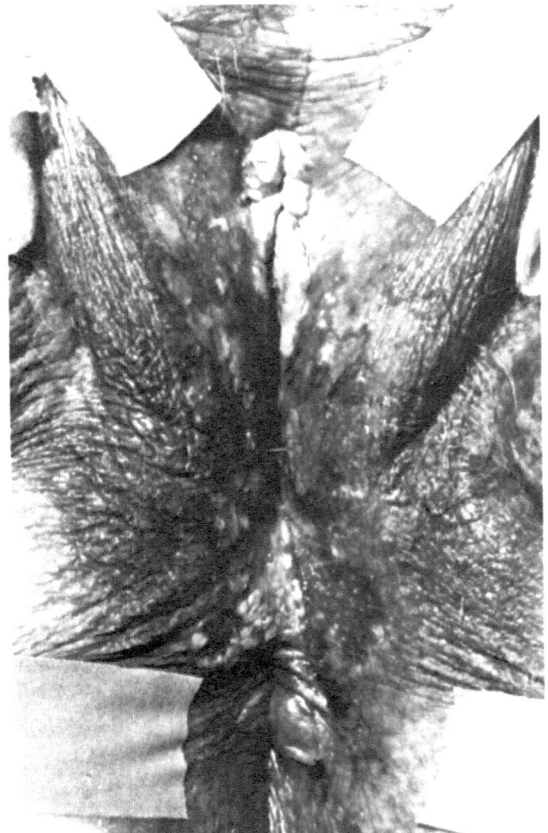

Figure 10-31. Bowen's disease of external genital area in 74-year-old female.

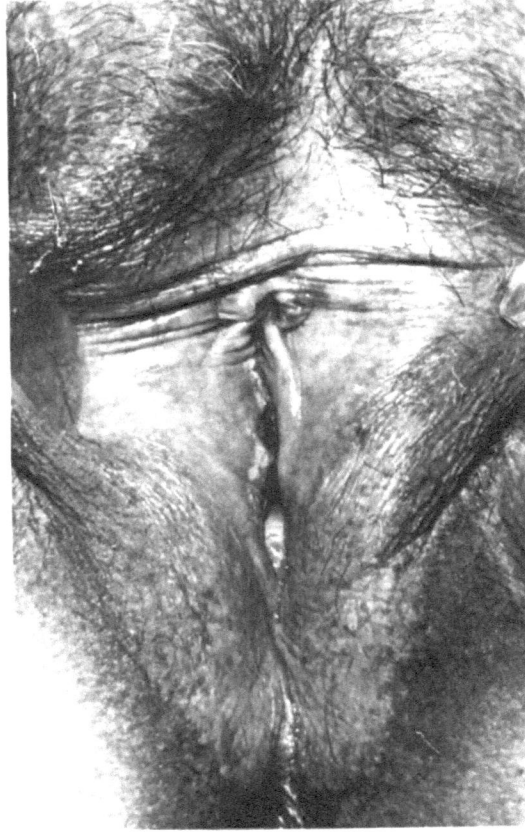

Figure 10-32. Residual lesion in introitus of vagina 5 months following first stage of radiation treatment.

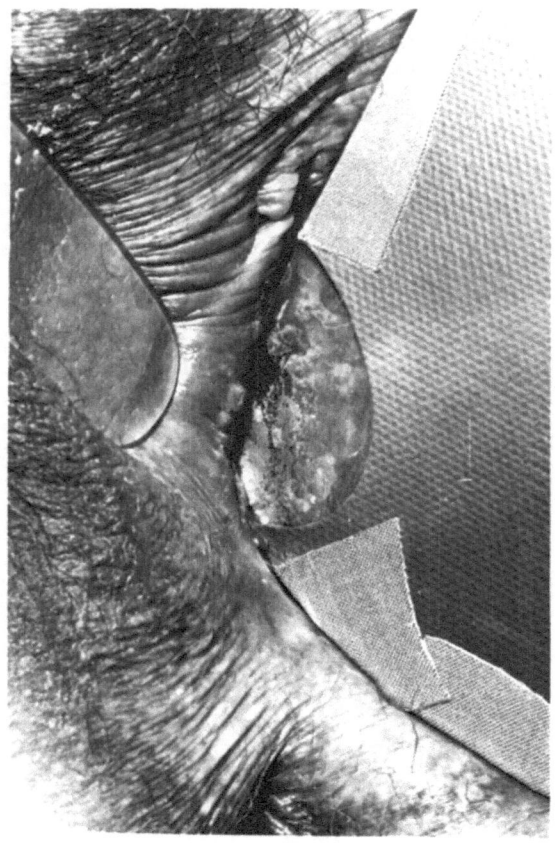

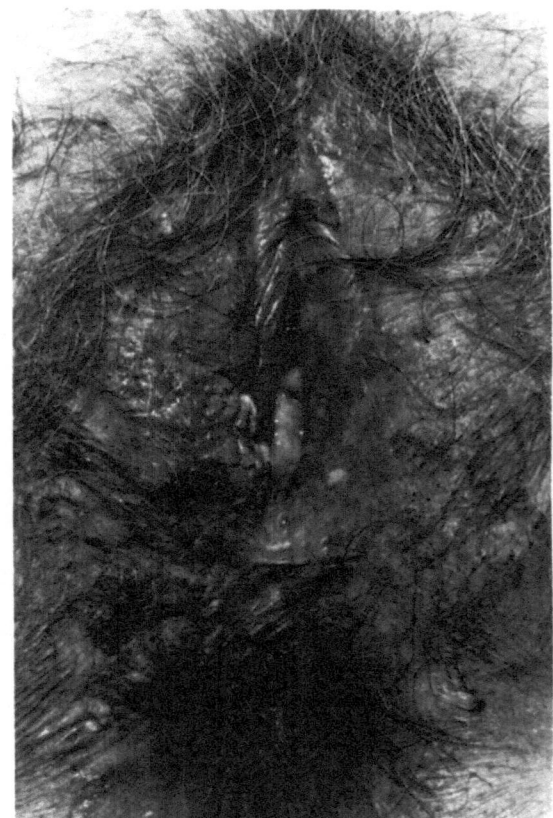

Figure 10-33. Plexiglass device with lead rubber shield positioned for second stage of treatment.

Figure 10-34. Bowen's disease of external genital area of 77-year-old female.

the clitoris and the urethral orifice to the external surface of both labia majora and the genito-crural fold, including even the perineal area and the anal ring (Fig. 10-31). The diagnosis of Bowen's disease was confirmed by microscopic examination.

The patient also showed evidence of a Candida infection which was eliminated prior to radiation therapy. Treatment was started in two stages with Dermopan step 2. In the first stage a field of approximately 55 cm² extending over the labia majora was demarcated with a piece of tape and treated in individual fractions of 250 R up to a total dose of 3250 R. Following the erosive reaction (acute radiodermatitis), the lesions healed 3 weeks later. A residual area on the left side of the introitus of the vagina could be visualized when the area was stretched (Fig. 10-32). We deliberately waited 5 months before we started the second stage of treatment. The

introitus of the vagina was again stretched with adhesive tape and two pieces of plexiglass (1-mm thickness), one each for the left and right side, were applied to the area. The previously treated and healed skin areas were shielded with lead rubber which was attached to the plexiglass. Figure 10-33 shows the positioning of the cone which also holds the plexiglass in place. With this special technique the area could be treated safely in daily fractions. Plexiglass absorbs approximately 25% of the incident radiation (exposure). The dose on the surface of the plexiglass resulting from 13 doses of 300 R is reduced to individual doses of 225 R (a total dose of 2925 R) at the surface of the tumor. The area cleared completely following treatment.

Case 16: 77-year-old female who noted a growth on the right labium of unknown duration (Fig. 10-34). Examination showed a polycyclic, partially erosive, verrucous lesion in the area of both labia majora, the clitoris, and the posterior commissure. Biopsy revealed the presence of Bowen's disease with carcinomatous degeneration. Treatment was started with Dermopan step 2. Again a plexiglass adaptor was used with an incident dose of 17 × 250 R (yielding a dose at the tumor surface of 17 × 187.5 R). Figure 10-35 shows the therapeutic results 2 months later.

Summary

Lentigo maligna presents a good indication for radiotherapy with ultrasoft x rays (grenz rays). In certain anatomic locations, and particularly in lesions of large size, radiation therapy can be considered the treatment of choice. Bowen's disease is also amenable to treatment with soft x rays. In contrast to lentigo maligna, slightly more penetrating x ray qualities are required (eg, Dermopan step 2: 29 kV; 0.3 mm Al filtration; HVL, 0.152 mm Al). Using special techniques (ie, flattening of convex or concave areas by compression with plexiglass), even inoperable lesions of Bowen's disease in the female genital region can be treated adequately. Our results indicate that radiation therapy with soft x rays can be used without hesitation in these special circumstances.

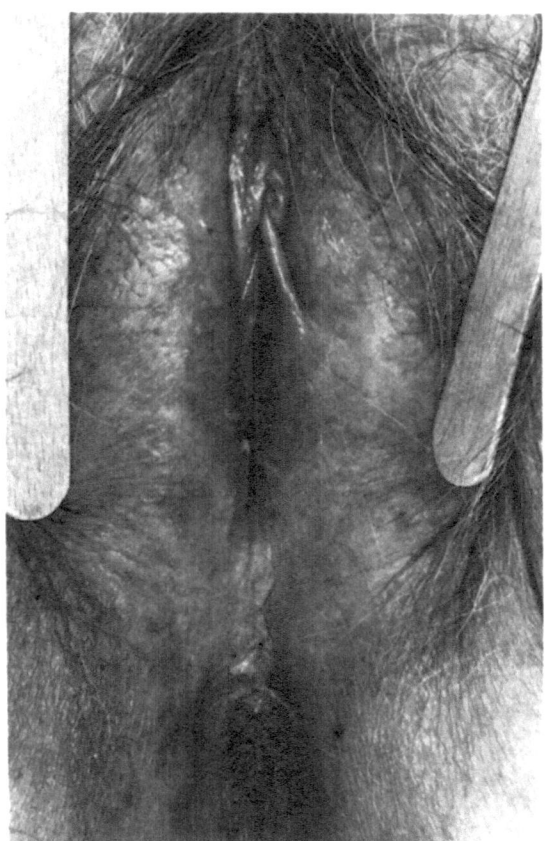

Figure 10-35. Same patient as in Fig. 10-34 2 months after radiation therapy.

References

1. Arma-Szlachcic M, Ott F, Storck, H: Zur Strahlentherapie der melanotischen Präcancerosen. Hautarzt 21:505, 1970
2. Braun-Falco O, Lukacs S, Schoefinius HH: Zur Behandlung der Melanosis circumscripta praecancerosa Dubreuilh. Hautarzt 26:207, 1975
3. Clark WH Jr: A classification of malignant melanoma in man correlated with histogenesis and biologic behaviour. Adv Biol Skin: 621, 1967
4. Clark WH Jr, Mihm MC Jr: Lentigo maligna and lentigo maligna melanoma. Am J Pathol 53:39, 1969.
5. Daeves K, Beckel A: Grosszahlmethodik und Häufigkeitsanalyse. II. Aufl. Weinheim, Verlag Chemie, 1958
6. Hauss H: Die Bedeutung des Geschlechts für die Entwicklung und die Prognose des Melanoms. Vortrag in Medizinische Gesellschaft Kiel, Sitzung vom 10. Mai 1973. Schleswig-Holsteinisches Ärzteblatt 26:594, 1973
7. Hauss H, Proppe A: Lokalisation und Geschlecht. Arch Dermatol Forsch 244:193, 1972
8. Kopf AW, Bart RS, Gladstein AH: Treatment of melanotic freckle with x rays. Arch Dermatol 112:801, 1976
9. Little JH: Histology and prognosis in cutaneous malignant melanoma in melanoma on skin cancer. In Proceedings of the International Cancer Conference. Sydney, 1972, pp 107–119
10. Markus B: Über den Begriff der Gewebeäquivalenz und einige "wasserähnliche" Phantomsubstanzen für Quanten von 10 KeV bis 100 MeV sowie schnelle Elektronen. Strahlentherapie 101:11, 1956
11. McGovern VJ: Melanoma. Growth patterns, multiplicity and regression in melanoma and skin cancer. In Proceedings of the International Cancer Conference. Sydney, 1972, pp 95–106
12. Miescher G: Über Klinik und Therapie der Melanome. Arch Dermatol Syph 200:215, 1955
13. Petratos MA, Kopf AW, Bart RS, et al: Treatment of melanotic freckle with x rays. Arch Dermatol 106:189, 1972

14. Proppe A: Spezielle Röntgenbehandlung. In Gottron H, Schönfeldt W (eds): Dermatologie und Venerologie. Bd. II. Stuttgart, Thieme-Verlag 1958, pp 26–132

15. Schirren JM: Zur Röntgentherapie des Morbus Bowen an der Vulva. Z Hautkr 45:297, 1970

16. Spier HW, Lucius K: Melanotische Präcancerose und Pseudo-Präcancerose. Zur Frage der Abgrenzbarkeit. Arch Dermatol Forsch 244:231, 1972

11

Electron Beam Therapy in Dermatology

John L. Fromer

Low megavoltage electron beam therapy has now been used for over 20 years to treat patients with various malignant and benign processes of the skin. Cooperating in this program have been the Department of High Voltage, Massachusetts Institute of Technology, and the Departments of Dermatology and Radiology of the Lahey Clinic. The modality was first used in August 1951 for a patient with widespread nodular mycosis fungoides who had been given considerable conventional x-ray therapy. To our knowledge, humans had never been exposed to regular courses of electrons for therapy. It was, therefore, most gratifying to find a modality which caused the suppression of previously intractable lesions when treated with conventional x rays.

The physical properties of monoenergetic and normally incident electrons with respect to the therapy of malignant and benign superficial cutaneous disorders have been described [1,3–6,8,10,12,13]. The electrons used in this study were obtained from a constant potential electrostatic generator of the Van de Graaff type, insulated in compressed gas. The electrons are collected and emerge into air from an evacuated accelerator tube through an aluminum window of 0.076-mm thickness, and are further scattered by an additional 0.38 mm of aluminum. The electrons emerge from the aluminum cone through a slit 45 cm in length and 1 cm in width. A recent modification eliminates the scattering foils and results in improved uniformity of the beam across the width of the slit. Masonite lines the lower and inner aspects of the distal part of the cone to reduce the roentgen ray emission. There is minimal γ radiation attendant to the electron beam treatment. Measurement of the electron dose is possible. Penetration of electrons is a function of the voltage applied at the source and calibrations are available for the range of electron energy from 1 to 4 MeV.

Treatments are given while the patient reclines on a motorized table that passes under the cone at a rate of 6 feet/min (Fig. 11-1). A patient may then receive total surface radiation using various port schemes depending on the extent and distribution of the lesions. Small fields may be conveniently treated with suitable shielding by low atomic number materials (e.g., 0.75-inch plywood). A suitable voltage is chosen depending on the relative infiltration of the lesions. This modality is particularly suitable for rapid large field treatment, since the radiation can be localized and the delivered entry dose to the desired depth is easily managed. With the treatment schedules used there is apparently no damage to underlying vital structures; patients have no evidence of radiation illness and may show transient minimal changes in the hemogram.

Another type of instrument in current use is the linear accelerator. While the Van de

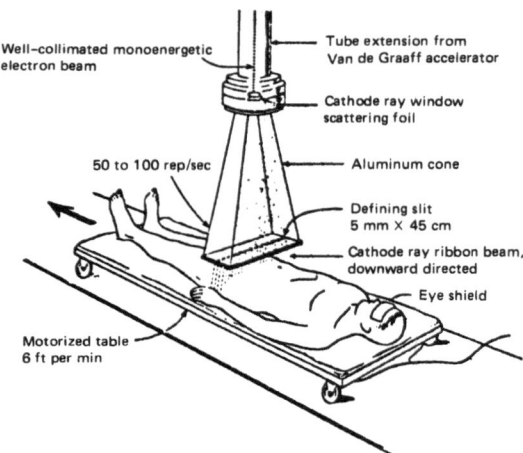

Well-collimated monoenergetic electron beam

Tube extension from Van de Graaff accelerator

Cathode ray window scattering foil

50 to 100 rep/sec

Aluminum cone

Defining slit 5 mm × 45 cm

Cathode ray ribbon beam, downward directed

Eye shield

Motorized table 6 ft per min

Figure 11-1.   Arrangement for treating extensive superficial dermatoses with high-energy cathode rays.

Graaff generator is a pressurized constant potential electrostatic machine, the linear accelerator incorporates a wave guide process. Electrons are injected and, using a wave guide principle, the electrons travel in a pulse fashion generating from 3 to 40 MeV. Usually a scanning device is used with the patient positioned at the side of the treatment room away from the emission source. Polystyrene (a tissue-equivalent absorber) is used to limit beam penetration in special instances, eg, in treatment of the scalp to avoid brain damage, in treatment of the chest wall to avoid lung damage, and in the management of ocular metastasis [2,9].

Methods and Materials

Our initial gross experience with electrons stemmed from the management of a patient with mycosis fungoides (malignant lymphoma) whose cutaneous condition with nodules and tumors was rapidly deteriorating. Suppression of lesions was achieved with a single course of treatment, and we extended our experience to other patients with malignant and benign disorders of the skin. Table 11-1 summarizes the cutaneous disorders treated. More than 500 patients with various malignant lymphomas have now been treated, the bulk of which have been mycosis fungoides. On initial examination in 1962, of 200 patients with mycosis fungoides, 40% were in the erythema and plaque stage, 40% were in the nodular tumor stage, and ap-

proximately 10% had advanced disease with ulceration and evidence of systemic involvement. The remaining 10% were in the early eczematous–erythematous stage and had never been given definitive treatment. There were relatively few contraindications to initiating electron beam therapy.

Treatment Results in Mycosis Fungoides

Patients with classical, biopsy-proven mycosis fungoides usually show generalized involvement and were either in stage 1, 2, or 3 when treatment was instituted. Various programs have been utilized. Most of the patients received 600 to 800 rads at 2 to 3 MeV over an 8- to 10-day period. As a rule, 200 rads to two opposing body surfaces were delivered. Various port schedules were used to avoid overlapping. The eyes and genital regions were shielded. The scalp was shielded if there were no lesions. Patients with known sensitivity to sunlight were given special consideration. Instead of concentrated courses, some patients were given fractional treatment over 2 to 3 months. This was especially useful in benign conditions such as atopic dermatitis. The high dose schedule of 2000 to 3000 rads is delivered in about 1 month. This schedule has been recently used in 15 patients with lymphoma. The penetration of electrons at 3.5 MeV (50% ionization at 1.3 cm depth) will control many infiltrative lesions. This can be supplemented with 2 MeV x-ray radiation for deeply infiltrative lesions using a dose of 400 to 1200 rads given in fractions.

Maximum improvement is noted 2 to 4 weeks after a course of irradiation. Since all therapy for lymphoma cutis is palliative, recurrences are to be expected. Some patients remain in remission for 6 to 12 months; the longest remission was 6 years following a single course. Retreatment for as long as 18 years has been possible in some patients with the production of minimal radiation changes in the skin. Alternating radiation with selective cytotoxic agents has been the most effective method of management to date. When lesions become resistant to electron irradiation, it is important to implement the standard chemotherapeutic methods used for treating Hodgkin's disease and other forms of lymphoma.

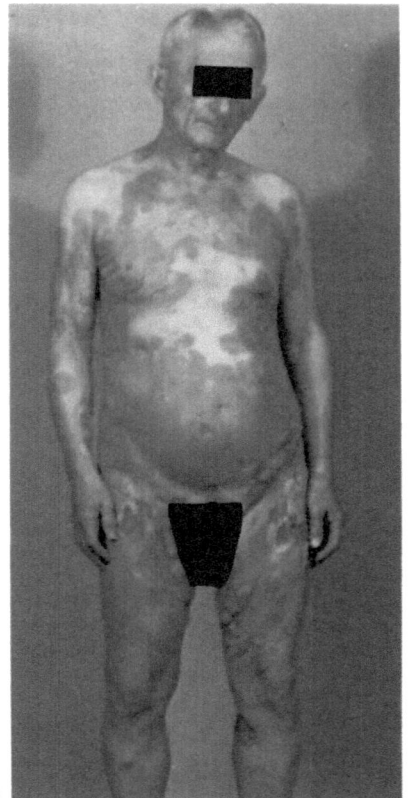
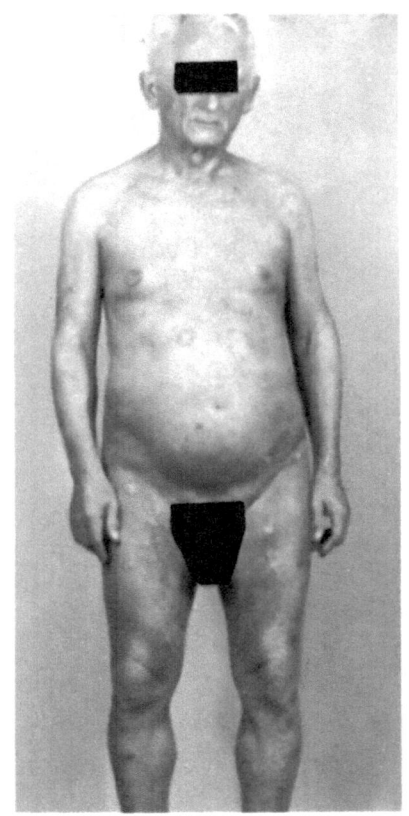

Figure 11-2. A 68 yr old white male in the advanced eczematous-plaque stage of mycosis fungoides, before (*a*) and after (*b*) treatment with electron beam.

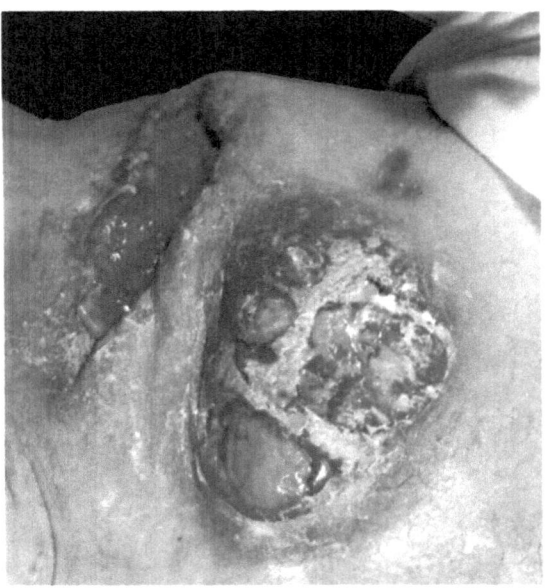
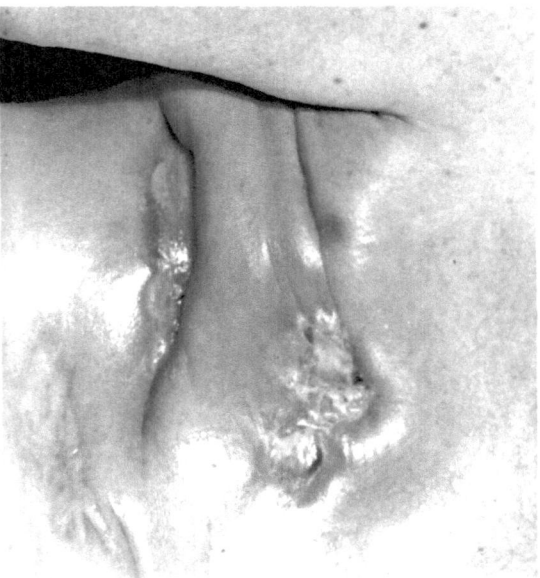

Figure 11-3. Lesions of advanced tumor ulcerative stage of mycosis fungoides. *a*. No previous treatment. *b*. Six weeks after electron beam therapy. The more infiltrative lesions received two million volt gamma radiation.

Table 11-1 *Treatment with Low Megavoltage Electrons 1951–1960*

		No. of Patients
Malignant Cutaneous Disease		400
Lymphoma cutis		271
Mycosis fungoides	220	
Lymphosarcoma	27	
Hodgkin's disease	13	
Lymphoma, not specified	5	
Reticulum cell sarcoma	3	
Leukemia	3	
Primary skin carcinoma		47
Basal cell	28	
Epidermoid	15	
Bowen's disease	4	
Skin metastases of breast carcinoma		28
Kaposi's disease		25
Miscellaneous		29
(Metastatic carcinoma from parotid, gingiva, tongue; melanosarcoma; hidradenocarcinoma; choriocarcinoma; Ewing's tumor; meningioma)		
Benign Cutaneous Disease		122
Generalized dermatoses		43
(Atopic, exfoliative, neurodermatitis; seborrheic psoriasis)		
Keloids		52
Miscellaneous		27
(Fox–Fordyce disease, furunculosis, granulomas, histiocytosis X, Hansen's disease, neurofibroma, neurogenic anhidrosis, papilloma, pemphigus, poikiloderma, undiagnosed, verruca vulgaris)		
	Total	522

From Smedal et al [10].

Figures 11.2 and 11.3 are before and after electron beam treatment pictures of two patients in two different stages of mycosis fungoides.

Treatment Results in Other Malignant Diseases

Lymphomas other than mycosis fungoides with cutaneous manifestations have been treated with total surface, low megavoltage electrons. These include reticulum cell lymphoma, Hodgkin's disease, leukemia, and lymphosarcoma. The itching and discomfort of cutaneous lesions in lymphoma may be as annoying and troublesome to the patient as is the primary visceral process. Regardless of the stage of lymphoma, the cutaneous lesions are radiosensitive and most patients achieved good to excellent suppression of cutaneous lesions and subjective itching. A total dose of 800 to 1200 rads is delivered in 8 to 10 days.

Kaposi's Sarcoma

Over a 20-year period we have treated more than 50 patients with Kaposi's idiopathic hemorrhagic sarcoma. Most of these patients had had irradiation with conventional techniques elsewhere and the response to electron therapy was similar to the response of patients with mycosis fungoides. Suppression of widespread cutaneous lesions can be expected. Infiltrative lesions, however, must be treated with other techniques and 2 MeV x-ray radiation was effective in these patients. In general, Kaposi's idiopathic hemorrhagic sarcoma has a more benign course than does mycosis fungoides and visceral involvement appears late in the disease. The disease may occur simultaneously with other lymphomas, and it is of interest that the same amount of electron irradiation will suppress lesions of exfoliative erythroderma (lymphoma) as well as papules and nodules of Kaposi's sarcoma in the same patient. Dosage schedules and remission rates are comparable to treatment for mycosis fungoides.

Cutaneous Implants of Breast Carcinoma

In spite of surgery, hormonal treatment, chemotherapy, and/or radiation, skin metastasis from breast carcinoma may occur. Isolated nodules may be treated with conventional superficial radiation. However, when the distribution of superficial nodules is scattered, large fields may then be easily treated with electrons. Regression of lesions in 50% of patients persisted for 6 months or longer. Dose range delivered fractionally was similar to that used in conventional x-ray therapy.

A number of patients with basal cell carcinoma, epidermoid carcinoma, and Bowen's disease were treated with protracted exposure to electrons. Shielding techniques are easily applied. Follow-up studies showed results comparable to those with conventional x-ray therapy.

Tapley and Fletcher [11] treated 156 patients with squamous and basal cell carcinomas of the skin and lips using electron beam sources. Most patients (86%) received primary control of lesions and were followed for 2 to 8.5 years. Additional salvage to 95% was achieved with follow-up surgical treatment.

Benign Disease

Various erythrodermas involving total surface areas were treated. This group included primary and secondary exfoliative dermatitis, atopic dermatitis, psoriatic erythroderma, and some universal erythrodermas that defied classification. All patients in this group had been previously treated unsuccessfully using conventional topical modalities. Intolerable pruritus was the main problem. Some patients were treated with schedules similar to those used in mycosis fungoides, while others received small daily or weekly protracted doses. A favorable response was obtained in 50% of patients. Some patients may have been photosensitive and intolerable itching and burning occurred while under treatment. It was of special interest that psoriasis and psoriatic erythroderma usu-

ally showed a good initial response but recurred within a month following termination of treatment.

Keloids

Doses of 1000 to 2000 rads were given to a number of patients in whom keloids had been excised. Good cosmetic results were seen in 75% of patients. Some symptomatic improvement was seen in about 50% of patients in whom keloids were not excised.

Miscellaneous Dermatoses

Temporary or permanent suppression of lesions occurred in a number of benign dermatoses including histiocytosis X, tuberculoid leprosy, granuloma annulare, pemphigus foliaceus, and pityriasis rubra pilaris.

Summary

Our primary interest with electron beam therapy has been directed toward management of mycosis fungoides. In general the total dose delivered in 8 to 10 days has been on the order of 800 to 1200 rads to the total skin surface. Fuks and Bagshaw [7] reported a group of 107 mycosis fungoides patients treated by total skin irradiation with 2.5-MeV electrons. Eight patients were free of disease 3 to 11 years after a single course of electron beam radiation. Dosage for some patients was increased to 3000 rads delivered in 40 days. An analysis of the results suggests that early treatment, before the occurrence of plaques or tumors, may result in prolonged suppression of disease. This has occurred in 2 of our 500 patients with a single course of electron therapy in the conventional range mentioned above. Our experience with the higher dose in 15 patients (some in the nodule and plaque stage) showed no better suppression of disease or improvement in recurrence rate than with the more conservative dose schedules.

Our 20-year experience with this modality indicates that it is an ideal radiation procedure for the management of radiosensitive cutaneous lesions over large surface areas. The electron dose can be applied readily and conveniently to large surface areas, and the electron penetration can be adjusted to the infiltration of the lesions with resultant sparing of underlying normal structures. In this way, adverse side effects are avoided and, especially in malignant disease, retreatment has been possible without major side effects over many years.

References

1. Campbell FW, Fromer JL: Surg Clin North Am 39:585, 1959
2. Chu F, Nisce L, Baker AS, et al: Radiology 89:216, 1967
3. Cyr DP: Rev belgePathol 24:296, 1955
4. Fromer JL, Johnston DO, Salzman FA, et al: South Med J 54:769, 1961
5. Fromer JL, Smedal MI, Salzman FA, et al: Proceedings of the XII International Congress of Dermatology, 1962, pp 643–650
6. Fromer JL, Smedal MI, Trump JG, et al: Arch Dermatol 71:391, 1955
7. Fuks Z, Bagshaw MA: Radiology 100:145, 1971
8. Johnston DO, Smedal MI, Wright KA, et al: Surg Clin North Am 39:579, 1959
9. Keith A: Clin Bull 1(3):111, 1971
10. Smedal MI, Johnston DO, Salzman FA, et al: Am J Roentgenol 88:215, 1962
11. Tapley NduV, Fletcher GH: Radiology :423, 1973
12. Trump JG, Wright KA, Evans WW, et al: Am J Roentgenol 69:623, 1953
13. Wright KA, Granke RC, Trump JG: Radiology 67:553, 1956

12

Teleroentgen Therapy of Mycosis Fungoides and Benign Dermatoses

Stefan Lukacs and Herbert Goldschmidt

The term teleroentgen therapy denotes treatment with x rays at long target–skin distances (as required for effective treatment of the entire body surface in one exposure). Teleroentgen therapy has been used for cutaneous lymphomas and also for generalized benign dermatoses.

Modern advances in other fields of therapy have limited the use of ionizing radiation in skin diseases. Among the few widely accepted and unchallenged indications is the presence of mycosis fungoides and other malignant lymphomas. New developments in systemic and topical chemotherapy [16,17] have added promising new therapeutic approaches but have not made radiotherapy obsolete. Mycosis fungoides is a highly radiosensitive skin disorder and it responds to relatively small doses of ionizing radiation [15]. Limited small plaques or isolated tumors usually disappear after a course of 3 to 4 weekly doses of 100 to 200 R. These courses can be repeated safely several times, even beyond the maximum cumulative dose of 1000 R per lifetime and area. In many cases, however, the lesions are not limited to small areas and involve large regions of the body surface.

Until 20 years ago patients with generalized eruptions could not be treated satisfactorily because the available radiation modalities were not useful for large body surfaces. Penetrating x-ray qualities could not be adminis-

tered to large body areas because of the resulting systemic effects (radiation syndrome); very soft x rays (grenz rays) had the disadvantage of limited field sizes. This was partially overcome with multiple exposure techniques that required very long total treatment times and often resulted in overlapping exposures. These problems were largely solved when Schirren [10,12] described his technique of teleroentgen therapy with soft x rays 20 years ago. Similar dermatologic techniques for the treatment of large body surfaces with soft x rays at different target–skin distances were described by Wiskemann [19], Proppe [8,9], and Wagner [18]. Since Schirren's initial report his teleroentgen technique has been used successfully in many dermatologic centers [7]. The purpose of this chapter is to review its indications, modifications, and limitations and to present our results in 26 patients with mycosis fungoides. Electron beam treatment of mycosis fungoides is discussed in Chapter 11 (see also 3, 4, 5).

History

Penetrating x rays were used in the treatment of widespread extensive cutaneous manifestations of lymphomas as early as 1931. Beneficial results in the treatment of leukemia (using radiations with a 3 to 4 mm Al HVL) encouraged Teschendorf [14] to employ similar x-ray qualities in the treatment of mycosis fungoides using a form of "roentgen bath." These penetrating radiations affect the hematopoietic system (in leukemia a desirable effect, as evidenced by the modern use of total body cobalt radiation). Even with small individual doses of 5 to 15 R at 3- to 10-day intervals up to a total dose of 50 R, severe leukopenia and other hematologic side effects were unavoidable.

Superficial x-ray machines with a HVL of 1 to 2 mm Al were also used. Since total body irradiation in one exposure was not possible for technical reasons, the total body had to be divided into 8 to 12 different areas which were treated individually with proper shielding of the remainder of the body. Treatment with grenz-ray machines was equally time-consuming for the same reason and often less satisfactory because of the limited penetration of ultrasoft x rays. Daily treatment times could last as long as 1 hour per patient when multiple overlapping fields were used.

The introduction of beryllium-window machines eliminated many of these disadvantages. Due to the enormous output of these units total body treatments with relatively soft x rays were now possible at longer target–skin distances. Schirren was the first to suggest total body irradiation at a distance of 2 m. He also emphasized the relative safety of this superficial form of radiation which does not affect the hematopoietic system due to its limited penetration.

Methods

Total Body Irradiation

Beryllium-window Units at 25 mA and 50 kV

The original method described by Schirren utilized beryllium-window machines with high milliamperage (25 mA) at 50 kV (Siemens Dermopan units). Under these conditions 50 R can be delivered in 6 min to the entire frontal or dorsal body surface at a TSD of 2 m; even the periphery of the body (scalp and feet) receive no less than 70% of the dose at the center of the body (Fig. 12-1). Accurate direction of the beam can be secured with the aid of a light pointer inserted into the window opening. The central beam should be directed to the area between symphysis pubis and umbilicus. At a 2 m TSD the HVL of this radiation is 0.1 mm Al and the $D_{1/2}$ is 1 to 2 mm of skin. This penetration is ideally suited to treatment of stage 1 and 2 lesions of mycosis fungoides. Figure 12-2 compares percentage depth doses achieved with the teleroentgen technique with the $D_{1/2}$ of grenz rays, conventional superficial x rays, and total body electron beam treatment.

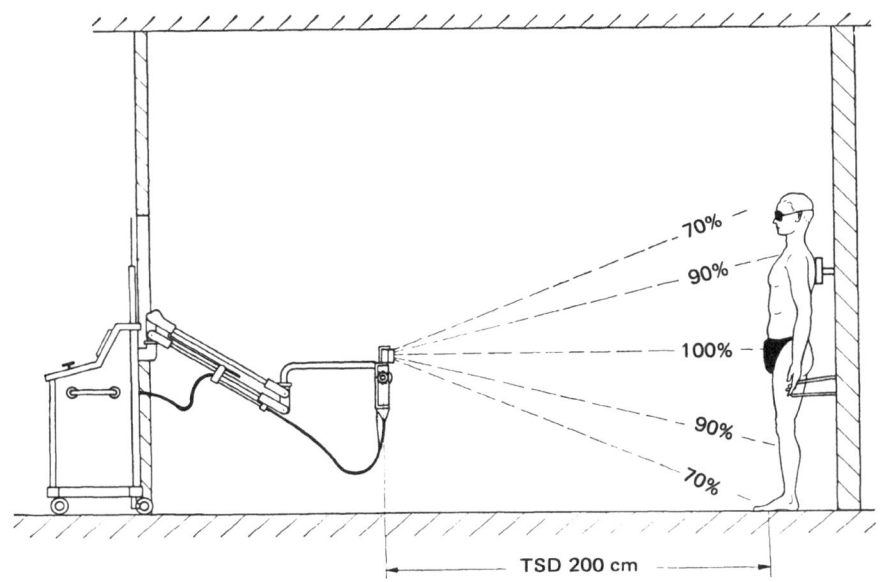

Figure 12-1. Positioning and shielding of patient for teleroentgen therapy.

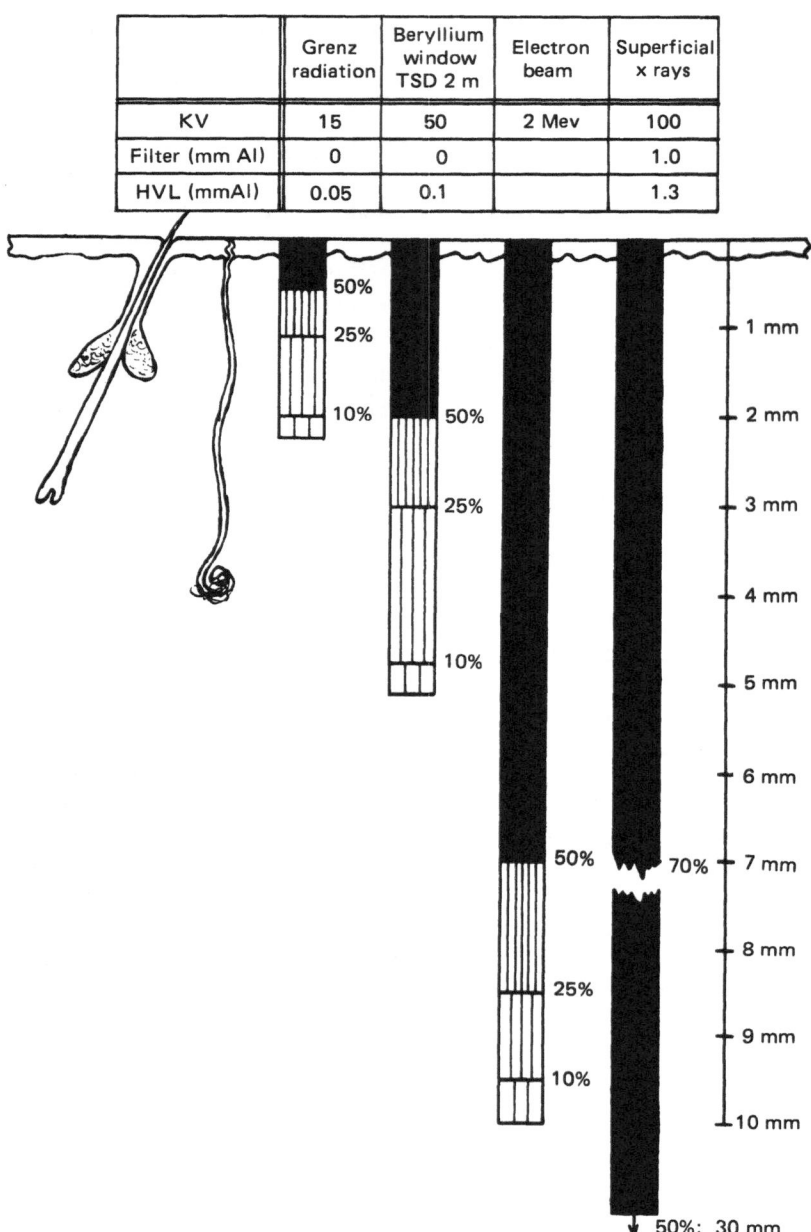

	Grenz radiation	Beryllium window TSD 2 m	Electron beam	Superficial x rays
KV	15	50	2 Mev	100
Filter (mm Al)	0	0		1.0
HVL (mmAl)	0.05	0.1		1.3

Figure 12-2. Comparison of percentage depth doses for different radiation modalities used in the treatment of widespread mycosis fungoides.

Beryllium-window Units at 5 mA and 100 kV

Some beryllium-window machines cannot be operated at a milliamperage higher than 5 mA (eg, GE Maximar 100). At 50 kV, exposure times would be too lengthy. At the University of Pennsylvania Hospital we have calibrated our 5 mA machine at 100 kV; this allows 50 R to be delivered in only 15 min. The slightly increased penetration ($D_{1/2}$, 2 to 2.5 mm) due to the increased kV is of no practical consequence. Unfiltered radiation from a beryllium-window source is relatively independent of changes in kV due to its higher percentage of characteristic radiation (in contrast to bremsstrahlung).

Half- or Quarter-body Irradiation

Beryllium-window Units at shorter TSDs with Overlapping Fields

The soft radiation qualities of beryllium-window machines can also be utilized at shorter target–skin distances. Wiskemann [19] recommended a TSD of 120 cm. Wagner [18] and Proppe [9,10] used TSDs of 90 cm. The resulting radiation qualities are slightly less penetrating (because of the reduced absorption of longer wavelengths in air compared to a 2 m TSD); the $D_{1/2}$ is approximately 1.4 mm. At a 90 cm TSD, 8 different exposures are necessary to treat the entire skin surface. The treated areas are deliberately overlapping; adjacent areas are not shielded. The authors used higher individual doses (300 to 400 R once or 3 to 4 times) at 50 kV, 25 mA, without added filtration.

Treatment of Large Areas at 80 cm TSD (without overlapping)

The main advantage of teleroentgen therapy at 2 m lies in the fact that the entire anterior or posterior surface of the body can be treated in one sitting. When the TSD is decreased several treatments become necessary, resulting in prolonged treatment times, particularly since meticulous shielding of the other areas is usually necessary to avoid overdosage resulting from overlapping treatment areas. Some radiotherapists use glass-window or beryllium-window x-ray machines at a distance of 80 cm and divide the length of the body into three equal fields (80 cm); therefore 6 different treatments are necessary in order to irradiate the entire body (3 anterior and 3 posterior). One of the advantages of this method is that the patient can be treated in a horizontal position.

Glass-window Machines at 130 cm

Because of their high output and limited penetration beryllium-window machines are clearly quite advantageous for teleroentgen therapy. However, in some cases glass-window (Pyrex) machines can also be adapted for treatment of large body areas. Domonkos [1] has reported favorable responses with a technique utilizing 60 kV and 20 mA at a target–skin distance of 130 cm. The resulting HVL of 0.8 mm Al is significantly more penetrating than that of the techniques described above.

Dosage

Both the anterior and posterior surfaces of the body are treated in 1 day. In obese patients, additional treatments can be given to the lateral body surfaces. Schirren [10] originally recommended daily doses of 100 R 5 times per week up to a total of 1000 to 1500 R. His dosage schedule for benign generalized dermatoses (50 R 3 times per week up to a total of 500 R) was adapted by the New York Skin and Cancer Unit for the treatment of mycosis fungoides [7]. These authors felt that higher total doses per course of treatment are required only in exceptional cases and that less frequent treatments and lower doses give equally satisfactory results.

Since the limited penetration of soft x rays has no harmful systemic effects (particularly not on the hematopoietic system), a course of radiation can be repeated in case of a recurrence that is severe enough to warrant radiation therapy. In the majority of patients this will not be necessary until 3 to 6 months following initial therapy. Since mycosis fungoides cannot be considered a benign disease, the total dose limits per lifetime recommended for benign dermatoses (ie, a maximum dose of 1000 R) do not apply. In some of our patients a course of 500 to 1000 R was repeated 2 to 3 times up to a total dose of 2000 R within a period of 3 years without any noticeable changes in the hematopoietic system and without cutaneous sequelae. Doses over 2000 R should be administered with caution since chronic radiodermatitis must be expected at a later time. Schirren (13) noticed marked telangiectasia and atrophy in 3 unusual cases with otherwise intractable mycosis fungoides and severe pruritus that were treated with several courses of teleroentgen therapy up to a total of 6000 to 8000 R over a period of 8 years. Even though the skin showed signs of chronic radiodermatitis, no hematologic or other systemic changes could be noted. As expected from the treatment of individual lesions of mycosis fungoides, the response of recurrent generalized mycosis fungoides is less satisfactory and recurrences occur more rapidly after the first 2 to 3 courses of teleroentgen therapy.

Radiation Protection

Even though very soft x rays (only slightly more penetrating than grenz rays) are used, certain radiation protection measures are necessary. Shielding of the eyes is mandatory. In younger patients gonad protection (abdominal and sacral lead shields for women: lead bags around the scrotum for men) and thyroid shielding is advisable (Fig. 12-1). Even though the operator is protected behind the instrument panel and its lead glass shield, installation of the instrument panel outside the treatment room is preferable.

Indications

At present, teleroentgen therapy of mycosis fungoides is limited to severe and generalized cases which have not responded to other forms of therapy or when other therapeutic modalities are not advisable. In our more recent cases, topical treatment with nitrogen mustard [16,17] was always the first therapeutic choice and x rays were used only in resistant cases with severe pruritus or in progressively worsening cases. Because of its lack of side effects, teleroentgen therapy is particularly useful in patients who have experienced side effects from systemic chemotherapy or in patients sensitive to nitrogen mustard. Teleroentgen therapy can be given in the office of any dermatologist whose office is equipped with a beryllium-window machine operating at 50 to 100 kV [6].

Best therapeutic results can be attained during the premycotic, eczematous, and plaque stages (Figs. 12-3 and 12-4). Response to treatment is delayed in many patients. Two weeks after the last treatment marked improvement can be noted; complete disappearance of visible skin lesions may require up to 8 weeks. Due to the limited penetration of the radiation, response in the tumor stage is less satisfactory,

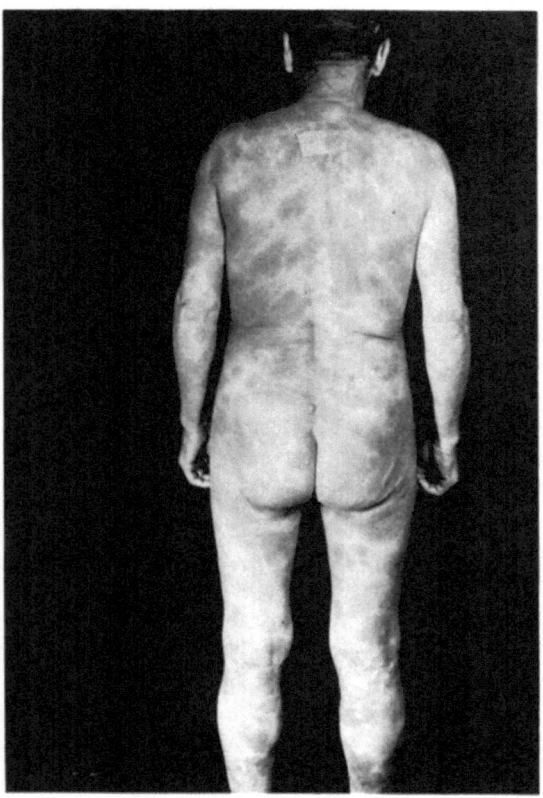

Figure 12-3. Widespread mycosis fungoides before teleroentgen therapy.

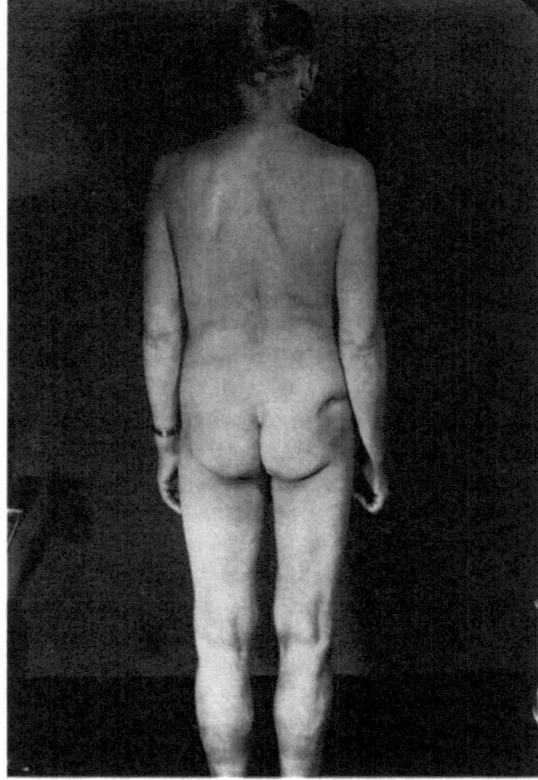

Figure 12-4. Same patient as in Fig. 12-3 4 weeks after a course of 1200 R.

particularly when markedly elevated tumors are present. In the presence of large tumors total body electron beam therapy yields better results because of its deeper penetration [3–5,15]. Residual tumors following teleroentgen therapy can be treated with additional superficial x-ray therapy to the individual lesions until disappearance occurs. In most instances these tumors are highly radiosensitive and require only small doses (200 to 300 R once or twice a week up to 1000 R; the $D_{1/2}$ of the radiation should match the estimated depth of the tumor).

Side Effects

Asymptomatic temporary erythema usually disappears shortly after treatment. Hyperpigmentation of the treated area is a common side effect of teleroentgen therapy; it usually subsides after several months. Numerous laboratory investigations in patients and animals have failed to demonstrate any negative effect on hematopoietic or other organ systems. Radiation syndrome–like changes have never been observed and are not expected due to the very superficial penetration of soft x rays. For the same reason, however, indications for teleroentgen therapy should be limited to patients with cutaneous mycosis fungoides. Except for palliative treatment of severe pruritus or severely disfiguring lesions other forms of treatment are preferred in the presence of systemic lesions of mycosis fungoides.

Summary of Therapeutic Results in 26 Patients

This retrospective study was carried out at the Department of Dermatology of the University of Munich, where Schirren developed his teleroentgen technique as head of the section of dermatologic radiotherapy. Even though a larger number of patients were treated with this modality, our records permitted detailed analyses of 196 patients treated between 1959 and 1972 with teleroentgen therapy. Twenty-six of these patients had generalized mycosis fungoides.

Patients presented with different stages of mycosis fungoides. The diagnosis was confirmed by microscopic examination in all patients. Age and sex distributions are given in

Table 12-1 *Age and Sex Distribution of 26 Patients with Mycosis Fungoides*

Age	Male	Female	Total
20–29	—	1	1
30–39	1	1	2
40–49	—	2	2
50–59	3	4	7
60–69	5	4	9
70–79	2	2	4
80–89	—	1	1
Total	11	15	26

Table 12-1. The course of these patients is summarized in Table 12-2. Ten patients were followed for several courses of treatment but were eventually lost to follow-up. The technical conditions of treatment are listed in Table 12-3. In most patients individual doses of 80 to 100 R were administered daily, 5 times per week, to both the anterior and posterior body surfaces. The total dose per course of treatment varied from 700 to 2000 R. Some patients received several courses of treatment. The highest cumulative total doses in 4 patients were 9200, 4500 (2 patients), and 3400 R. In the majority of patients teleroentgen therapy was the only form of treatment; in some patients other forms of therapy were administered in recurrent cases but rarely concomitantly with radiotherapy.

Results

Response to Treatment
Therapeutic results are summarized in Table 12-4. Of 26 patients, 81% showed marked improvement, and 19% showed only slight or no improvement.

Duration of Remission
The mean interval between termination of therapy and the appearance of new lesions was 7.3 months (evaluation of 41 courses of therapy in 24 patients). The median duration of remission was 6 months.

Table 12-2 *Course of Disease in 26 Patients*

	Male	Female	Total
Died of mycosis fungoides	5	7	12
Died of other causes	—	1	1
Lost to follow-up	6	4	10
Surviving	—	3	3

Table 12-3 *Teleroentgen Therapy with Soft X Rays: Technical Data*

Quality	Beryllium tube
	50 kV (Siemens Dermopan) *or*
	100 kV (GE Maximar 100)
	No added filter
TSD	2 m
HVL	0.1 mm Al
$D_{1/2}$	2 mm tissue
Dose Rate	20 R/min (Siemens Dermopan)
	(25 mA; 50 kV)
	10 R/min (GE Maximar 100)
	(5 mA; 100 kV)

Survival Rate After Biopsy Diagnosis

The survival time was calculated from the availabe data of 24 patients for the first 6 years following biopsy diagnosis. The percentage data are presented in Table 12-5. Twelve patients died during the observation period, 11 as a direct consequence of mycosis fungoides. The average time until death following biopsy diagnosis in these patients was 3.02 years.

Survival Time After Onset of Skin Lesions

The average survival time after onset of cutaneous lesions (in contrast to survival rate after biopsy diagnosis) was 16 years for men and 10 years for women.

Discussion

Mycosis fungoides is one of the most serious diseases seen by the dermatologist. The National Cancer Institute [2] estimates that there are 2000 new cases of mycosis fungoides each year and that over 70 patients in the United States die of this lymphoma every year. Fortunately, several new and promising therapeutic modalities are now available to combat this awesome disease. To date, however, all treatment methods have only palliative value.

In their large study involving 144 patients with mycosis fungoides seen at the National Cancer Institute, Epstein et al [2] were unable to demonstrate that any treatment method had

significantly prolonged life. These authors also stressed the importance of using survival after biopsy as a more useful parameter than survival after onset of cutaneous lesions.

Our results are based on similar criteria and parallel those found in the large NIH study. The mean survival time of our group of patients was 3.02 years; in the NIH group 50% of all patients had died of mycosis fungoides after 3.5 years. It should be emphasized in this context that all patients in our series had severe involvement with widespread lesions requiring total body irradiation.

The mean duration of remission following each course of therapy was 7.3 months. The median duration of remission was 6 months. This palliative effect is at least similar to that of other treatment modalities. For total body electron beam therapy the duration of remission is given as ranging from 2 to 6 months or longer; precise statistical data for other modalities are not available. Since the therapeutic effect of teleroentgen therapy is similar to that of other treatment methods it can be used in any patient where other forms of treatment are not indicated, not available, or too risky. The advantages of teleroentgen therapy include its complete lack of systemic effects, its easy availability in any department or office equipped with a beryllium-window x-ray unit, and the relatively prompt response to treatment. Its disadvantages include the potential development of chronic radiodermatitis after frequent courses of treatment, and shorter remissions following repeated courses of therapy (this also applies to other forms of therapy). Teleroentgen therapy is most suitable for the premycotic, infiltrative, and plaque stage of mycosis fungoides, and is less effective in the tumor stage because of the limited penetration of soft x rays.

Teleroentgen Therapy for Generalized Benign Dermatoses

Indications

The main indication for teleroentgen therapy with soft x rays is mycosis fungoides. In some cases, however, it is also considered a valuable adjunct in the treatment of generalized benign dermatoses. Table 12-6 lists diagnoses of 196

Table 12-4 *Response to Teleroentgen Therapy in 26 Patients*

	Male	Female	Total (%)
Marked improvement	8	13	21 (81)
Slight or no improvement	3	2	5 (19)

Table 12-5 *Survival Rates of 24 Patients for First 6 Years Following Biopsy Diagnosis*

No. of Years	Number of Patients Surviving (%)
1	23 (95.8)
2	19 (79.2)
3	17 (70.8)
4	15 (62.5)
5	13 (54.2)
6	12 (50)

patients that were treated with teleroentgen therapy between 1954 and 1972 at the Department of Dermatology of the University of Munich. In addition to mycosis fungoides and other cutaneous lymphomas, the most important current indications are resistant erythroderma of various origins and selected refractory generalized cases of psoriasis, seborrheic dermatitis, atopic eczema, and intractable senile pruritus.

Dosage

As recommended by Schirren [12], 50 R are given 3 times a week to the anterior and posterior body surfaces. The total dose per course usually does not exceed 400 to 600 R. Most radiosensitive dermatoses respond promptly to this treatment schedule. A similar course of treatment can be repeated after several months. In contrast to treatment of mycosis fungoides, it is mandatory not to exceed a total cumulative dose of 1000 R in benign dermatoses, since higher doses may result in minor radiation sequelae which cannot be tolerated in the treatment of any nonmalignant cutaneous disorder. Radiation protective measures are essential, including shielding of eyes, gonads, thyroid, and other radiosensitive organs [11].

Table 12-6 *Indications for Teleroentgen Therapy 1954–1972 (University of Munich)*

Indication	No. of Patients	%
Mycosis fungoides	26	13.2
Chronic exfoliative dermatitis	59	30.1
Erythrodermas of various origin	38	19.4
Senile pruritus	26	13.3
Psoriatic erythroderma	25	12.7
Lymphomas (reticulum cell)	9	4.6
Generalized lichen planus	9	4.6
Generalized seborrheic eczema	4	2.1
Total	196	100%

References

1. Domonkos AN: Andrews Diseases of the Skin. Philadelphia, Saunders, 1971
2. Epstein EH Jr, et al: Mycosis fungoides. Survival, prognostic features, response to therapy, and autopsy findings. Medicine 51:61, 1972
3. Fromer JL, et al: Management of lymphoma cutis with low megavolt electron beam therapy. Nine-year follow-up in 200 cases. South Med J 54:769, 1961
4. Fuks Z, Bagshaw MA: Total skin electron treatment of mycosis fungoides. Radiology 100:145, 1971
5. Fuks Z, Bagshaw MA, Farber EM: Prognostic signs and the management of the mycosis fungoides. Cancer 32:1385, 1973
6. Goldschmidt H: Teleroentgen irradiation in dermatological therapy. In Proceedings of XII International Congress of Dermatology, Washington, DC, 1962. International Congress Series No. 55. Amsterdam, Excerpta Medica, 1963, p 643
7. Petratos MA: Current practice of teleroentgen therapy. Cutis 4:716, 1968
8. Proppe A: Fortschritte in der Methodik der dermatologischen Röntgentherapie. Klin Teil Arch Dermatol Syph 200:107, 1955
9. Proppe A: Die Bewertung alter und neuer Röntgengeräte in der dermatologischen Röntgentherapie. Dermatol Wochenschr :259, 1957
10. Schirren CG: Roentgen irradiation at a distance using the soft radiation from beryllium-window tubes in treating cases of generalized dermatoses, Ro.-Fernbestrahlung. J Invest Dermatol 24:463, 1955
11. Schirren CG, Haumayr W, Dittmar R: Zum Problem des Strahlenschutzes. Die genetische Strahlenbelastung des Patienten bei der Hautröntgentherapie. Strahlentherapie 108:127, 1959
12. Schirren CG: Totalbestrahlung, Röntgen-Fernbestrahlung der Haut und Indirekte Bestrahlungsmethoden Zur Beeinflussung von Dermatosen. In Marchionini A (ed): Jadassohn's Handbuch der Haut- und Geschlechtskrankheiten, Vol V/2. Berlin, Springer-Verlag, 1959, p 599
13. Schirren CG: Personal Communication, 1962
14. Teschendorf W: Uber Bestrahlung des ganzen menschlichen Körpers bei Blutkrankheiten. Strahlentherapie 26:720, 1927
15. Trump JG, et al: High energy electrons for the treatment of extensive superficial malignant lesions. Am J Roentgenol 69:623, 1963
16. Van Scott EJ, Winters PL: Responses of mycosis fungoides to intensive external treatment with nitrogen mustard. Arch Dermatol 102:507, 1970

17. Van Scott EJ, Kalmanson JD: Complete remissions of mycosis fungoides lymphoma induced by topical nitrogen mustard (HN2). Control of delayed hypersensitivity to HN2 by desensitization and by induction of specific immunologic tolerance. Cancer 32:18, 1973

18. Wagner G: Die Grossfeldtechnik in der dermatologischen Strahlentherapie. Z Haut 22:267, 1957

19. Wiskemann A: Röntgen-Oberflächentherapie mit beryllium-gefensterten Röhren. Hautarzt 2:456, 1951

13

Radiotherapy of Benign Dermatoses

Mark Allen Everett

General Considerations

Throughout the first half of the 20th century, x-ray therapy was an essential, if not indispensable, therapeutic modality used by every dermatologist. Since 1950, however, there has been a marked decline in the employment of radiation therapy by dermatologists, particularly for benign dermatoses. This greatly diminished use of x rays in the treatment of benign cutaneous disorders is largely attributable to the utilization of corticosteroids and antibiotics in various cutaneous conditions. In addition, recognition of the undesirable local and general effects produced by improperly utilized radiation during the early part of the century contributed to its decreased use.

Advances in scientific knowledge have led to greater understanding of the tissue effects of radiation and have increased appreciation of not only the potential undesirable limitations, but also the unique value of ionizing radiation when administered with discretion in selected disorders of the skin. Specifically, information regarding undesirable side effects and maximal safe tissue dosage, as well as radiation protection, has led to modification of the concept of the total amount of radiation permissible for use in any one area, tissue, or organism.

Two basic considerations determine the safety of dermatologic radiation therapy: the amount of radiation absorbed by tissues other than skin and the effects on the skin itself. Three principle factors limit the skin's tolerance to radiation.

The first factor is the total cumulative dose administered to any given field. The incidence of cosmetically undesirable side effects from radiation, such as telangiectasia, atrophy, hyperpigmentation, and depigmentation, were reported by Sulzberger et al [13] following an observation period of 5 to 23 years. Late radiation effects did not occur when the total dose did not exceed 1000 R. If the total dose was in the range of 1000 to 2630 R, relatively mild cosmetic sequelae were observed in approximately 1.5% of patients. Such sequelae were more frequently observed in skin which had previously received considerable actinic radiation. Malignant changes were not observed when total doses were less than 2000 R (see also Chapter 5). Borak et al [2], in a study of 102 patients treated for hyperhidrosis of the axillae, palms, and soles with a total of 1600 R administered in 6 divided doses over a period of 8 weeks from superficial therapy machines with a HVL of 2 to 4 mm Al and a single dose not exceeding 300 R, found that over a follow-up period of 2 to 18 years there was no evidence of radiation damage. Rowell [11] studied 136 patients who had received radiation for benign disease and found that 1600 R was the lowest dose at which sequelae had been observed, when treatment factors were 100 R per treatment with approximately 3 treatments per month from a superficial therapy machine of 90 kV and a HVL of 0.7 mm Al. He suggested 1200 R as a safe upper limit for a total dose administered in benign dermatoses. Cipollaro and Crossland [4] state that from their experience with conventional superficial x rays, "We know that it is risky to employ weekly doses of more than 100 R for longer than 12 weeks." Domonkos [6] stated that maximum permissible radiation values for benign dermatoses range from 500 to 2200 R, but suggested a dose of 800 R as a reasonable limit. Accordingly, we may consider that 1000 to 1200 R approximates the maximum safe cumulative tissue dose for administration in benign conditions.

Since grenz rays are almost completely absorbed in the outer 2 mm of skin, they are "safe" at the deeper levels (below the hair bulb) to which they do not penetrate. Accordingly, Goldschmidt has proposed a maximum cumulative dosage of 5000 R for grenz rays [8]. Cipollaro and Crossland [4] state that conservative authorities on grenz-ray therapy use doses smaller than 300 to 400 R weekly. The minimal penetration of grenz rays beyond 2 mm of skin renders them particularly suitable for treatment of such areas as the eyelids, scalp, and scrotum.

The second factor governing the development of sequelae is the size of the individual dose administered to any given area. It is be-lieved that with a cumulative dose of 1000 to 2000 R, visible sequelae appear primarily when the individual dose exceeds the erythema dose of the skin. As may be seen in Fig. 13-1, the erythema dose is related to the quality of radiation and lies between 250 and 500 R for superficial therapeutic techniques. The individual dose most frequently used in treatment of benign dermatoses is considerably less than an erythema dose. Erythema dose values have been reported by Wansker [14], Cipollaro and Crossland [4], and Glasser [7] (Table 13-1).

The third factor modifying the incidence of radiation sequelae is the quality of radiation, ie, the depth of tissue penetration. The occasional sequelae reported with cumulative doses less than 2000 R have been in those instances when harder, more penetrating radiation was employed, or where actinic degeneration was prominent.

Effects of X Rays on Tissues Other Than Skin

With regard to the amount of radiation received by tissues other than skin, if radiation for benign dermatoses is administered with properly calibrated equipment, the field demarcated by a shield of lead or an appropriate substitute, and the radiation confined to the treatment area by a cone, then penetration of superficial radiation to distant tissues is minimal or insignificant. As has been shown by Goldschmidt et al [9], with

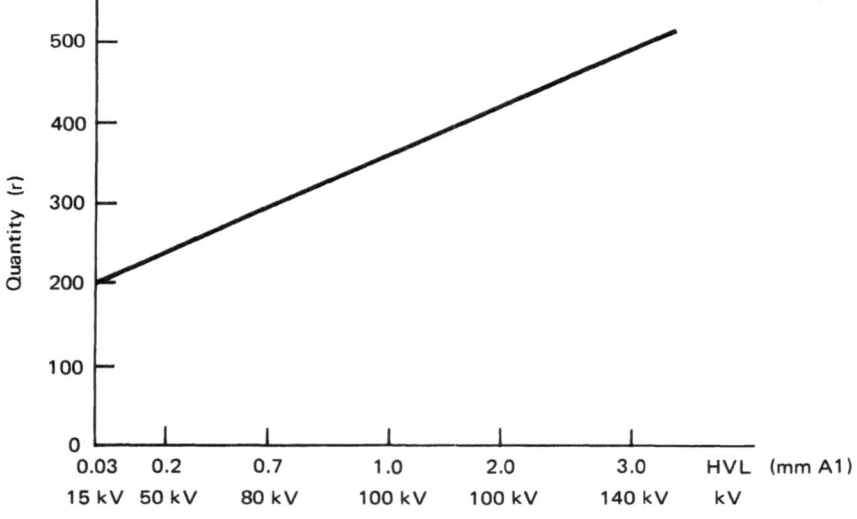

Figure 13-1.   Erythema production by a single dose of radiation.

Table 13-1 *Erythema Threshold by Quality of Radiation*

kV	HVL (mm)	Erythema Threshold (R) (Includes Backscatter)
15	0.03 Al	200
50	0.2 Al	250 or less
100	1.0 Al	270 to 300
140	3.0 Al	500
140	0.4 Cu	525
200	0.9 Cu	680
700	7.0 Cu	800
1000 or radium	3.8 Pb	1000

such techniques, and *without* additional gonadal shielding, 100 R to the face with a HVL of 0.3 mm Al results in a gonadal exposure of only 0.007 mR in a recumbent man, 0.005 mR when the foot is similarly irradiated, and 3 R when the anus is irradiated. If the testicles are shielded by lead during anal radiation, the gonadal exposure is reduced from 3 R to 147 mR. Further, studies by Alden [1] showed that a gonadal dose was 0 when 40 R with a cone were applied to the ankle (HVL, 0.75 mm Al).

These figures for radiation exposure should be taken in the context that background radiation in the United States is in the vicinity of 1.0 mR per day or 340 mR per year to the entire body [4]. The much greater exposure from diagnostic as opposed to therapeutic x rays is illustrated by the fact that gonadal doses approaching 20 mR are received from one ordinary chest x ray. In other words, diagnostic radiation often represents a significantly increased body exposure over background radiation while properly administered radiation therapy does not.

Routine safety precautions should include treatment-field demarcation by a shield and confinement of the beam with a cone. Minimal additional shielding should include the lens of the eye and the thyroid gland when irradiating the head, trunk, or upper extremities, and

shielding of the gonads when irradiating the trunk, thighs, or perineal areas. Further shielding may be presumed to be primarily of psychologic rather than a physiologic value. Therapy of pregnant females should be undertaken with special considerations of the fetus. Further details of radiation protection are discussed in Chapter 4.

In actuality, public attitudes play as important a role as do the above facts in determining the uses of radiation therapy by physicians. The current attitudinal climate may all but preclude the use of radiation for disorders other than malignant disease.

Technical Considerations

The depth of the process to be treated determines the quality of radiation employed. The quality of radiation is in turn determined by the characteristics of the x-ray machine (Table 13-2) [10].

Grenz ray tubes with beryllium windows have an intrinsic filtration of 0.01 to 0.04 mm Al. At 10 kV the $D_{1/2}$ is in the vicinity of 0.1 to 0.3 mm; at 15 kV, approximately 0.2 to 0.4 mm; and at 20 kV, approximately 0.5 to 0.7 mm of skin. The depth for 90% absorbency is approximately 1.5 mm of skin at 10 kV and 3 mm at 20 kV [3].

Superficial x-ray machines have an intrinsic filtration of approximately 0.3 to 0.5 mm Al for Pyrex-window units. Operated at 40 kV, the $D_{1/2}$ is approximately 5 to 7 mm of skin and the 90% absorbency level is 2.5 to 3 cm of skin. At 80 to 100 kV, the $D_{1/2}$ is 5 to 14 mm and the 90% absorbency level is 3.5 to 5 cm [10].

For grenz-ray therapy 150 to 300 R are administered at weekly intervals, while for therapy with a conventional superficial machine, usually 60 to 100 R are administered at 7- to 14-day intervals 3 to 10 times. The cumulative dose maxima are as described previously.

Table 13-2 *Characteristics of Superficial X-Ray Equipment*

Characteristic	Picker Zephyr	Universal Treatmaster	Universal Grenz Ray	Siemens Dermopan II
Type	Superficial	Superficial	Grenz ray	Soft x ray
kV	70–120	40–100	10–20	10–50
mA	5	5	10	25
Window	Pyrex	Pyrex	Beryllium	Beryllium
HVL (mm Al)	0.56–1.5	0.4–1.4	0.017–0.037	0.02–2.0
$D_{1/2}$ (mm tissue)	8–20	5–15	0.15–0.57	0.5–2.0

Field Size

In addition to other factors, field size will influence a decision regarding the employment of radiation in the treatment of benign dermatoses. With the exception of teleroentgen therapy, radiation is now administered with the beam confined by a cone and therapy is limited to small areas demarcated by a shield. The larger the dermatosis, the less likely that radiation therapy will be seriously considered as a therapeutic possibility.

Traditional Indications for Radiation Therapy

Dermatitis–Eczema

X-ray therapy is primarily useful in chronic, recalcitrant, localized, eczematous processes such as lichen simplex, hand eczema, or nummular disease which have not responded to intralesional or topical steriods. Studies by Crissey and Shelley [5] showed conclusively that chronic eczematous lesions respond significantly and promptly. Very acute dermatoses, such as vesicular contact dermatitis, also improve, but only slightly faster than do untreated areas. Atopic eczematous disease is usually not treated with radiation therapy because of the chronicity of the process, its almost certain recurrence, and the frequently wide extent of the disorder.

Chronic eczematous dermatoses usually are treated with 70 to 100 R at a HVL of not greater than 0.3 to 0.4 mm Al at weekly intervals for 3 to 5 treatments. Some eczematous lesions are sufficiently superficial to respond to grenz radiation (Chapters 14 and 15).

Hypertrophic Lichen Planus

Although lesions of lichen planus respond well to radiation, such therapy has largely been replaced by intralesional steroids. Occasionally, hypertrophic lichen planus is benefited by the utilization of both modalities.

Psoriasis

As with atopic dermatitis, the tendency for widespread involvement and frequent recurrences militates against the use of radiation therapy in psoriasis, even though the lesions themselves often respond promptly to such treatment. Currently, radiation is employed only in persistent, localized psoriasis which has not responded to intralesional steroid therapy. Such lesions might include palmar or plantar patches, or psoriatic nail involvement. For palmar–plantar involvement, we employ dosages and radiation qualities similar to those used in eczematous disease. For involved nails, a HVL of 0.4 to 0.5 mm Al is employed and individual doses of 150 to 200 R are administered at weekly intervals up to a total of 500 to 700 R. Also, radiation is useful in lichen simplex–psoriasis of the occiput in those individuals who fail to respond to intralesional steroids or topical steroids with occlusion. In other forms of psoriasis, the extent and tendency to recur preclude the use of x rays in most instances. Grenz radiation has been utilized by some therapists with some benefit in thin plaques of psoriasis. Indications for grenz-ray therapy are discussed in Chapters 14 and 15.

Parapsoriasis

Parapsoriasis does not respond to radiation therapy unless a transition to early lymphoma has occurred, in which case it is no longer a benign process.

Infectious Skin Disorders

Because of their influence on inflammatory disease, x rays were once widely used in the treatment of bacterial infections such as folliculitis, furunculosis, and other cutaneous infections; but now, in nearly every instance, radiation has been completely supplanted by appropriate antibiotic therapy. Only in certain chronic pyodermas, where mechanical and other tissue factors limit the effect of antibiotics, is radiation employed effectively. These include chronic paronychia and early hidradenitis suppurativa. For paronychia, a HVL of 0.5 mm Al ($D_{1/2}$, 8 mm) is employed at 75 to 100 R given weekly for 5 or 6 weeks. In hidradenitis, 2 to 3 weekly exposures of 100 to 200 R with a HVL of 1.5 mm Al ($D_{1/2}$, 20 to 25 mm) are employed. Occasionally, recurrent herpes simplex on non–sun exposed areas may respond to grenz radiation ($D_{1/2}$, 0.05 mm) when other measures have failed. With regard to verrucae, other therapeutic modalities are used in nearly every instance.

Acne Vulgaris

Strauss and Kligman [12] demonstrated that the effect of radiation on acne was principally due to reduction in the size of sebaceous glands. Because after several months (ie, 3 to 18) there is evidence that gland size returns to pretreatment levels, employment of radiation is reserved for older age groups (above 17 years) where the likelihood of recurrence is less. Careful patient selection is indicated for severe, nodular, cystic, scarring acne unresponsive to antibiotics, intralesional steroids, and other appropriate therapy. A cumulative dose of at least 500 R is necessary to obtain a suppressive effect. Ordinarily, 70 to 100 R are given weekly to a total of 500 to 800 R. Radiation is usually administered to two fields, one centered over each cheek, with the area to be treated demarcated by lead–rubber shielding. Radiation protection is very important (see Chapter 4). The quality of radiation ($D_{1/2}$) corresponds with the depth of the lesions and ordinarily would be approximately 5 to 8 mm (HVL, 0.4 to 0.5 mm Al). Severe involvement of the upper back and chest may be similarly treated, but in these instances tissue scatter requires meticulous attention to protection of surrounding and distant areas.

Keloids

Experience has shown that keloid development is restricted and young keloids are flattened by either intralesional steroid therapy or radiation. Inasmuch as the therapeutic effect of both methods is significant but not coincident, it is possible to employ radiation either with or following intralesional steroid therapy. Two to 3 treatments of 140 to 200 R with a $D_{1/2}$ of 10 to 12 mm of skin at weekly intervals are usually sufficient.

Lymphocytoma Cutis

Radiotherapy ordinarily promptly causes reso *lution of lymphocytoma cutis lesions. A single treatment dose of 150 to 200 R with a $D_{1/2}$ of 5 to 8 mm (HVL, 0.4 to 0.5 mm Al) is usually sufficient.

Lichenification in Pruritus

As with psoriasis, atopic dermatitis, and extensive eczematous disease, neurodermatitis, when widespread, is not treated with radiation because of the large field and high recurrence rate. However, for severe pruritus vulvae, pruritus ani, and pruritus scroti (which has not responded to a combination of steroids, sedation, systemic antipruritic drugs, and proper local care), grenz-ray therapy, in doses of 75 to 100 R administered in 4 to 8 weekly intervals, may be beneficial. Appropriate shielding and field demarcation should be utilized.

Hirsutism and Hyperhidrosis

In the past, hirsutism and hyperhidrosis were treated with x rays, but suppression of hair growth and sweating requires radiation in quantities that exceed the cumulative "safe" dose. Consequently, x-ray therapy is contraindicated in these conditions.

Hemangiomas

Hemangiomas, both capillary and cavernous, are rarely treated by radiation therapy. The natural history of the capillary lesion (strawberry mark) suggests spontaneous resolution, while most cavernous lesions are not radiation sensitive. Hence, surgery is the treatment of choice where aggressive therapy is indicated. Capillary hemangiomas that produce symptoms of mechanical obstruction or ulceration are currently treated by systemic steroid therapy rather than x-ray therapy.

Summary

Superficial x-ray therapy plays a limited and decreasing role in the management of certain benign cutaneous disorders. Specifically, x rays are useful in a few cases of chronic, localized eczematous dermatitis, occasional scarring and cystic acne unresponsive to other measures, occasional patients with chronic paronychia or hidradenitis suppurativa, and sometimes in keloids. Grenz radiation has been particularly useful in the management of neurodermatitis of the perineum, anus, or vulvar areas and possibly in the treatment of recurrent herpes simplex. Practically, public attitudes toward environmental radiation hazards have virtually limited the use of radiation therapy by most dermatologists to malignant lesions.

References

1. Alden HS, Weens HS, Youmens HD: Observation on radiation exposure in dermatologic x-ray therapy. Arch Dermatol 79:159, 1959
2. Borak J, Eller J, Eller W: Roentgentherapy for hyperhidrosis. Observation of one hundred and twenty-two patients. Arch Dermatol Syph 59:644, 1949
3. British Institute of Radiology: Depth dose tables for use in radiotherapy. Br J Radiol (Suppl) 10:96, 1961
4. Cipollaro AC, Crossland PM: X-rays and radium in the treatment of diseases of the skin. Philadelphia, Lea & Febiger, 1967
5. Crissey JT, Shelley WB: A controlled clinical study of the effect of x-ray therapy in certain non-malignant dermatoses. N Engl J Med 247:965, 1952
6. Domonkos AN: Andrews' Diseases of the Skin, 6th ed. Philadelphia, Saunders, 1971
7. Glasser O, Quimby EH, Taylor LS, et al: Physical Foundations of Radiology, 2nd ed. New York, Hoeber, 1952
8. Goldschmidt H: Dermatologic radiation therapy. In Moschella, Pillsbury, Hurley (eds): Dermatology. Philadelphia, Saunders, 1974
9. Goldschmidt H, Betetto M, Bonse G: Die Röntgentherapie von Dermatosen. In Jadassohns (ed): Handbuch der Hauf-und Geschlechtskrankheiten, V/2. Berlin, Springer-Verlag, pp 464–598
10. Jennings WA: Physical aspects of the roentgen radiation from a beryllium-window tube, operated over a range of 2–50 KVP for clinical purpose. Acta Radiol 33:435, 1950
11. Rowell NR: A follow-up study of superficial radiotherapy for benign dermatoses. Br J Dermatol 88:583, 1973
12. Strauss JS, Kligman AM: Effect of x-rays on sebaceous glands of the human face. Radiation therapy of acne. J Invest Dermatol 33:347, 1959
13. Sulzberger MB, Baer RL, Borota A: Do roentgen-ray treatments as given by skin specialists produce cancers or other sequelae? Arch Dermatol 65:639, 1952
14. Wansker BA: X-ray and Radium in Dermatology. Springfield, Ill, Thomas, 1959

14

Ultrasoft X Rays, Including Grenz Rays

Mark B. Hollander [†]

Physical and Technical Considerations

After many previous workers had tried to construct an apparatus which would produce ultrasoft x rays, Bucky succeeded in devising a tube to produce such rays in 1923. It had long been known that the interaction of x rays and living tissue always produced damage of some degree to the tissue. How much damage is done, whether the tissue can repair the damage, and how complete the repair may be will vary with the quality and dosage of radiation as well as with the tissue, but the damage per se is inevitable.

Since one objective of sound radiotherapy is to minimize injury to univolved tissues or structures, there is an immediate constraint on the quality of radiation used to treat conditions limited to the skin, whose maximal normal thickness is only about 3 mm. To treat such conditions with x rays capable of passing through the entire body in significant proportions is to overshoot the mark badly. When a process is not limited to the thickness of the skin, it must then be evaluated in terms of its depth, but the general principle remains the same. It is good practice to select a quality of radiation appropriate for the depth or thickness of the condition to be treated, with due regard for whatever other organs or structures that may lie in the path of the beam.

Quality is the term applied to the penetrating power of an x-ray beam. It is determined primarily by the voltage at which the beam is generated. The part of the electromagnetic spectrum referred to as ultrasoft x rays is generated entirely at or below 30 kilovolts peak (kVp), yielding HVLs of or below 0.2 mm Al. That portion of the ultrasoft spectrum identified as grenz rays by Bucky inclues beams with HVLs of or below 0.036 mm Al and, in most contemporary beryllium-window tubes, is generated at or below about 18 kVp. These grenz rays are so soft that they are absorbed to a significant extent in air.

Quality is influenced by filtration, inherent and added, as well as by voltage. Filtration increases the average penetrating power of the photons comprising the beam by absorbing their softer components. While the harder rays are also weakened to some extent, the net result is to increase the average penetrating power. By "inherent filter" we mean the tube window, plus oil or whatever else that is an inherent part of the tube. Added filter represents whatever absorbing material is added from the outside. In the grenz-ray range, target–skin distance (TSD) also affects the quality of the beam, since grenz rays are filtered by air. Consequently, the inverse square law, which states that the intensity of the beam, or dose rate, varies inversely with the square of the distance from a point source, cannot be applied to grenz rays, although conventional x rays follow it closely. The tube of a grenz-ray machine must be calibrated specifically for each distance at which it is to be used. Table 14-1, a recent calibration sheet, demonstrates this point, and also indicates the different qualities available in this portion of the x-ray spectrum. The inherent filter of this tube, the original Machlett AEG-50-A, is 1 mm Be.

For heterogeneous x-ray beams, the most intense absorption occurs within the half-value depth ($D_{1/2}$). The rays that pass beyond this point are the harder components of the beam, whose softer photons have been absorbed in the previous tissue layers. These harder photons interact with tissue more gradually than do the less energetic ones.

Grenz rays are absorbed predominantly through the photoelectric effect (Chapter 1). Since their energy is small at the outset, the path of the photoelectron is short, on the order of 0.05 to 0.1 μ, so that its entire quantum of energy is absorbed within one cell. Thousands of collisions occur, however, along that short path. The atoms from which either photoelectric or scattered electrons are removed are left in an "excited" state, for they now have a positive charge. They, or the molecules that contain them, are able to enter into chemical combination with free radicals or other molecules to form new molecules, sometimes bizarre, and of unpredictable effect on the tissue. Further information regarding these matters may be obtained elsewhere [4].

Field size and care in measuring TSD have been emphasized appropriately in Chap-

ter 15. The original beryllium-window tubes, the AEG-50 series, were designed by Machlett for industrial radiographic applications, so their target angles were only 19°. This small target angle restricted field size to 75% of the target–skin distance, and caused distortion at the anode side of the field due to heel effect. Machlett's latter OEG-60 tubes were designed for therapy and were built with a much wider target angle, i.e., more than 30°. Although this made the effective field size equal to the TSD and diminished the heel effect considerably, there was still an inevitable fall-off in intensity at the edges of the field due to the inverse square law. Diagrams of the fields of both tubes are shown in Fig. 14-1.

Most machines built in this country have voltmeters which can be set at any point along a continuous, wide voltage range. The voltmeter we use, for example, can be set anywhere from 0 to 30 kVp. One of the earlier beryllium-window units, no longer in production, could be operated anywhere from 0 to 100 kVp. This machine was inherently dangerous, as are all others of similar design, for the accidental omission of a filter at the upper voltages could be disastrous. In addition, its tube has an inherent filter of 3 mm Be, so that it could not produce grenz rays in useful amounts.

As an illustration of the danger involved, in 1950 I omitted a filter in treating a 2.5-cm squamous cell carcinoma of the dorsum of the hand at 25 kVp. The filter omitted was 0.15 mm Al, and the time was set for a single exposure of 5000 R. The omission of the filter increased the intended exposure dose to an estimated 18,000

Table 14-1 *Calibration Date for X-R-M Grenz Ray Model G-1-B # G-240 Tube: Machlett AEG 50 # 05314*

KV (load on)	mA	Filter	HVL (mm Al)	$D_{1/2}$ (mm tissue)	TSD (cm)	R/min in Air	Deliver Time (sec)		
							100 R	200 R	500R
15	7	none	0.021	0.5	10	1440	4	8.5	21
	15	none	0.023	0.5	15	1080	5.5	11	28
16	10	none	0.024	0.5	15	960	6	12	31
	20	none	0.026	0.6	20	840	7	14	35
18	10	none	0.027	0.6	15	1200	5	10	25
	20	none	0.029	0.7	20	1080	5.5	11	28
16	20	3 poly	0.029	0.7	15	1440	4	8.5	21
		3poly	0.030	0.7	20	750	8	16	40
18	20	3 poly	0.032	0.8	15	1920	3	6	16
		3 poly	0.033	0.8	20	1020	6	12	29
25	15	0.2 Al	0.13	3.1	10	1140	5.5	11	26
29	10	0.2 Al	0.14	3.2	10	1020	6	12	20
	20	0.2Al	0.14	3.2	15	840	7	14	35

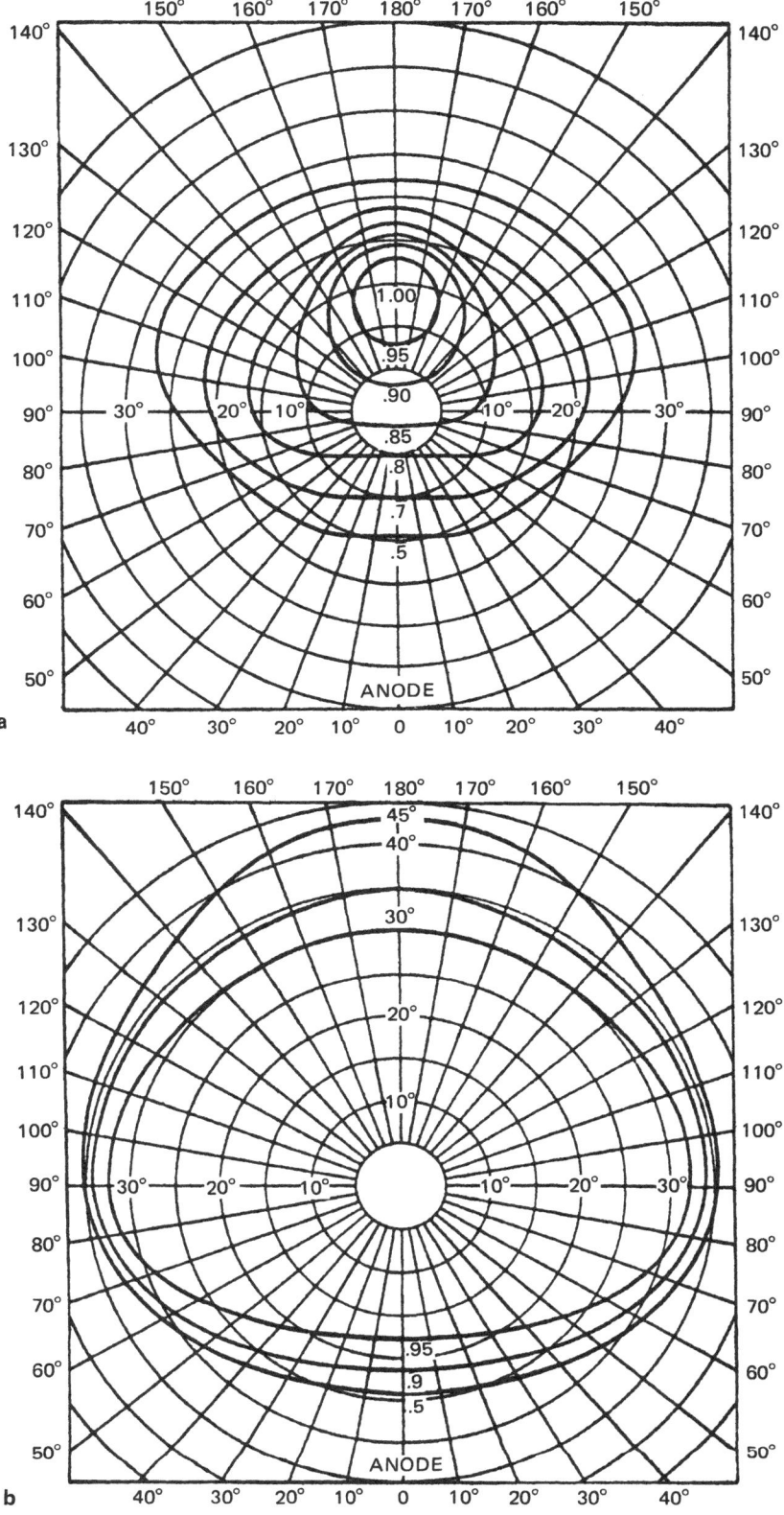

Figure 14-1. *a.* Fields of radiation for Machlett AEG-50. *b.* OEG-50 tubes.

or 19,000 R. The excess consisted chiefly of the very soft rays which would have been absorbed by even so thin a filter, so the irradiated area healed spontaneously in 4 or 5 weeks, instead of the anticipated 3 or 4 weeks, with no more than a slight increase in atrophy and telangiectasia.

Some of the current European units are built with interlocks which can be operated only if an appropriate filter is in place. While these machines are vastly safer than those that are operable over a continuous range of voltage, they lack the flexibility that is desirable in the ultrasoft portion of the x-ray spectrum. The most popular of these units can be operated at only 4 voltages; 10, 29, 45, and 50 kVp. This arrangement straddles the ultrasoft range, which probably extends from 12 or 14 kVp to 29 or 30 kVp. I prefer the continuous-spectrum units extending to a maximum of 30 kVp, although they demand much more meticulous care in use. While the hardness of the beam rises directly with increasing voltage, the dose rate increases approximately with its square, so such care is imperative at energies much above 18 kVp.

Proper calibration of machines designed to produce ultrasoft x ray still poses a problem. Most radiation physicists are neither trained nor equipped to perform such measurements, probably because there is not sufficient demand for these services at present. Target-chamber distances must be accurate within 1 or 2 mm, and the window of the ionization chamber must be truly air-equivalent. While the thimble-chambers used in calibrating conventional x rays are accurate in that range, their walls absorb ultrasoft rays unpredictably and excessively, resulting in apparent hardening of the beam and too-low measurement of quantity. Qualified radiation physicists do exist, however, and the Radiological Society of North America can provide a list of them.

This situation calls for a precise understanding of the international R. The R is a measurement of ionization in air, and tells nothing about the energy flux in the beam nor about energy absorption in tissue. Although a biologic unit would be preferable, no accurate or reproducible unit has been devised as yet. In the x-ray range below 1000 kVp the R is reasonably exact, so it must serve until a satisfactory biologic unit is established. The rad, the unit of absorbed dose, must be calculated from the exposure dose in roentgens at present.

The question of the half-value depth of ultrasoft x rays is in a similarly unsatisfactory state. Recent measurements made in skin by Grisewood [3a] are almost twice those indicated by Jenning's absorption curves in aluminum. Though the $D_{1/2}$ of any therapeutic beam of radiation is of critical importance, only a possibly misleading approximation can be given now. Work on hopefully accurate $D_{1/2}$ measurements in tissue is currently in progress, but it seems preferable to speak of half-value layers in alumium until the new work yields more reproducible data.

Backscatter is not of material concern in the ultrasoft range. The energy of the photoelectron is low in the grenz-ray range, and its path is so short that all of its energy is absorbed within a single cell. While the secondary electron at the upper end of the ultrasoft spectrum is somewhat more energetic, the difference is not great. I have made experimental exposures of sensitive dental x-ray film, using a cone and sharp-bordered, chrome-plated brass ports, exposing the film to 500 R at its surface. Up to 16 kVp, the border of the exposed portion of the film was sharp. Above that level, and with appropriate filters, the border was hazy, but only for about 1 mm. It is thus evident that, while some ultrasoft rays are absorbed by scatter, the path of the scattered beam is too short to constitute a problem or a threat to treatment.

Radiation Side Effects

None of the preceding statements can be construed as representing complete safety for grenz ray use, much less for use of the harder ultrasoft rays. As has been described in considerable detail elsewhere [4], ultrasoft rays are much safer than are conventional x rays only because their comparatively low energy limits their depth of penetration and their scatter. In sufficiently high overdosage, they can cause the same damage as can conventional x rays, but at lesser depth. The only readily apparent exception to this broad statement is that grenz rays have not been reported to cause epilation of the scalp, where the hair bulbs lie at a depth of about 4 mm. Where the hair bulbs are closer to the surface, as are those of the eyelashes, they are vulnerable. Experimental epilation of laboratory rodents, whose skins are thin and whose hair bulbs are much closer to the surface than are those of the human scalp, is clear evidence of this. In 1926, Bucky [1] exposed 2 1.5-cm areas on the flexor surface of each of his forearms to very high doses of grenz rays, recorded in terms of kVp, mA, TSD, and time. When the international R was introduced 1 year later, calibration of his machine indicated that the HVL had been about 0.036 mm Al and that the single exposure to each area had been on the order of 23,000 R. When he showed me his forearms, in 1947, each of the triangular irradiated areas showed complete epilation, with mild atrophy and telangiectasia. At my suggestion, one area was excised for biopsy in 1950. The other three were excised and sent to me at his death, in 1963. The sections all showed similar patterns of thinning of epidermis and dermis, with almost complete absence of appendages. A photomicrograph of a representative section is shown in Fig. 14-2.

Harder rays, toward the upper end of the ultrasoft spectrum, can do still more damage. Figure 14-3 shows a photomicrograph of a section of a biopsy taken in January 1964, from the site of a squamous cell carcinoma of the buttocks exposed in September 1957 to 5 × 2000 R at a HVL of 0.10 mm Al (25 kVp, 10 cm TSD, 0.15 mm Al added filter) in 2 weeks. Damage to the upper dermis is obvious, but the deep artery appears unaffected.

Pigmentation occurs frequently and, to a large extent, parallels that following high expo-

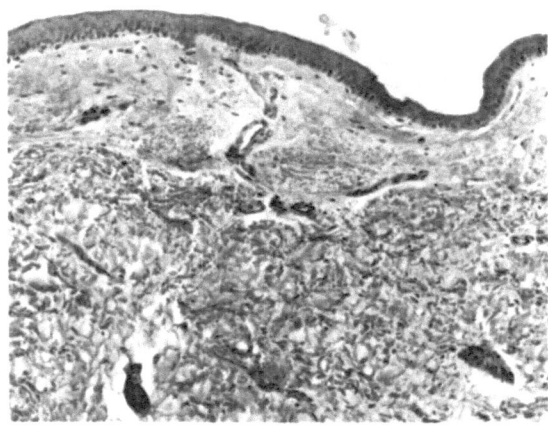

Figure 14-3. Squamous cell carcinoma, 15 × 12 mm², on upper buttock exposed to 5 × 2000 R (25 kVp; 0.15 mm Al added filter; 10 cm, TSD; HVL, 0.10 mm Al) between August 31 and September 13, 1957. Section of biopsy taken on January 27, 1964. Superficial radiodermatitis is obvious; deep artery is apparently unaffected.

sure to ultraviolet radiation. In general, a therapeutic dosage induces both erythema and pigmentation somewhat later than does ultraviolet radiation and appears to pigment darker skins more than fair ones (again, similarly to ultraviolet radiation). Pigmentation induced by exposure to large doses of ultrasoft rays lasts somewhat longer than does that from ultraviolet rays, hut is permanent only very rarely.

In general, it is desirable to use the softest quality which will reach adequately the base of the lesion under treatment, and, especially in treating benign disease, to fractionate total exposure into increments of about 200 to 300 R weekly. The testes should be protected, sometimes with lead foil or leaded vinyl, although the slight to clinically absent scatter in this range makes proper direction of the beam highly protective. Except when one is planning high dosage to a granuloma, a keloid, or a malignant lesion, close shielding is not needed. It may even be undesirable, because of the possibility of causing a sharp line of hyperpigmentation. All medication, especially powders and pastes, should be removed, because it will absorb significant amounts of radiation. The growth centers of the bones of infants are in no danger from grenz rays, which will be absorbed readily by the bone cortex, though I would not use the harder ultrasoft rays in such situations. Nor would I use grenz rays, much less the

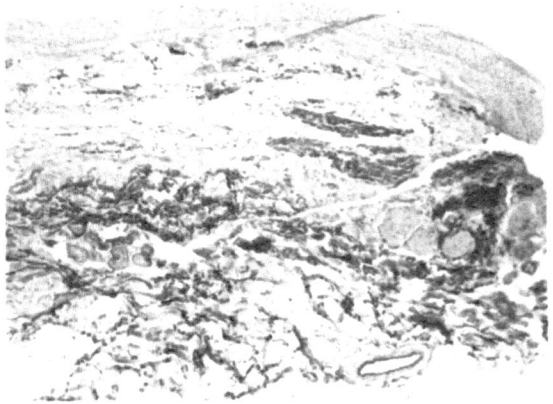

Figure 14-2. Photomicrograph of section from specimen removed from Dr. Bucky's forearm in 1963. Slight atrophy and flattening of epidermis. Appendages sparse.

harder rays, to treat a pregnant woman. Although we know that little, if any, radiation in that energy range could reach the uterus or its contents, it might be difficult to convince a lay jury of this.

In general, most modern authors limit the total cumulative dose of ultrasoft x rays (administrated to the same body region in fractional doses) to 5000 R. I and others, however, have given cumulative totals of 15,000 to 20,000 R without serious sequelae.

In our discussion, we will consider use of the harder ultrasoft rays (also known as soft x rays) for treatment of malignant disease and use of grenz rays for benign processes. Although all grenz rays are exceedingly soft in comparison to conventional x rays, there are differences among grenz rays themselves. For convenience, then, grenz rays will be referred to as soft (HVL up to 0.02 mm Al), medium (HVL, 0.023 to 0.029 mm Al), and hard grenz rays (HVL, 0.030 and 0.036 mm Al), and will be identified merely as s, m, or h, repectively.

Indications for Radiotherapy

The indications for radiotherapy of skin conditions have shrunk drastically since the advent of antibacterials and antibiotics, topical and systemic steroid therapy, chemotherapy, psychopharmacologic therapy, and more or less direct psychotherapy. Consequently, many conditions formerly treated almost routinely by radiotherapy will be omitted from discussion, others will be mentioned as responsive to radiation but, currently preferably treated by other approaches, and some will be discussed in full detail. Documentation will not be offered for radiotherapy of most conditions, all of which are discussed fully elsewhere [4].

Dermatitis

Acute and subacute dermatitis are treated preferably with topical, occasionally systemic, steroids. While most instances of chronic dermatitis will also respond well to such agents, some, especially the lichenified lesions, may not. The patient may frequently become emotionally involved in such situations, and it becomes worthwhile to use something more dramatic. Grenz rays, s or m, usually do an excellent job here. There is a buzzer built into my machine, which operates silently otherwise, and that buzzer informs the patient that he is receiving strong treatment indeed.

However, the response of lichenified dermatitis to grenz rays is not entirely psychotherapeutic. Figure 14-4 shows a photomicrograph from a biopsy taken through the border between the treated and untreated halves of an inveterate plaque 1 week after exposure of half of the lesion to 3 × 450 R at a HVL of 0.018 mm Al, at weekly intervals, in 1951. Pigmentation after the first treatment made it possible to duplicate shielding fairly closely. The junction between treated and untreated halves of the lesion is readily identifiable microscopically.

Psoriasis

Grenz rays, of quality varying with the thickness of scale, are an outstanding therapy for psoriasis. By no means does every patient respond well to topical steroids, and, if the disease is not too extensive, ultrasoft radiotherapy is much preferred to steroids with occlusion, which are a nuisance to the patient and sometimes a cosmetic danger to the skin, or to methotrexate. The response is faster, 3 or 4 weekly exposures usually sufficing, and safer, a consideration to both patient and therapist. Strong exposures to radiation should be avoided, for recklessness can lead to a Koebner reaction. Ordinarily, such treatment can be repeated every 4 to 6 months, apparently for years, without sequelae. It is imperative to use the softest quality possible, for grenz rays will no more

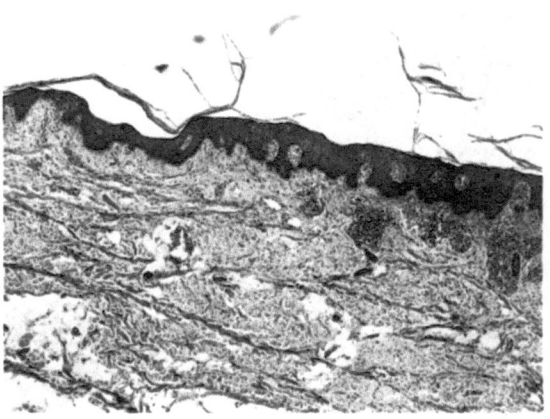

Figure 14-4.   Section of biopsy taken through junction of treated and untreated halves of plaque of lichenified dermatitis, exposed to 3 × 450 R at a HVL of 0.018 mm Al, at weekly intervals, in 1951. Biopsy 1 week after third treatment.

cure psoriasis than will any other currently known agent.

Seborrheic Dermatitis

Although topical steroids or the time-honored sulfur–salicylic acid–resorcin formulations are usually adequate for treatment of seborrheic dermatitis, resistant patients or lesions will usually respond quite well to grenz rays, s or m. This appears to be merely another of the as yet unexplained overlappings between seborrheic dermatitis and psoriasis.

Lichen Planus

The inflammatory infiltrate hugging and sometimes invading the basal layer of the epidermis makes lesions of lichen planus an inviting target for grenz rays, s or m, in selected cases. Early lesions have been seen to disappear within 2 to 3 weeks with as little as 2×300 R, s. Responses seen repeatedly in hypertrophic lesions with exposures of 300 to 400 R, s, twice a week (in the early 1950s), suggest that smaller doses of medium rays once a week might do as well. Deplorably, such responses bring us no closer to understanding the disease or its cause.

Herpes Simplex

Surprisingly good results have been seen many times in treatment of herpes simplex, within the first 24 hours, with even single exposures of 300 R, s. In 2 or 3 patients with herpes usually recurrent in the same location, permanent relief or marked reduction in frequency of recurrence has been obtained.

Keratosis Follicularis

Keratosis follicularis is highly responsive to grenz rays. The condition is quite photosensitive, so it is advisable to limit exposures to 100 or 150 R, s, once a week. Improvement up to complete clearing has been seen after 2 to 4 exposures.

Benign Familial Pemphigus

The benign familial pemphigus of Hailey and Hailey has also responded quite well, with remissions lasting for as long as 4 to 14 months. Atrophy and telangiectasia can be induced eas-

ily with excessive treatment, especially high single exposures, of so responsive a condition. I once exposed a plaque of Darier's disease to a single dose of 500 R at a HVL of 0.018 mm Al. The immediate response was severe erythema, lasting for almost a week. When the reaction subsided, the lesion had disappeared. It may be that the superficial location of the disease process makes it more sensitive to superficial radiation, most of which is absorbed on the surface, than to more penetrating rays, even in the ultrasoft range.

Poikiloderma Atrophicans Vasculare

In 1957, many lesions of poikiloderma atrophicans vasculare were exposed to 8×350 R, s, at weekly intervals, without much clinical change, but with distinct diminution of infiltrate in a biopsy taken 1 year later. In and after 1960, there was noticeable reduction of atrophy in treated areas. This did not stop progression of the disease, however, and the patient died of mycosis fungoides in 1972. Today, I would use harder grenz rays, but would still be merely hopeful about arrest of the disease process.

Cavernous Hemangioma

There is a great difference of opinion regarding the management of the familiar capillary or cavernous hemangioma known popularly as "strawberry mark." Since about 75 to 80% of such lesions involute spontaneously before age 5 years, obstetricians, pediatricians, and most surgeons advocate strongly that they be merely "observed." There are two valid objections to this attitude. One is that no one has found a way to predict which 20 to 25% will fail to involute spontaneously; the other is that no allowance is made for the anxiety and other feelings of the parents. Some of these tumors continue to spread, and all become increasingly radioresistant with age, even within the first year.

The vessels comprising this lesion are lined by a highly immature endothelium which appears impressive under the microscope, and which is almost acutely sensitive to ultrasoft x rays. One such tumor, growing rapidly on the radial surface of the proximal phalanx of an infant's third finger, was exposed to 6 or 8 × 500 R, h, weekly, in 1950. In 1966, the mother phoned to ask on which hand the lesion had been. I saw the boy in 1971, and could find neither sign of tumor nor evidence of radiation sequelae. Yet, in terms of my experience since 1950, the lesion was overtreated. That experience has shown that the first exposure, of 500 R at a HVL of 0.033 mm Al (18 kVp, 20 cm TSD, 3 layers of polyethylene film added filter), usually arrests the growth of the tumor and initiates the process of involution. After 2 weeks, the lesion is expected to be its original diameter and to show gray streaks on its surface, indicative of thrombosis of the superficial vessels. If there is an increase in diameter or absence of graying of the surface, a second exposure of 500 R is given. Whether or not the second treatment is needed, another examination is made 4 weeks after the first treatment. At that time, the surface is found to have become uniformly gray, with a much duller red color beneath it and no further growth. The patient is then seen at monthly intervals, and the tumor is measured and examined. Involution is allowed to proceed spontaneously, further treatments being given only when regression seems to have slowed unduly. Ordinarily, a total of 3 or 4 × 500 R suffices. The parents are relieved, the skin shows no evidence of damage, and the child's body economy is not impaired as it might have been after systemic therapy. Proper shielding procedures are essential.

Nevus Flammeus

The flat hemangioma known as port-wine stain or *nevus flammeus* does not respond in any such gratifying fashion. The endothelium lining its capillaries is adult in appearance, and cannot be injured without parallel injury to the skin in which it occurs. Grenz radiation in sufficiently high dosage has been reported to make nevus flammeus fade, but only with a corresponding degree of atrophy, which is unacceptable.

Keloids

Since young fibroblasts are highly radioresponsive, early keloids and hypertrophic scars can be treated successfully with medium to hard grenz rays, depending, as usual, on the thickness of the lesion. An exposure of 500 R once a week, for a total of 5 to 15 treatments, usually suffices (Fig. 14-5). One caveat, however, is in order, especially in surgical scars. The radiation that inhibits young fibroblasts from multiplying excessively also prevents solid scar from forming, so it is imperative that the wound be protected from spreading. When a surgeon is to operate on a known keloid-former or a patient who is suspected of being likely to rub the scar excessively, it is requested that the wound be supported from below by a layer of closely placed fine subcuticular sutures.

This problem, of course, does not exist with older scars. Mature scar tissue is resistant to x rays of any quality. While it can be flattened to some extent at times, the response is inadequate, regardless of degree of overdosage. It is best either to have the scar excised or to bring it down to skin level with solid CO_2, fulguration, and curettage, or intralesional steroids, and then to treat with hard grenz rays,

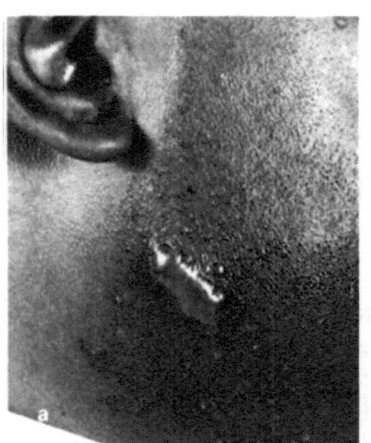 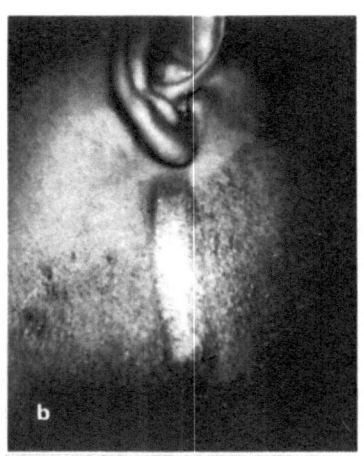 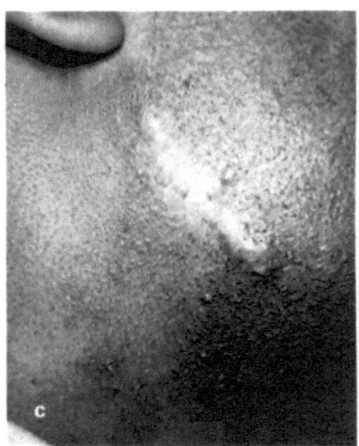

Figure 14-5.   Keloid at angle of jaw. *a.* 11-17-61. *b.* 6-6-62. *c.* 5-14-63.

500 R weekly, to prevent a new keloid or hypertrophic scar from forming. Results with this approach have been excellent. Destruction of the mature scar tissue by any of the noncutting methods merely brings the scar down to skin level, but does not weaken the holding power of the scar left in the cutis. Excision demands preradiation support, as mentioned above.

The described treatment will bring the scar down to the level of the surrounding skin, and will usually keep it there. It will not do away with the scar, however, as some patients may wish. In addition, it is apparent that digital trauma, in the form of rubbing or squeezing, causes ordinary scars to thicken. It is also related to the recurrence of keloid.

Precancerous Tumors and Skin Cancers

Actinic keratoses, superficial epithelomatosis, and lesions of Bowen's disease respond very well to 12 exposures of 500 R each. While it may be desirable to treat Bowen's disease 3 times a week, the other two conditions will behave equally well on treatment once a week, with significantly better cosmetic results. Radiation of any quality sufficiently penetrating to deliver adequate dosage to the base of the lesion is capable of causing some degree of atrophy, which can be minimized or even prevented at the visible level by protraction of treatment. The lesions of Bowen's disease will disappear, leaving minimal atrophy, but Bowen's disease usually looks a good deal more aggressive than do the other two conditions. They involute, after more protracted therapy, usually with no visible sequelae.

Contrary to the belief of the 1920s and early 1930s, seborrheic keratoses are not radiosensitive. It is far preferable to remove them with a sharp curette, with healing approximating restitution to normal.

Basal and squamous cell carcinomas are lesions of a different order of seriousness. The purpose of treatment is to destroy the lesion. Cosmetic results still deserve consideration, but are distinctly secondary. Grenz rays are not sufficiently penetrating to reach the bases of such tumors in adequate proportion, so ultrasoft rays with a HVL of approximately 0.14 mm Al (25 to 30 kVp) must be employed. My routine, barring certain exceptions, is to use 12 × 500 R (25 or 29 kVp, 10 cm TSD, 0.2 mm Al added filter), 6 times a week, although 3 times a

week can be used if the patient cannot come in every day. A margin of apparently normal skin at least half as wide as the diameter of the tumor is included in the field of exposure, which is sharply shielded otherwise. Because of the frequent errors reported in differentiating keratoacanthoma from squamous cell carcinoma, I prefer to keep that differentiation at an academic level. Biopsy through the center of the lesion suffices for academic distinction, but the tumor is treated as a squamous cell carcinoma. Response of the two to radiotherapy is about the same. Tumors of the eyelid are sometimes treated with 6× 500 R at a HVL of 0.14 mm Al plus 6× 500 R at a HVL of 0.032 mm Al (18 kVp, 15 cm TSD, 3 layers of polyethylene film added filter). The end result is usually permanent disappearance of tumor, with some mild but varying degree of atrophy and telangiectasia (Fig. 14-6).

Lentigo Maligna

Recently reported work [6] indicates that the malignant freckle of Hutchinson (lentigo maligna) responds well to radiotherapy. The previous accepted difficulty seems to have been failure to recognize that the anaplasia may extend down hair follicles, so that one must use a quality of radiation sufficiently hard to deliver an adequate dose to the hair bulb. Rays with a HVL of 0.14 mm Al, as used for malignant tumors of the skin, are called for. A total exposure dose of 12 × 500 R should suffice.

Mycosis Fungoides

Mycosis fungoides is one of the most radioresponsive of all skin neoplasms. The problem is merely to deliver an adequate dose to the base of the lesion. Grenz rays will suffice in the premycotic and early plaque stages, but the tumor stage is usually too thick for any rays in the ultrasoft range. Here, the work with electron beams, started in 1952 as a collaborative effort of the Lahey Clinic and the Massachusetts Institute of Technology [3], has yielded brilliant results, (Chapter 11).

Swimming Pool Granuloma

Plaques of *Mycobacterium marinum* (swimming pool) granuloma respond surprisingly well to radiation. Grenz rays, in a total exposure

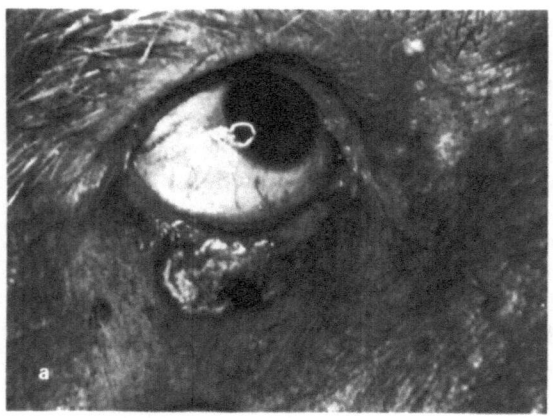 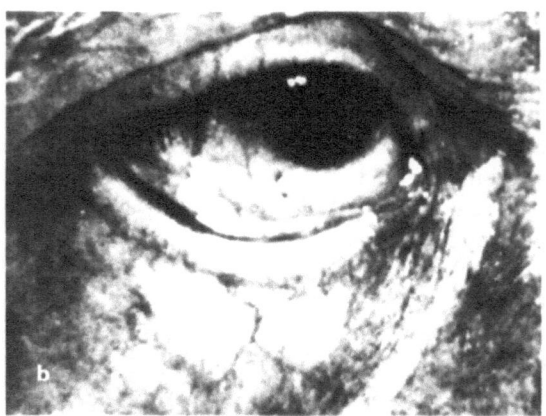

Figure 14-6.   Basal cell carcinoma of eyelid, involving 16 mm of eyelid margin. *a.* 5-29-61. *b.* 9-18-62, 15.5 months after 8 × 1000 R at a HVL of 0.10 mm Al (25 kVp, 0.15 mm Al added filter, 10 cm TSD) administered between May 29 and June 7, 1961.

dose of 12 × 500 R, administered once a week, suffice for those of ordinary depth, but the harder ultrasoft rays are needed for thicker lesions.

Leishmaniasis

Cutaneous leishmaniasis does not occur in the Western world, and is seen only in an occasional traveler coming (or returning) from the Middle East or parts of East Africa. It is worth mentioning, nonetheless, since it is still seen frequently in those areas, grenz rays were reported in 1942 as effective in treating it, and no other satisfactory treatment for it has been found as yet.

Indications for Superficial X-ray Treatment

There are some more or less common skin diseases for which ultrasoft x rays are not effective. These are conditions in which more penetrating rays are needed. It is in such conditions that the ''superficial x rays'' upon which dermatologists used to depend so strongly prior to 1950 are still invaluable. These rays are generated at energies between 60 and 100 kVp in tubes with glass windows. The usual glass windows absorb far more of the ultrasoft rays than does beryllium, and thus produce, in the voltage range specified, beams with a HVL of 0.5 to 0.9 mm Al. The depth doses of these beams are known with considerably greater accuracy. They range from a $D_{1/2}$ of approximately 5 to

more than 10 mm, depending in part on field area and, consequently, on backscatter.

Acne

While x rays are now seldom used in the treatment of acne, there is the occasional case of cystic acne which will not respond to topical therapy, systemic antibiotics, or both, and which is disfiguring both the patient's skin and his emotions. In such cases, conventional superficial x rays will usually control the acne both safely and effectively. Exposure dosage consists of 12 to 16 weekly treatments, with 60 to 75 R at 60 kVp to each side of the face and to whatever other areas need it. The fields overlap sufficiently so that a midline exposure to the face is not necessary, and may result in overdosage. Such treatment should not be given earlier than age 20, for it cannot be repeated without grave danger of late sequelae.

Recurrent Skin Cancers

Recurrence of basal or squamous cell carcinoma, especially on the forehead, after removal by excision or by curettage and fulguration, is often too deep for use of ultrasoft x rays. Such cases must be evaluated carefully. If there is reason to suspect a depth of more than 2 mm, it is preferable to administer 12 × 400 R, to a field at least wide enough to include possible lateral subepidermal projections, at 80 kVp and at the rate of 5 or 6 exposures a week.

Melanomas

It has been shown [1a] that excision of a primary melanoma, in cases in which that seems feasible, yields better long-term results if preceded or followed by radiotherapy at 100 kVp to the area between the site of the graft and the satellite nodes.

Hidradenitis Suppurativa

When the response of hidradenitis suppurativa to systemic antibiotics has been exhausted, epilation with a single application, most often of 500 R at 80 kVp, is usually effective [9]. Here, again, the depth dosage of ultrasoft x rays would be altogether inadequate.

Conclusion

Grenz rays, like x rays of higher energy, are capable of causing serious damage if used in excessive dosage. It also appears that repeated small exposure doses over a long period of time are more likely to cause serious late sequelae than are very large cumulative total doses given in a short period. The reason may be that large doses probably cause irreversible damage and cell death, whereas small individual exposures produce reparable damage, in the course of which mutations can occur. There are at least three reports [2,7,8], previously overlooked [4], of induction of a squamous cell carcinoma in laboratory rodents by repeated exposure to grenz rays. There are also four known cases of induced squamous cell carcinoma, three included in my review [4] and one found later [5], in humans. Of the four, two were in patients with psoriasis and two in dermatologists who had exposed their hands unwisely while treating patients. It is evident, then, that while grenz rays are far safer than are conventional x rays they are nonetheless ionizing radiations, and deserve all the respect accorded to rays of greater energy.

These results clearly demonstrate that radiotherapy, of a quality appropriate to the depth of the process under treatment and in dosage adequate for that condition, is a valuable part of the dermatologist's armanentarium. This means not only that the office must be equipped with adequate apparatus, but that the dermatologist must be equipped with the technical knowledge necessary to help the patient in a safe manner. It is unfortunate that this point requires so much emphasis. Some of the present teachers of dermatology appear impervious to its importance. It could be said, in extenuation, that in many teaching institutions all of the apparatus producing ionizing radiation is under the control of the departments of radiology, that trainees in dermatology do not have access to the apparatus available for therapy, and that the radiologists and radiotherapists know little about either the skin or superficial radiotherapy. Such apologia, however, is not sufficient. In actuality, most teachers do not display much interest in the matter, and, as a result, the new generation of dermatologists will know painfully little about radiotherapy of the skin. Apart from the fact that this will reduce the stature and status of dermatology, it will be a great loss to the ultimate helpless victim, the patient.

Synopsis: Ultrasoft X Rays

Quality Range

HVD, 0.02 to 0.25 mm tissue (HVL, up to 0.2 mm Al)
Voltage range, 14 to 30 kVp
Selection of quality based on nature and thickness of lesion

Dosage Range

For ordinary superficial dermatoses, 200 to 300 R weekly for 4 or 5 exposures
For granulomas, hemangiomas, keloids, and plantar warts, 500 R weekly for 10 to 15 exposures
For superficial epitheliomatosis, 500 R weekly for 8 to 10 exposures
For granulomas, 500 R weekly for 10 to 15 exposures
For Bowen's disease and other intraepidermal carcinomas, 500 R daily or 3 times a week for 10 to 12 exposures.
For carcinomas less than 2.5 mm, in thickness, 12 × 500 R daily or 3 times a week

Indications

Ordinary dermatitides, psoriasis, seborrheic dermatitis, lichen planus, erythema annulare centrifugum, granuloma annulare, and perhaps lichen nitidus
Deeper lesions, including plantar wart, strawberry mark, keloid, mycobacterial granuloma, intraepidermal carcinomas
Basal and squamous cell carcinomas less than 2.5 mm in thickness

Sequelae

Pigmentation, more marked in dark than in fair
    skins
Superficial atrophy and telangiectasis, varying
    with locus and exposure dosage

References

1a. Dickson RJ: Malignant melanoma. A combined
    surgical and radiotherapeutic approach. Am J
    Roentgenol Radium Ther Nucl Med 79:1063, 1968
2. Epstein JH: Carcinogenic and cocarcinogenic effects of grenz radiation. J Invest Dermatol 54:439,
    1969
3. Fromer JL, Smedal MI, Trump JG, et al: High-
    energy electrons for generalized superficial dermatoses. Arch Dermatol Syph 71:390, 1955
3a. Grisewood, EN, personal communication
4. Hollander MB: Ultrasoft X Rays. An Historical
    and Critical Review of The World Experience
    with Grenz Rays and Other X Rays of Long
    Wavelength. Baltimore, Williams & Wilkins,
    1968
5. Lagerholm B, Skog E: Squamous cell carcinoma
    in psoriasis vulgaris. Acta Derm Venereol
    (Stockl) 48:128, 1968
6. Proppe A: Discussion at meeting of American
    Academy of Dermatology, December 1973
7. Shapiro EM, Knox LM, Freeman RG: Carcinogenic effect of prolonged exposure to grenz rays.
    J Invest Dermatol 37:291, 1961
8. Zackheim HS, Krobeck C, Langs L: Cutaneous
    neoplasia in the rat produced by grenz rays and 80
    kVP x rays. J Invest Dermatol 43:519, 1964
9. Zeligman I: Temporary x-ray epilation therapy of
    chronic axillary hidradenitis suppurativa. Arch
    Dermatol & Syph 92:690, 1965

15

Grenz-Ray Therapy: Regimens and Results

Henry M. Lewis

Grenz rays, properly employed for those disorders aided by this extremely superficial ionizing radiation, provide a greater benefit/risk ratio than does any other dermatologic modality. This chapter will attempt to highlight those disorders in which grenz rays are preeminently beneficial, and to elucidate the author's therapeutic regimens and results.

Unfortunately, an alarming number of novice dermatologists receive only cursory training in radiotherapy. X-ray equipment is usually housed and safeguarded in the radiology department, often far removed from the dermatology unit, and the separation between radiology and dermatology departments is frequently more than merely geographic. Recognizing that some radiotherapy training is essential for completing dermatology specialty examinations, radiologists may tolerate the presence of dermatology residents for demonstration of superficial therapy technique. However, because the primary concern of radiologists lies deeper than the first millimeter of skin in which 75% of grenz rays are absorbed, no grenz-ray units may be available.

In a recent survey of the Task Force on Ionizing Radiation of the National Program for Dermatology [10], *practical* clinical instruction in dermatology departments was indicated as "poor" in 22% or "not given" in 18% of the 2271 questionnaire replies. Even *theoretical* instruction by dermatologists was "poor" in 20%

and "not given" in 12% of training programs. In only 15% of responses was the practical clinical instruction given by radiology departments considered "good." This questionnaire did not specifically isolate grenz-ray therapy instruction.

Upon entering practice, radiotherapeutically naive dermatologists are logically skeptical of the role of ionizing radiation in dermatology. As their practices grow they may begin to feel that adequate dermatologic care can be administered without it. Confirming this ominous trend, grenz-ray therapy of psoriasis is mentioned in neither of two recent dermatologic textbooks [7,8], although Baer and Witten [3] specify psoriasis as one of the principal indications for its use. This abdication of radiotherapy by the neodermatologist obviously constricts his armamentarium. But, more importantly, it deprives the patient of that maximal care he rightly deserves, and to which he is fully entitled.

Technical Considerations

Since Chapter 14 thoroughly detailed the physical principles involved in grenz ray production, mensuration, and absorption, this chapter will emphasize practical matters.

At the Denver Skin Clinic. two grenz-ray machines are currently in use. Table 15-1 is a simplified calibration chart for our technical

Table 15-1   *Calibration Chart for Universal X-Ray Equipment (kVp, 15; mA; 10; HVL, 0.028 mm Al)*

Localizer	TSD (cm)	R/min	100 R	200 R	300 R	1200 R	1500 R	2000 R
Glass cones	13.5	842	0′7″	0′14″	0′21″	1′25″	1′46″	2′22″
Open field	13.5	872	0′6″	0′13″	0′20″	1′22″	1′43″	2′17″
Metal cone	25.5	196	0′30″	1′1″	1′31″	6′7″	7′39″	10′12″
Metal cylinder	27.0	170	0′35″	1′10″	1′45″	7′3″	8′49″	11′45″
Open wire frame	25.5	184	0′32″	1′15″	1′37″	6′31″	8′9″	10′52″

personnel of the equipment manufactured by Universal X-ray Products, Inc, Chicago, Ill. Table 15-2 is a similar chart of the unit manufactured by the International Medical Research Co, New York, NY. Our technicians prefer the rail-mounted Universal equipment over the modified dental x-ray unit arm of the portable International Medical Research machine for stability and ease of handling, despite the greater output of the latter.

When technical personnel operate radiotherapy equipment, scrupulous training and supervision are required, but opportunity for error must also be minimized. Preset target–skin distances (TSD) utilizing plastic-tipped metal cylinders, metal cones, and wire frames provide not only accurate TSDs, but are also designed to indicate the approximately 50% drop-off in field distribution at longer distances. At short TSD, as in treatment of small psoriatic plaques, peripheral dosage drop-off considerations are unimportant. For open field therapy at these distances, semicompressible measuring rods are employed. These are placed in contact with the tube center, extend perpendicularly to the skin surface, and are removed prior to open field irradiation.

Absolute precision in TSD is mandatory, for at a 10 cm TSD an error of 0.5 cm in either direction will alter the dosage by 10% or more [3]. Our plastic-tipped metal cylinders have a TSD of 13.5 cm. Shorter distances are not recommended, for at the high output of radiation at these short distances, minimal deviations in exposure time produce inordinate dosage variations. At 1000 R/min a 1-sec deviation results in

a dosage variation of slightly less than 10% [3].

Field distribution of radiation assumes increasing importance as the TSD enlarges. With early beryllium-window grenz-ray tubes there was a disturbing anode heel effect limiting the effective diameter of the irradiated area to approximately 75% of the TSD [14]; in newer units the effective field diameter and TSD are identical.

Shielding is essential when doses above 1200 R are delivered at longer TSD. Conventional lead sheets or thick leaded rubber are used either in an overlap fashion or by custom tailoring to the shape of the desired field (Fig. 15-1 and 15-2).

The problem of posttreatment hyperpigmentation has received much attention. It is seldom observed in doses greater than 1200 R, for erythema and subsequent superficial desquamation preclude its development. With doses less than the erythema dose, however, such posttreatment hyperpigmentation may be annoying. It is best to have this pigmentation blend imperceptibly into the skin. Any type of shielding, even the inadvertent presence of a short sleeve or wristwatch, may produce a disfiguring line of demarcation at the edge of the treatment site. Development of such pigmentation is roughly proportional to the intensity of the patient's normal melanin pigmentation.

In all exposures, the central beam must be perpendicular to the treatment site. This poses problems and necessitates special techniques when concave surfaces are treated. For example, a bowenoid superficial squamous cell carcinoma in situ involving the dorsal foot and

Table 15-2   *Calibration Chart for International Medical Research Equipment (kVp; 10)*

Localizer	TSD (cm	R/min	mA	100 R	200 R	300 R	1200 R	1500 R	2000 R	HVL (mm Al)
Glass cones	15	1060	5	0′5″	0′11″	0′16″	1′7″	1′24″	1′53″	0.034
Glass cones	15	1500	10	0′4″	0′8″	0′12″	0′48″	1′0″	1′19″	0.034
Metal cone	20	670	15	0′8″	0′17″	0′26″	1′47″	2′14″	2′59″	0.031
Open field	25	398	15	0′15″	9′30″	0′45″	3′0″	3′46″	5′1″	0.025

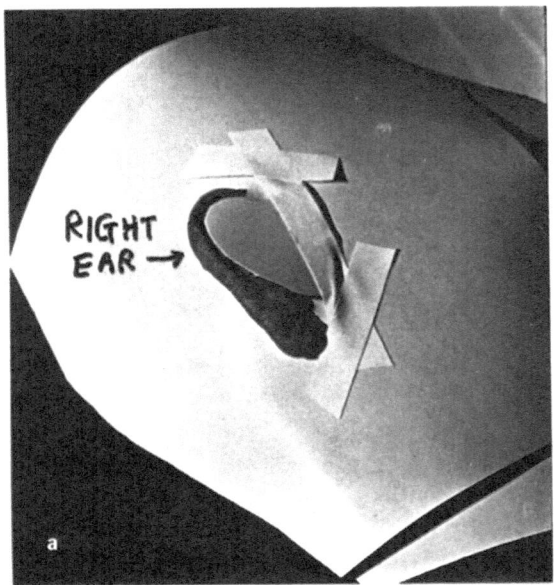 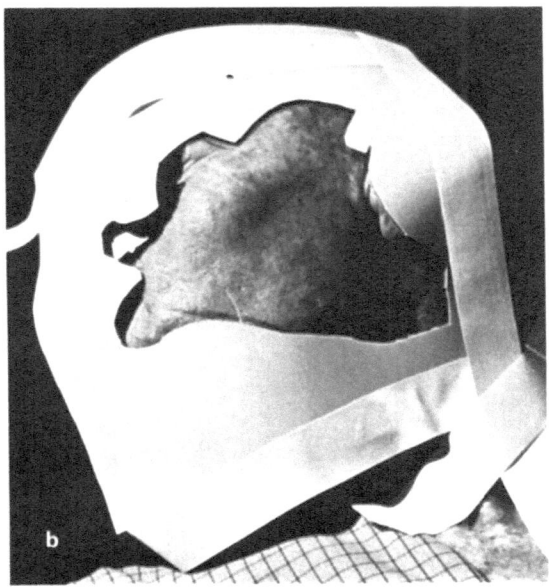

Figure 15-1. Shielding techniques for open field therapy. *a*. Actinic keratoses of left face, 25.5 cm TSD. *b*. Actinic keratosis of right helix, 13.5 cm TSD.

extending into the intertoe webs requires 3 separate exposures (Fig. 15-3): one to the dorsal foot and toe surfaces with the toes tightly apposed, and one to each lateral toe area with the toes forcibly separated. When larger concave surfaces of the axillae, genitocrural, and anal areas are treated, shielding is mandatory in order to protect the peripheral uninvolved zones which lie closer to the tube target than to the treatment site. Vulvar and anal lesions are best treated in two separate exposures with the patient in the Sims position. Testicles are always held out of the treatment field.

Special attention must be paid to removal of moisture, medication, cosmetics, sebum, crusts, and scales before therapy is adminis-

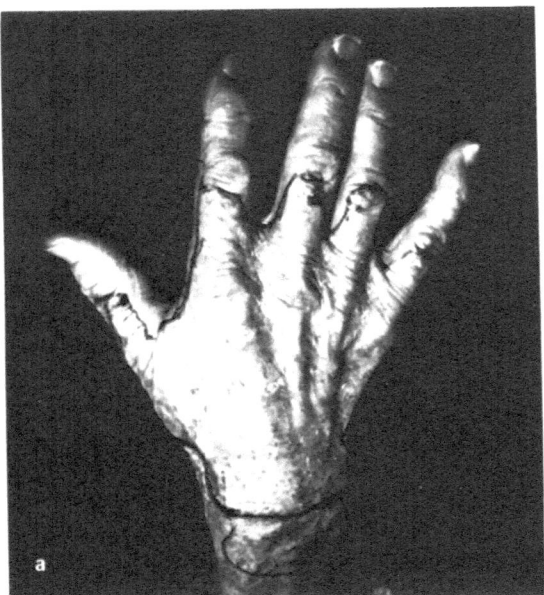 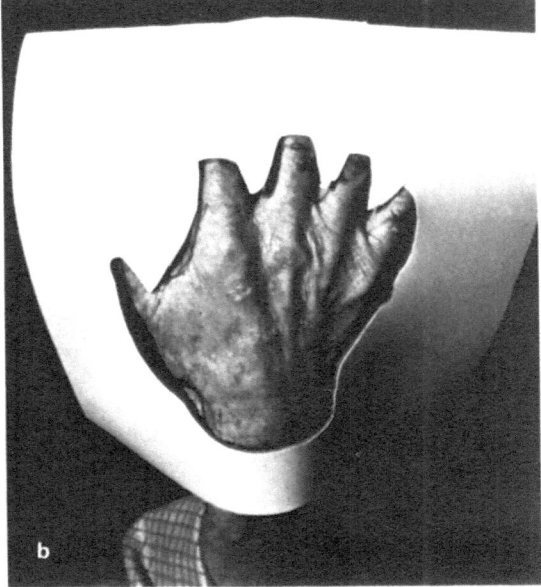

Figure 15-2. Shielding technique, closed metal cone therapy, 20 cm TSD. *a*. Demarcation of treatment sites. *b*. Lead shield in place.

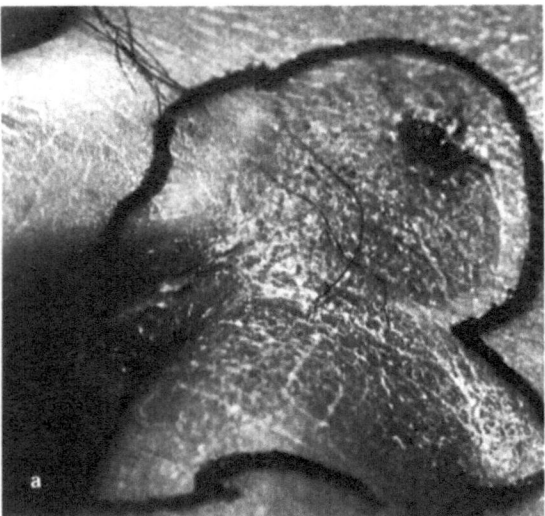

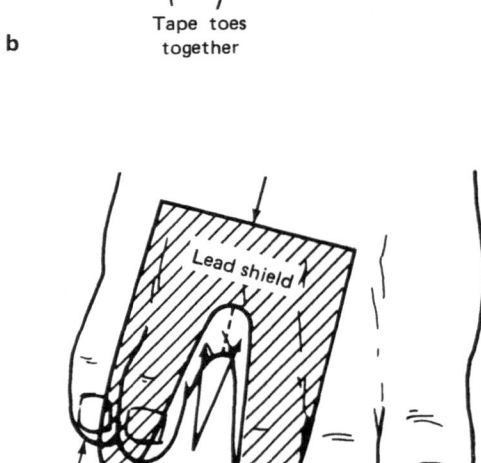

Figure 15-3. Technique for treating curved surfaces with perpendicular beam. Bowenoid squamous cell carcinoma in situ. *a.* Treatment areas delineated. *b.* Treatment diagram, beam directed to dorsal foot area. *c.* Toes forcibly separated. Lateral toes treated individually with short, closed cylinders.

tered. All of these will interfere with proper absorption of grenz rays and lead to imprecise dosages.

Sequelae

Properly used, the great advantage of grenz radiation lies in its lack of sequelae despite fractional doses exceeding 20,000 R administered over a period of years. Indeed, Meyer [15], using modern equipment, determined that a dose of 10,000 R administered in one session is necessary to produce epidermal necrosis. In 24 years, I have personally observed only one instance of development of atrophy and telangiectasia in a patient with perianal psoriasis treated with grenz rays over a 6-year period. This may, however, have resulted from undisclosed prior radiation administered elsewhere to this patient. I am currently seeing patients

whom I treated 22 years ago with 1500 R to the sides of the face for actinic keratoses; in none has there been any evidence of radiodermatitis, although these patients have had considerable sunlight exposure before and since such therapy. Recently, Arouete [2] declared that it is not only safe to administer 250 R weekly for 5 doses in psoriasis, but that after a delay of 3 or 4 months the maximum action of the rays is totally spent and one can irradiate the same sites without taking into consideration the previous doses.

When sequelae are reported, there is usually evidence of gross overdosage. The radiodermatitis, squamous cell carcinoma, and keratoses of Brodkin and Bleiberg's [5] patient's buttocks and thighs developed after she received 200 R weekly for a total of 4400 R (sic) to each site. Then, after only a 1-month lapse, another course totaling 5800 R was administered over an 8-month period and, after another lapse of 3 months, another 3400 R were administered over a 4-month period. The scrotal angiokeratoma of the patient of Abe et al [1] developed after he received single doses of 100 to 150 R twice a week for 3 months, once a week for 1 month, and every other week for 1 month for a total dose of 4200 R over a 5-month period. They report 3 additional cases of serious sequelae, all from extreme overdoses of grenz rays, in the Japanese literature.

Not all patients presenting with identical disorders will respond to grenz rays, and persistence in their use beyond accepted therapeutic dosage schedules is both hazardous and unconscionable.

Clinical Applications

Actinic Keratoses

At the Denver Skin Clinic, during the past 22 years, more than 40,000 grenz-ray treatments for actinic keratoses have been administered. The usual dose for face lesions is 1500 R in one exposure [6]. This may be reduced to 1300 R for patients with fair, "transparent" skin or increased to as much as 2000 R for thicker lesions in swarthy individuals when small, isolated areas are being treated. Short, closed treatment cylinders with TSDs of either 13.5 or 15 cm, depending upon the equipment employed, are used. These constitute the majority of lesions treated, for most patients report annually or semiannually and present with relatively fresh, discrete, small areas.

Patients volunteer their preference for grenz radiation over either cryotherapy or electrodesiccation and curettage, for both of the latter modalities may leave permanent posttreatment leukoderma, a cosmetic blemish which has received no discernible mention as an anticipated, albeit mild, sequel. Grenz-ray therapy of actinic keratoses leaves no discernible pigmentary alteration, and may be employed safely in sites such as the upper eyelid, where either of the other two modalities might be inconvenient.

For patients who present initially with innumerable facial actinic keratoses, treatment sites are delineated with a toothpick dipped in a solution containing 2% gentian violet and 20% acetone in alcohol. This penetrates sebum adequately, is readily removed after treatment

with ordinary rubbing alcohol, and is preferable to all the marking devices I have attempted to use. Most of these pens or pencils will not write on sebum. The "writes on any surface" variety is difficult to remove following treatment. After involved areas have been indicated, they are carefully isolated from uninvolved skin before treatment is administered (Fig. 15-2b).

After therapy, about 5% of patients will experience a mild transient erythema that evening; this persists for only 1 or 2 days. Between the seventh and eleventh posttreatment day, all patients begin to notice a more lasting reaction (Fig. 15-4). This peaks between days 17 and 22, gradually diminishes, and is gone by day 50, leaving grossly normal–appearing skin.

Open field grenz-ray therapy may be safely combined with conventional x-ray therapy (Fig. 15-5) when histologic examination dictates the latter modality for deeper malignant lesions.

Although the erythema produced by grenz radiation is similar to that provoked by 5-fluorouracil, the grenz-ray reaction is more precise in onset and metamorphosis, and there is considerably less patient discomfort. Only one treatment is needed and that is performed in the dermatologist's office. For both patient and physician, this approach has proved more expedient, economical, and therapeutically predictable than any other in the management of actinic keratoses.

Hand and forearm lesions are treated with 1500 to 2000 R in one sitting (Fig. 15-6). Here the advantages over 5-fluorouracil are even more pronounced. Occlusive nocturnal waps are required for 5-fluorouracil to be effective on these areas. These are uncomfortable, time consuming, and odorous on removal; consequently, patients may treat themselves inadequately or defect entirely. Besides yielding superior results, grenz-ray therapy circumvents the discomfort and unpredictability of 5-fluorouracil with occlusion.

A recurrence rate of about 5% may be expected after 3 years; such lesions may be safely retreated with 1500 R. Often, precise mapping of preexisting lesions is difficult and it is uncertain whether a new or recurrent lesion is being treated. Occasionally, patients who have not been treated for a number of years will develop fresh lesions and present a striking contrast between previously treated and untreated areas (Fig. 15-7).

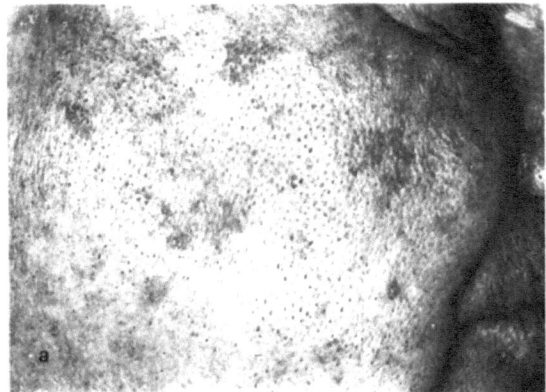

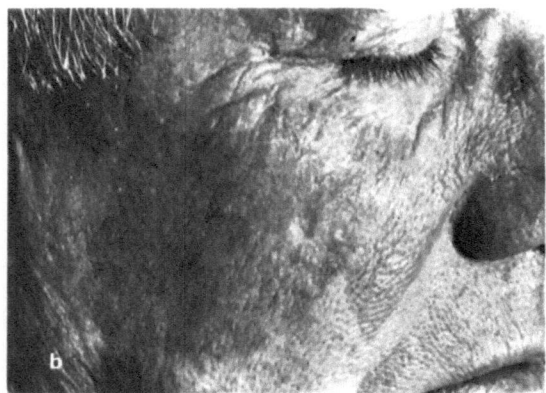

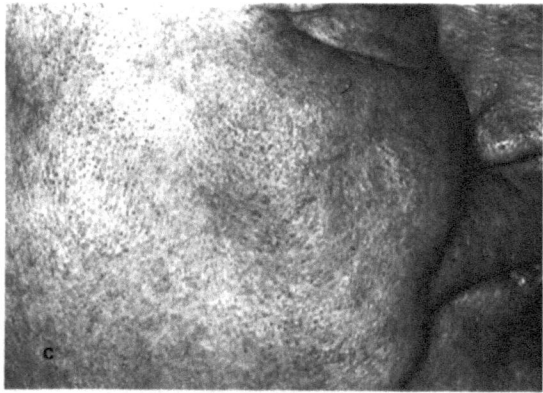

Figure 15-4.   Multiple facial actinic keratoses. *a*. Before treatment. *b*. Peak reaction, 20 days after treatment. *c*. Eight weeks after treatment.

Leukoplakia and Leukokeratosis

Although lingual and buccal lesions have been treated with grenz rays by others [6], I have found it difficult to obtain a vertical beam or maintain immobility of treatment şites during the required exposure times, and have abandoned attempts at intraoral therapy.

The single dose for lip lesions is 2000 to 2500 R, depending upon the microscopic depth of the lesion. Reactions are violent (Fig. 15-8), and patients are reassured that such reactions are both intentional and desirable. Topical corticosteriod ointments are provided for relief if these reactions become intolerable. I had found no clinical evidence that the application of topical corticosteroids to ameliorate severe reactions reduced the cure rate and this was confirmed in the recent study by Breza et al [4]. After 8 weeks, when these reactions have subsided, there is no visible scarring other than deep biopsy sites, in contrast to conventional x-ray therapy or various surgical approaches.

Bowen's Disease and Superficial Squamous Cell Carcinoma

Microscopic examination determines the susceptibility of these lesions to grenz rays, for the depth of each lesion and the thickness of its overlying stratum corneum create much therapeutic divergence. Consideration of tissue depth doses is most important, for they enable one to approximate absorbed quantities at different levels. Because the radiation absorbed by the stratum corneum is biologically inert, stratum corneum thickness must be discounted when considering that 75% of grenz rays are absorbed in the first millimeter of tissue. Since it is frequently difficult to estimate stratum corneum thickness in many skin sites, grenz-ray therapy for the disorders mentioned is employed only in areas where prejudging stratum corneum thickness does not unduly complicate dosage estimation.

Small specimens for biopsy are always taken from both the deepest and the most inflammatory portions of the lesion. Usually 2 doses of 3000 R are given with a 2-week interval between treatments. For more inflammatory lesions, this may be reduced to 2000 R on alternate weeks for 3 doses (Figs. 15-9 and 15-10). A different radiotherapeutic technique for Bowen's disease is discussed in Chapter 10.

Superficial Multicentric Basal Cell Epitheliomas of the Trunk

This generally employed term is a dangerous misnomer for these frequently arsenical-induced lesions. Instead of being superficial, an

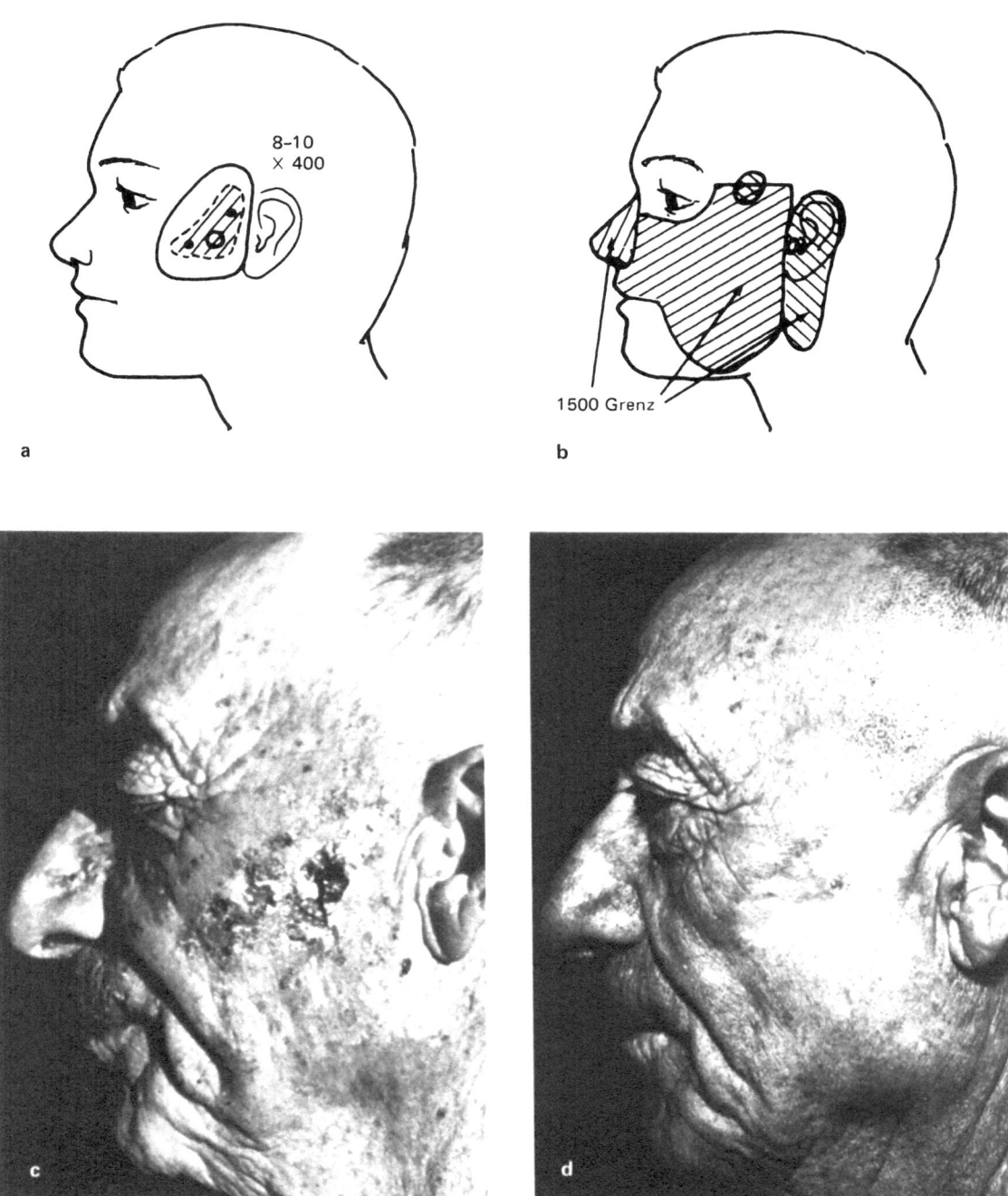

Figure 15-5.   Combined grenz-ray and x-ray therapy for sclerosing basal cell carcinoma and multiple actinic keratoses. *a*. Treatment diagram of x-ray therapy. *b*. Treatment diagram of grenz-ray therapy. *c*. Reaction 20 days after 2000 R of grenz rays, fractionated x-ray therapy in progress. *d*. Ten weeks after completing x-ray therapy, 10 × 400 R, 110 kVp, 3 times a week, to area delineated in treatment diagram.

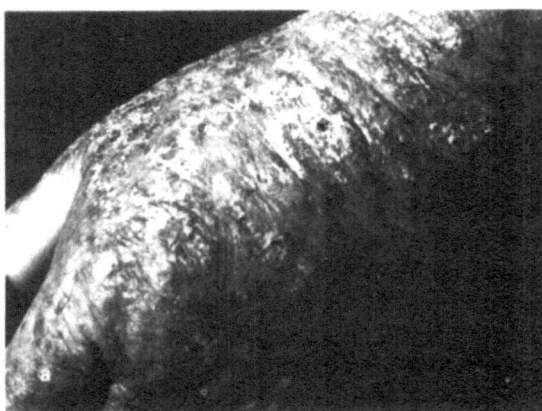 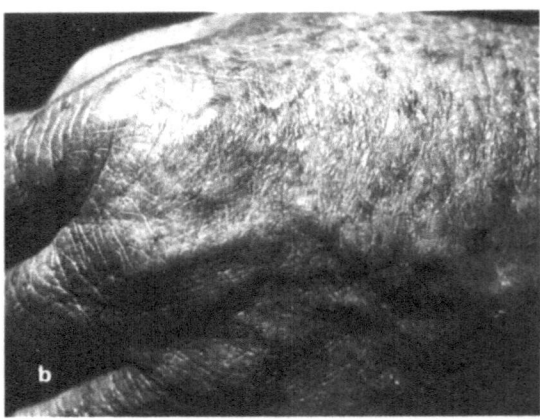

Figure 15-6. Multiple actinic keratoses of dorsal hand surface. *a*. Reaction of left dorsal hand 17 days after 1500 R of grenz rays. *b*. Thirteen weeks after treatment.

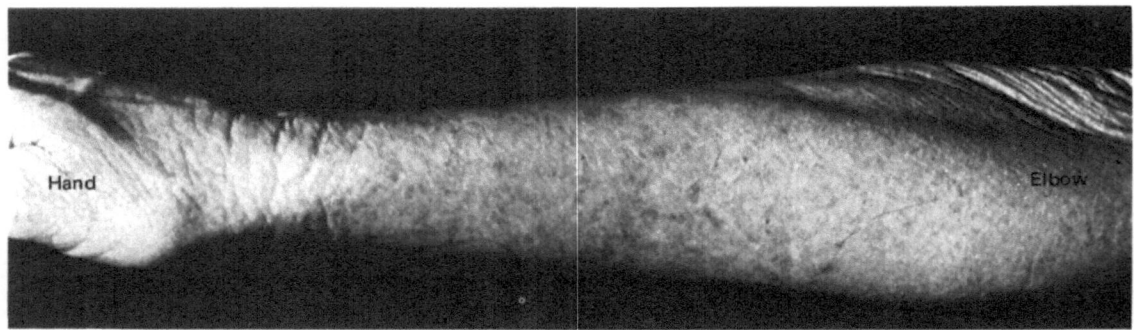

Figure 15-7. In this patient, the dorsal hand and forearm areas were treated with 1500 R of grenz rays 6 years previously. Note the sharp demarcation with untreated volar forearm surface, which has developed actinic keratoses in the interim.

occasional lesion may contain a deceptively deep fibroepitheliomatous component readily overlooked with either electrodesiccation and curettage or liquid nitrogen therapy; or portions of actual tumor may extend deep into the dermis. For such lesions, topical 5% or 20% 5-fluorouracil with occlusion is preferable, and any residuals should be managed by topical immunotherapy.

If biopsy specimens satisfy criteria for confident superficiality of lesions, the dosage of grenz rays is the same as that employed for Bowen's disease and very superficial squamous cell carcinomas (Fig. 15-11).

Psoriasis

The shallowness and accelerated turnover time of psoriasis combine to render it quintessentially susceptible to grenz-ray therapy (Fig. 12). Arouete [2] authoritatively explores minutiae

and concludes that grenz radiation "should be considered as one of the most useful external therapeutic agents in psoriasis. Apart from the results obtained, it outclasses other local therapy by its convenience in application."

Arouete [2] evaluated 309 patients. Poor results were defined as either irritation, exacerbation, absence of benefit, or rapid relapse. Thirty-nine of the 309 patients had poor results; these were patients with thick, lichenified hyperkeratotic plaques. Favorable results were defined as blanching of lesions for a minimum of 2 to 3 months. Of 309 cases, 207 had favorable results. The remainder had mediocre results. Frain-Bell and Bettley's [9] controlled paired comparison study of 86 cases concluded that grenz-ray therapy was effective. Harber [12] found grenz rays and conventional x rays to be equally effective in 76 unselected patients, as did Hanfling and Distelheim [11].

All patients are advised to bathe and remove scales before treatment, and lesions must be free of moisture or grease, for these will modify grenz-ray penetration. The major variables in dictating treatment technique are thickness of lesions and whether the psoriasis is "upswing" or stable.

Widespread lesions receive 200 R twice weekly for 4 or 5 doses, open field therapy. Witten [17] states that such a course of 800 to 1000 R may be repeated after an interval of 4 to 6 months, and he declares that this is probably conservative. Since in newer grenz-ray units the effective diameter of the field is essentially identical to the TSD, points 25 cm apart are treated without shielding when the TSD is 25 cm. Anterior and posterior extremities are treated at one sitting and lateral extremities are treated at the following sitting. Isolated discrete plaques may be treated at shorter distances with either open or closed techniques, depending upon anticipated posttreatment pigmentation.

Because of their thicker stratum cor-

neum, palms and soles may be safely given 400 R in each dose. Elbow and knee lesions, which are usually quite hyperkeratotic, respond to 300 R per treatment, as do hypertrophic pretibial plaques. Conversely, ear lesions are especially susceptible; they may clear with only 1 dose of 200 R. Open field treatment is given at a short distance to cover the external ear. Then the ear canal, after proper cleansing, is treated with a small-aperture closed cylinder at the same sitting. Anogenital lesions are especially susceptible to small doses of grenz rays [1]. In these areas particular care must be exerted to insure flat fields, vertical beams, and appropriate shielding techniques.

Pustular psoriasis and nail psoriasis do not respond to grenz-ray qualities. Because scalp lesions respond variably and effective topical scalp regimens are available, I do not employ grenz rays for scalp psoriasis, except when the lesions transgress onto glabrous skin.

Although grenz-ray therapy is probably safer, cleaner, cheaper, and more economical

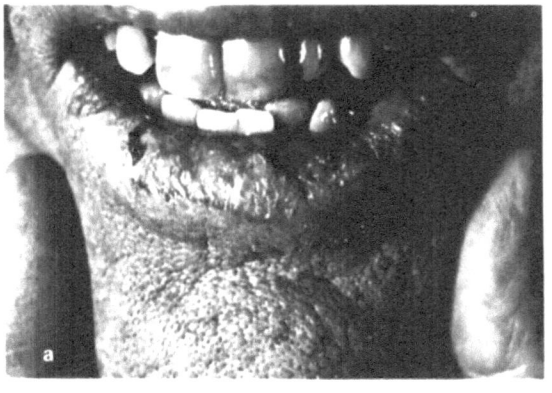
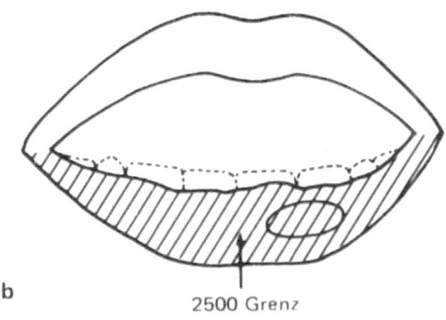
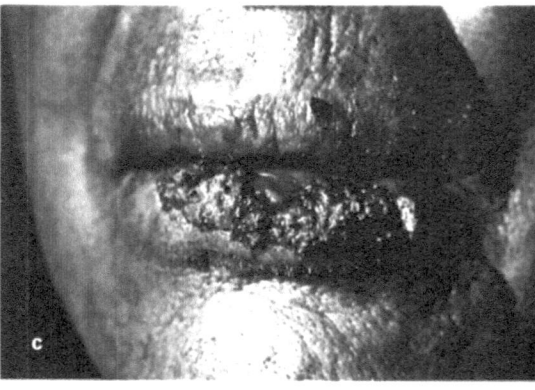
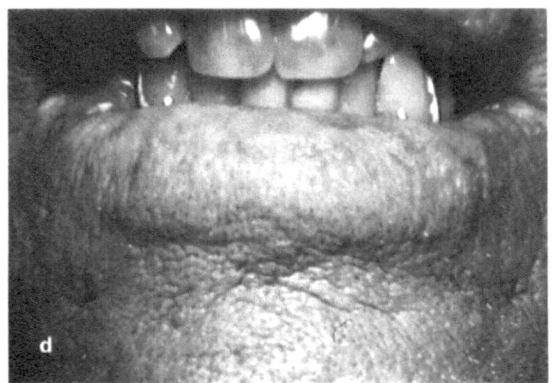

Figure 15-8. Extensive leukoplakia and leukokeratoses of the lower lip. *a*. Before treatment. *b*. Treatment diagram. *c*. Reaction 18 days after 2500 R of grenz rays. *d*. Fifty days after treatment.

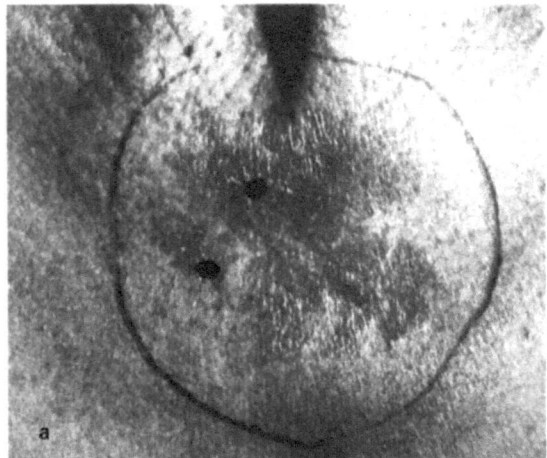

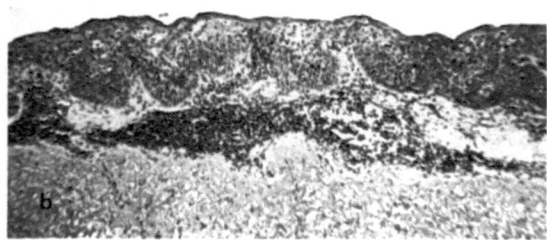

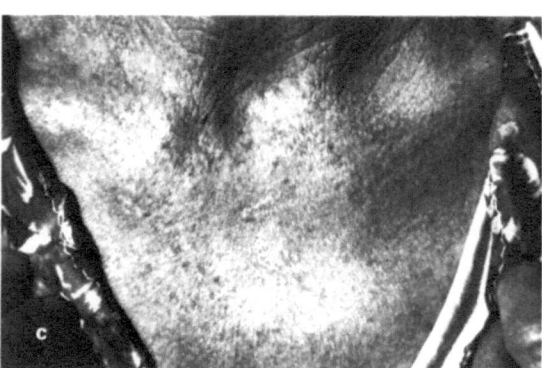

Figure 15-9.   Intraepithelial squamous cell carcinoma of supramanubrial area. Biopsy specimens were taken from the deepest and the most inflammatory areas. *a*. Before treatment. *b*. Superficiality of deepest area indicating susceptibility to grenz-ray therapy. *c*. Three months after 2 × 3000 R of grenz rays biweekly.

in time and effort for the patient, a major drawback to its widespread employment is its time consumption in a busy physician's office. A total body treatment may occupy 90 minutes of a technician's time, and tie up a treatment room for that long, so that appointment schedules must be carefully anticipated. The number of

patients who can benefit from grenz rays in a dermatologist's office may be limited by the availability of his ancillary personnel and the size of his physical plant.

Nummular Eczema

Of all the benign dermatoses, nummular eczema is the most responsive to grenz rays (Fig. 15-13). Indeed, one must be cautious not

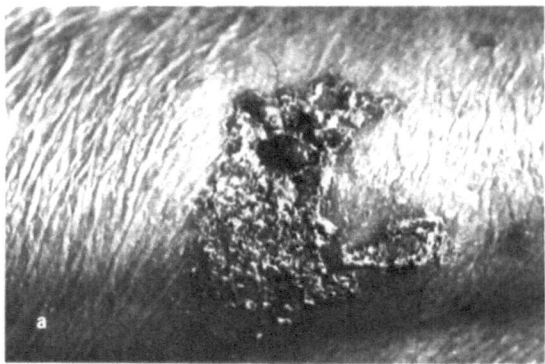

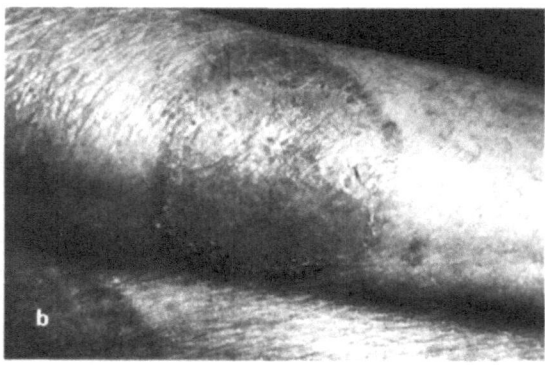

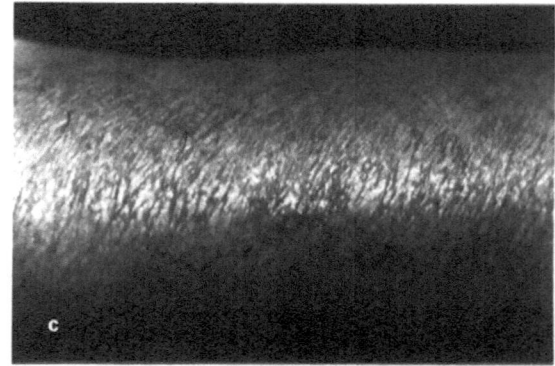

Figure 15-10.   Bowen's disease of left dorsal forearm. *a*. Before treatment. *b*. Six weeks after 3 × 2000 R of grenz rays biweekly. *c*. Six months later. Scars represent biopsy site.

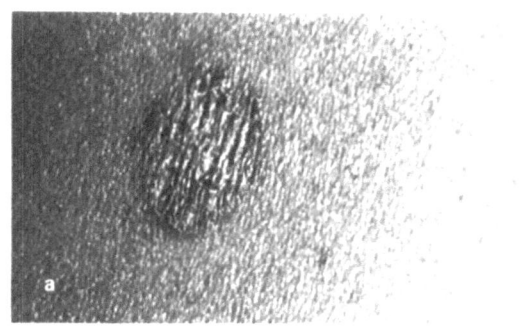

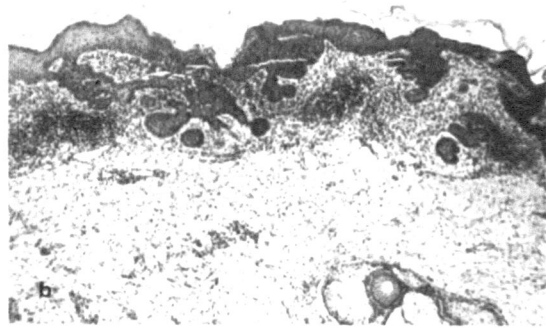

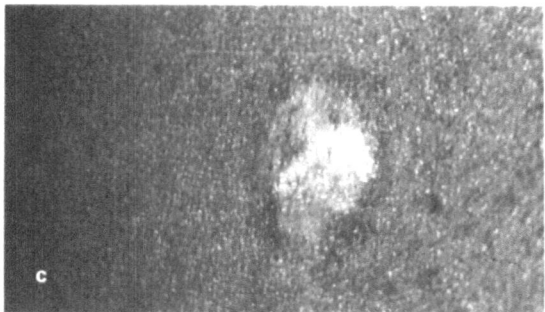

Figure 15-11. Superficial multicentric basal cell carcinoma of left arm. *a.* Before treatment. *b.* Microscopic appearance. Thin stratum corneum facilitates estimation of depth dosage. *c.* Nineteen months after 2 × 3000 R of grenz rays biweekly.

to overtreat, for even 300 R delivered in 1 dose to a susceptible lesion may produce intense vesiculation. The usual dose is 200 R once weekly; this is reduced to 100 to 150 R if the lesions are "juicy."

Atopic Dermatitis

Pruritic cubital and popliteal plaques resistant to topical measures respond well to 200 R once weekly for 3 or 4 doses, but other equally effective forms of therapy are available so that

this approach is seldom employed. Resistant chronic hand eczema, if a manifestation of adult atopic dermatitis, improves after 200 R to the dorsal hand and 300 R to the palmar surface delivered once weekly for 2 or 3 doses.

Immediate and remote results of treating chronic eczema, circumscribed neurodermatitis, and anogenital dermatitis with grenz rays were recently reported in the Russian literaure [16]. The authors concluded, after evaluating 385 patients, that "owing to greater efficiency and lack of complications, wider application of this simple method suitable for outpatient conditions is recommended in practical dermatology." However, most eczematous eruptions now respond adequatley to topical or intralesional therapy, so I have employed grenz rays only as an adjunctive measure in refractory cases.

Herpes Simplex

For many years, dermatologists have used small doses of grenz or x rays in an effort to abort early lesions of herpes simplex. Results were poorly evaluated and equivocal at best. However, Knight [13], in 1972, reviewed the literature on this subject and reported on 25 patients with recurrent herpes simplex who were treated with grenz rays, 200 R on alternate weeks for 4 doses, and assessed at intervals up to 2 years. Of the 25 patients, 50% were

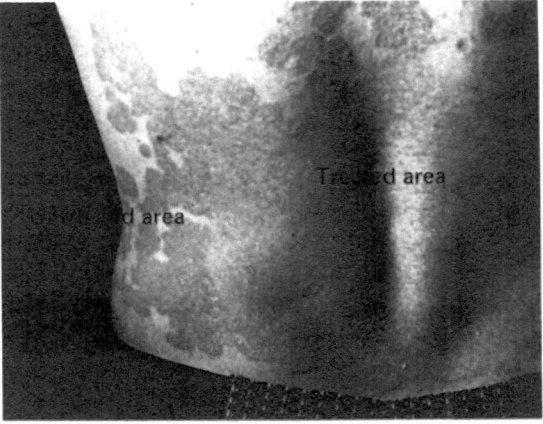

Figure 15-12. Psoriasis. Effect of 300 R of grenz rays administered to lumbar area 9 days previously. Closed cones were intentionally employed to demonstrate difference between treated and untreated areas.

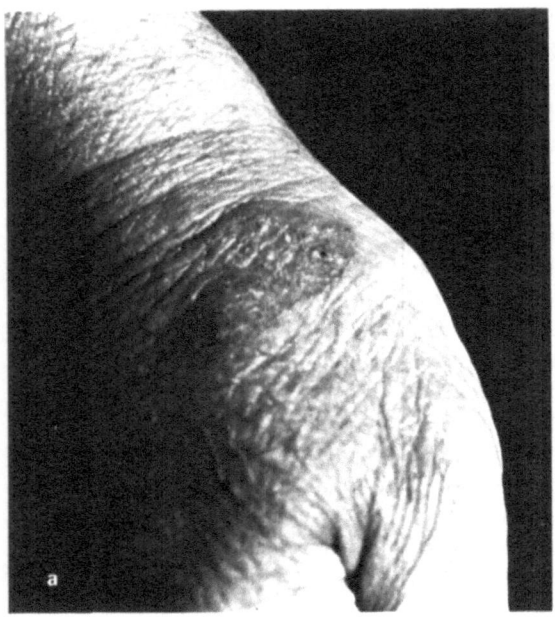 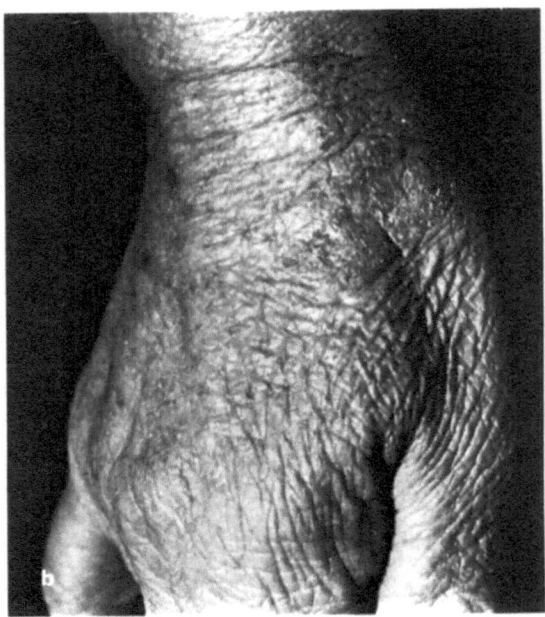

Figure 15-13. Nummular eczema, no topical therapy. *a.* Before treatment. *b.* One week after 200 R of grenz rays.

free of recurrences and a further 30% improved. In a control group of 10 patients, with no treatment whatsoever, the recurrence rate remained unchanged over this 2-year period. His results deserve confirmation by other investigators.

References

1. Abe Y, Sugai T, Saito T: Radiation angiokeratoma following grenz radiation. Arch Dermatol 100:294, 1969
2. Arouete J: Grenz-ray therapy. In Sidi E, Zagula-Mally ZW, Hincky M (eds): Psoriasis. Springfield, Ill, Thomas, 1968, pp 243–257
3. Baer RL, Witten VH: Selected aspects of dermatologic therapy with superficial x rays and grenz rays. In Year Book of Dermatology. Chicago, Year Book Medical, 1956
4. Breza T, Taylor R, Eaglstein WH: Noninflammatory destruction of actinic keratoses by fluorouracil. Arch Dermatol 112:1256, 1976
5. Brodkin RH, Bleidberg J: Neoplasia resulting from grenz irradiation. Arch Dermatol 97:307, 1968
6. Bucky G, Combes FC: Grenz-ray Therapy. New York, Springer, 1954, p 127
7. Demis DJ, et al: Clinical Dermatology. Hagerstown, Harper & Row, 1976
8. Fitzpatrick TB, et al: Dermatology in General Practice. New York, McGraw-Hill, 1971
9. Frain-Bell W, Bettley FR: The treatment of psoriasis and eczema with grenz rays. Br J Dermatol 71:379, 1959
10. Goldschmidt H: Ionizing radiation therapy in dermatology. Current use in the United States and Canada. Arch Dermatol 111:1511, 1975
11. Hanfling SL, Distelheim IH: Simultaneous symmetrical paired comparison method in evaluating results of grenz-ray and of x-ray therapy. J Invest Dermatol 16:65, 1951
12. Harber LC: Clinical evaluation of radiation therapy in psoriasis. Arch Dermatol 77:554, 1958
13. Knight, AG: Grenz ray treatment of recurrent herpes simplex. Br J Dermatol 86:172, 1972
14. Lewis HM, Mutscheller A: Quality, intensity, and field distribution of radiation emitted from a new type of low voltage roentgen therapy tube. J Invest Dermatol 12:324, 1949
15. Meyer J: Les rayons limites de Bucky en dermatologie. Ann Dermatol Syphiligr (Paris) 91:137, 1964
16. Torsoev NA, Murzenko DI, Dasheyskaya YA: Grenz ray treatment of itching dermatoses. Vestn Dermatol Venerol 44:35, 1970
17. Witten VH: The place of grenz radiation in dermatologic practice. Arch Dermatol 81:110, 1960

Introduction to Chapters 16 through 20

Hugh M. Crumay

In medicine, as in nature, modalities that promote healing of diseased body cells may be modified to destroy tissue. Physical agents may prompt anabolism or catabolism, soothe or irritate, sedate or stimulate nerves, slow or speed circulation, and retard or hasten growth of microorganisms, as well as cause physiochemical, electrochemical, and photochemical alterations.

Let us consider the phenomenon of heat. Heat may result from the conversion of all forms of energy; the degree of change may be modified to produce varied effects. Principle sources of heat are chemical reactions, mechanical actions (friction or vibration), electricity, and light. Of course, chemical activity in or outside the body, including cellular metabolic activity, produces heat. Conductors of electricity, such as filaments or wires in lights and heaters, become hot because they resist the flow of electric current. In somewhat the same fashion, body tissues are heated as they resist the passage of electromagnetic waves. Cells are injured or destroyed when limits of physiologic tolerance are violated.

In general, heat is transferred in 4 ways: (1) conduction: a colder body is warmed or burned by a hotter body through molecular collision (eg, skin is touched by hot metal); (2) conversion: other forms of energy are changed to heat (eg, electromagnetic radiations that are transformed to heat because of tissue resis-

tance); (3) convection: a limited portion of the atmosphere is placed in motion (eg, hot air rising in a heating system); and (4) radiation: a substance is warmed through an unaffected medium (as the earth is heated by the sun). Electrocautery surgery and electrosurgery produce heat by conduction and conversion, respectively, to destroy tissue.

Cold can be just as destructive, and beneficial, as heat. Tissue may be destroyed by freezing. If heat results from the internal vibration of body molecules, cold may be considered a negative condition resulting from a decrease in the amount of molecular collision [26]. In any event, all physical energy applied to the body exerts primary physical effects which cause secondary physiologic changes.

All of us recognize the need for accurate diagnosis and awareness of underlying pathology if we are properly to apply physical forces to treat disease. Some, however, fail to realize the importance of understanding our instruments, even though a complete knowledge of complex characteristics is usually not necessary. The dermatologic therapist and surgeon should be familiar with the elementary laws of electricity, the basic physical prinicples involved in the application of physical modalities, and the construction of simple generators, and should have an appreciation of how instruments work.

Among physicians, only the dermatologist is apt to understand the pathology of the skin. He should be best able to apply physical forces to treat integumentary disease, if he is properly informed. High frequency electric current (for surgical diathermy) is probably the most valuable physical agent available to the majority of dermatologists at present. It is of proven value in many conditions, procedures are established, and results are easily reproduced. Effects are visible and predictable. Use can be controlled as a "fine art," while rapidity and safety are desirable virtues. Acceptable cosmetic results are usually very good and often superior (Fig. I-1). This is also true of electrocautery and especially cryogens. Ideally, all dermatologists will be expert diathermy surgeons, electrocautery surgeons, and cryosurgeons.

Today, perhaps more than ever, all procedures must be examined from the economic standpoint. It is quite clear that office care costs less than either outpatient or inpatient hospital care. This is most evident when we compare the cost of office surgery to the cost of more expensive hospital surgery. All the modalities discussed in this book, with the exception of the laser beam and the plasma torch, can presently be applied in the office. Electrosurgery, electrocautery surgery, and cryogenic surgery greatly increase the scope of office practice, resulting in substantial reduction of medical cost.

References for Chapters 17 through 20 will appear at the end of Chapter 20.

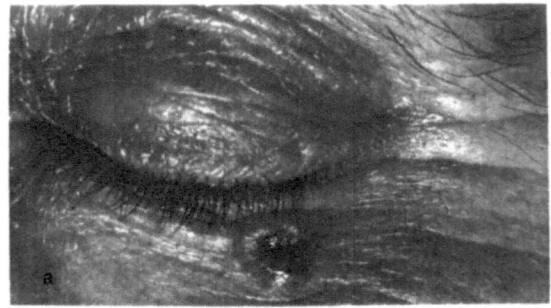

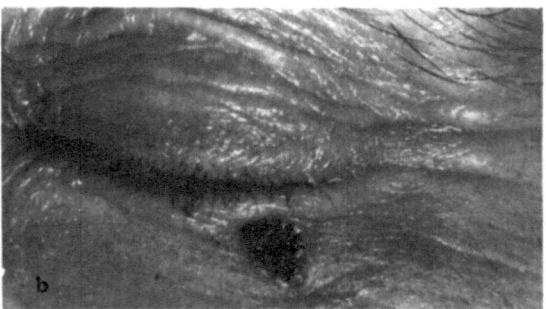

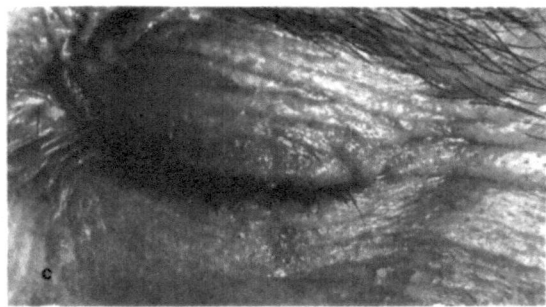

Figure I-1.   Removal of basal cell cancer. *a.* Cancer before surgery. *b.* Five days after electrosurgery (excision and electrocoagulation). *c.* Nineteen days after removal. Surgery resulted in cure and a superior cosmetic appearance comparable to that following plastic surgery. From Pillsbury DM, Shelley WB, Kligman AM: Dermatology. Philadelphia, Saunders, 1956. Courtesy of W. B. Saunders Co.

16

Electricity

Hugh M. Crumay

Electricity may be static (at rest) or dynamic (in motion). Dermatologists ordinarily do not use static electricity. On the other hand, they use dynamic electricity every day, in general much more so than any other physical modality, for electrotherapy and especially for electrosurgery. Understandably, we must stress the importance of the proper use of electricity.

Currently, the electron theory is used to explain electric phenomena: particles of matter, ie, atoms and molecules, may have a negative (excess of electrons) or positive (deficit of electrons) electric charge. Electrons are added to a body to give it a negative charge. Addition of these electrons entails work, represented by potential energy (electromotive force) expressed as volts. This force may be increased and held in a state of tension (stored) until it is released. Differences in electric potential may be generated by chemical energy, mechanical forms of energy (ie, friction and vibration), and heat.

A flow of electrons (transmission of energy), known as an electric current, permits us to make use of accumulated energy; this results when two bodies differing in potential charge are connected by a conductor. Good conductors are substances, such as electrolytes and metals, that contain electrons "free" of their atoms; they also conduct heat easily. Insulators are materials that resist the flow of electricity, eg, distilled water, rubber, glass, and porcelain.

Current flow continues until a difference in potential no longer exists between connected bodies. Obviously, flow can be maintained indefinitely if conductor terminals are connected to a functioning generator or battery.

Amperes are electrical units used to measure current transmission. Amperemeters, otherwise known as ammeters or, in medical applications, milliammeters, are used to measure intensity of flow. Amperage (flow of electrons) is dependent on the voltage (electromotive force) at the source and the resistance of the conductor expressed in ohms. Since a good conductor passes (conducts) current more easily than does a poor conductor, resistance is inversely proportional to current flow. Ohm's law expresses the relationship of the three factors: Intensity (amperage) is directly proportional to the electromotive force (voltage) and inversely proportional to the resistance ($I = E/R$ or $E = IR$).

Every complete electric circuit requires a continuous path from the generating source through all conductors back to the source. If current is direct (DC) the electron flow continues unchanged in the same direction (Fig. 16-1). In the case of alternating current (AC) the electron flow changes direction periodically, and the intensity varies continuously (Fig. 16-2).

Graphically, the voltage of direct current, ie, galvanic current, may be represented as a

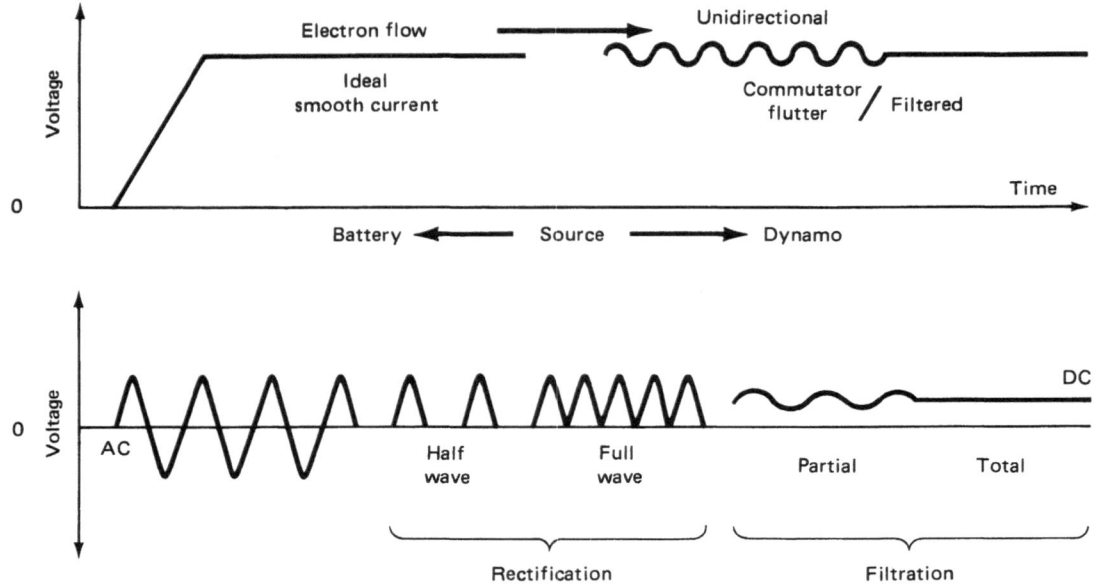

Figure 16-1.   Direct (galvanic) currents and their sources (battery, dynamo, and alternating current). Changes necessary to smooth dynamo currents (by filtration) (above) and alternating currents (by rectification and filtration) (below) so that they simulate ideal battery currents.

straight line above the zero (neutral) level. A battery is the simplest form of a direct current generator and current flow is "smooth." The graph of galvanic current produced by a dynamo is wavy due to commutator flutter. Current flow is smoothed by "filtration," accomplished by incorporating additional condensers and inductors (coils or choke coils) in the circuit. Alternating current, the form usually available commercially, may be changed (rectified) by thermionic tubes, commonly called vacuum tubes or valve tube rectifiers, and semiconductor rectifiers, substituted for tubes

in solid-state apparatus, to form a fairly smooth galvanic (direct) current. After proper rectification, flow can be made to mimic that of a battery by proper filtration. At present such rectifiers are usually used to change alternating current to direct current.

Alternating current voltage is diagrammatically depicted as two successive alternations (impulses) that make up a wave (cycle), one-half above and one-half below the neutral line. Today frequency is usually expressed in hertz (cycles per second). Arbitrarily, low frequency currents alternate at a rate below 100 kilohertz (100,000 hertz). Alternating current of a frequency less than 10 kilohertz (10,000 hertz), like interrupted direct current, stimulates nerves and muscles to contract spasmodically. Resulting convulsions may be fatal. High frequency currents, as one may expect, oscillate at a rate greater than 100 kilohertz. In dermatologic surgery, it is common to use high frequency current that oscillates at rates varying from 500 to 3000 kilohertz (0.5 to 3 megahertz). Practically speaking, any frequency in this range produces the same results. To heat body tissues medically (hopefully without any destruction) currents with frequencies ranging from more than 3 to 3000 megahertz are em-

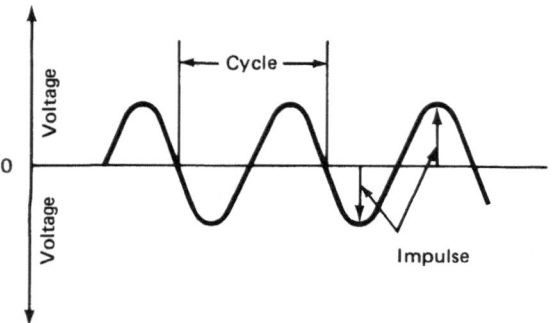

Figure 16-2.   Diagram of alternating current (sine wave).

ployed. With high frequency alternating current a form of dielectric heating (rapid and uniform heating caused by an electromagnetic field in a nonconducting material) replaces the contractions caused by low frequency current.

Some terms used to describe alternating currents in general, and diathermy currents in particular, may be confusing. We must remember that descriptions such as long wave and short wave—low frequency and high frequency—are meaningful only by comparison (Fig. 16-3).

When electric current flows the following phenomena always occur: (1) heat develops in all parts of the circuit, (2) a magnetic field develops, and, sometimes, (3) a chemical reaction takes place. Both alternating and direct currents produce thermal and magnetic effects. Only direct currents, practically speaking, induce net movements of ions (ion transfer) necessary to produce chemical effects. It is easy to comprehend that rapid changes in direction of current flow—a necessity with rapidly oscillating (high frequency) alternating currents—prevent ion transfer; hence, chemical reaction is impossible.

Rise of temperature in a conductor of electric current occurs in accordance with Joule's laws: it is directly proportional to the square of current strength (I^2), to resistance (R) and to the time that current flows (t). Both direct and alternating currents produce primary heating effects in all conductors, including body tissues. Secondary heating effects develop due to chemical reaction when direct current passes through electrolytic solutions, including body fluids.

It is not strange, therefore, that heating action of electric current in the human body is also governed by Joule's law (I^2Rt). Here the body is the conductor. But it is a "poor" conductor because it offers resistance and heats up. Body tissues vary in their resistance and one should expect those with higher resistance to become warmer or hotter. This may not be true if parallel paths of higher and lower resistance exist, because current tends to follow the path of least resistance.

The skin is a relatively poor conductor, largely because horny keratin is a good insulator. Body tissues vary in their conductivity. Those containing the most water are richest in ions and are the best conductors. Muscle and brain are the best conductors and subcutaneous tissues are relatively good conductors; but tendons are (as are fasciae) poor conductors. Bones are the poorest conductors. Complexity of tissues alters and confuses the picture. Peripheral nerves intrinsically conduct better than does muscle; however, surrounding fat and fascia, both poorer conductors, decrease the overall conduction.

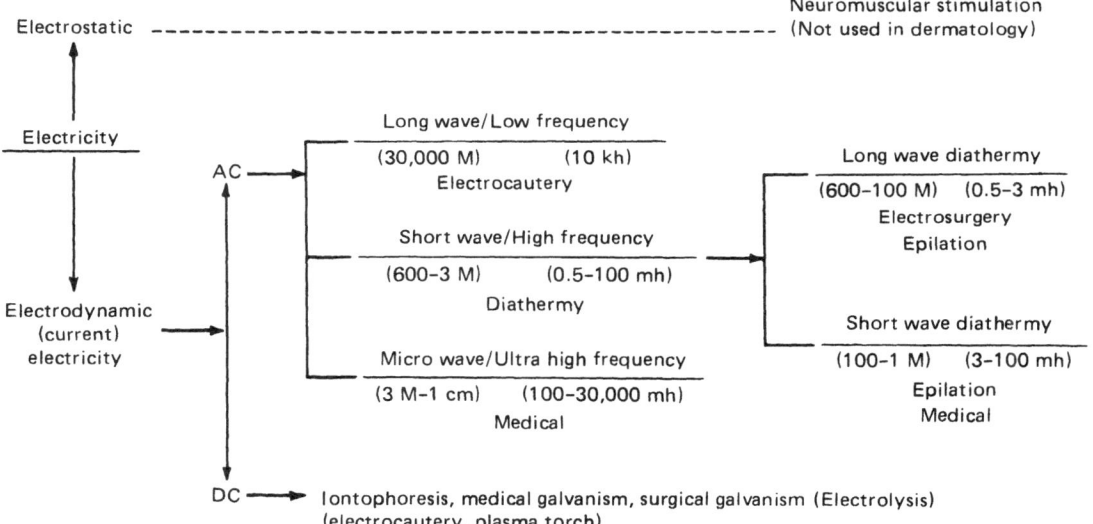

Figure 16-3. Dermatologic and medical uses of electricity. Types, wavelengths, and frequencies of alternating current. cm, centimeter; kh, kilohertz; M, meter; mh, megahertz. Courtesy of W. B. Saunders Co.

17

Direct Current: Iontophoresis and Galvanic Surgery

Hugh M. Crumay

Direct (galvanic) current may be used by dermatologists for ion transfer (medical galvanism, iontophoresis, and surgical galvanism) and to heat electrocautery terminals (Table 17-1); in the future we may use it to generate plasma for the plasma torch. Electrolysis (surgical galvanism) is currently used with decreasing frequency for hair removal and limited surgery. It results in dissolution of tissue caused by the formation of chemical caustic (sodium hydroxide) following ion transfer. Electrocauteries may be heated by either direct or alternating current to perform limited or extensive surgery. Heat is conducted from red-hot cautery tips (cf, branding irons or soldering irons) to comparatively cold bodies and tissue destruction follows.*

A battery of adequate voltage is the simplest source of direct current. Batteries are composed of a series of galvanic cells, each consisting of two metals and an electrolyte (Fig. 17-1). When metals enter a chemical solution electrons are liberated and electricity is chemically produced. In the galvanic cell ions flow from the negative (cathode) to the positive (anode) pole; current flows (by definition) in the

opposite direction from the positive to the negative pole. Negative ions flow in the same direction as electrons, from the negative to the positive battery terminal; positive ions flow in the same direction as the current flow, from the positive to the negative battery terminal. A common single dry cell using a zinc container for the negative electrode and a central carbon rod for the positive electrode produces about 1.5 V. The average resistance encountered in the human body approximates 1000 ohms [25]. According to Ohm's law, the amperage produced in the body by 1.5 V is 0.0015 A (1.5 mA). A battery of 45 V may be made by connecting 30 galvanic cells (dry cells) in series.

Battery weight and replacement cost usually make it more practical to use current from power lines (power mains) as a source of direct current. When a direct current main is accessible, a shunt resistance may be used to reduce current to a satisfactory therapeutic level. Such current is rarely supplied in the United States, and a rectifier is employed to change the usually available alternating current into direct current. The vacuum or valve tube rectifier uses thermionic tubes (eg, diodes, triodes, pentodes) to produce half-wave or full-wave rectification. Increasingly solid-state metallic rectifiers (semiconductor rectifiers) are preferred to tubes. In either case, the resulting direct current is not smooth as is a battery current. Filters consisting of capacitors (condensers) and

---

*Low frequency alternating current, as well as direct current, is used for electrocautery. High frequency alternating current, on the other hand, is used for surgical diathermy; destruction of tissue by conversive heat results when a comparatively warm body resists passage of high frequency oscillations emitted by a cold electrode.

190

Table 17-1 *Dermatologic Uses of Direct Current and Techniques of Application*

Purpose or Use	Method of Treatment	Agent	Electrode	Time (min)	Current (mA)
Terminate hyperhidrosis	Medical galvanism (experimental)	Tap water	Anode (+)	15+	15–20
Produce anhidrosis		Tap water	Anode (+)	15+	15–20
Decrease edema	Iontophoresis (experimental and possibly therapeutic)	Hyalouronidase	Anode (+)	20	20
Cause vasodilation		Histamine (1% jelly)	Anode (+)	3–5	2–10
Treat varicose ulcer		Methacholine	Anode (+)	20	5–30
Treat tinea pedis		Copper sulfate (1% solution)	Anode (+)	10–15	5–15
Surgery (destruction)	Surgical galvanism (including electrolysis)	Needle	Cathode (−)	0.5–1.0	0.5–2.0
Epilation (destruction)		Needle	Cathode (−)	0.5–1.0	0.5–1.5
Surgery (destruction)	Cautery	"Hot wire"	No polarity	Varies	15 A
Surgery (destruction)	Plasma torch	Torch: hot flame	None	Does Not Apply	

Modified after Moschelle SL, Pillsbury DM, Hurley HJ: Dermatology, Vol 2. Philadelphia, Saunders, 1975.

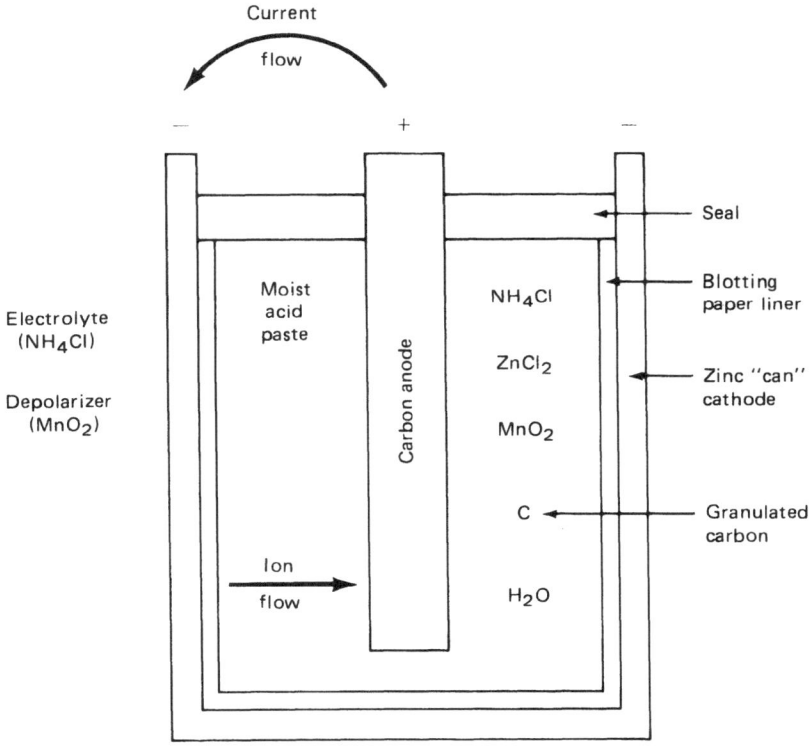

Figure 17-1. Diagram of dry cell, a simple source of galvanic current (DC) for therapeutic purposes. Wet cells are not suitable because of polarization (gas deposited on electrodes increases resistance, setting up a counter electromotive force). Note that current flows (by definition) from the positive pole to the negative pole, while ions flow (as expected) from the negative pole to the positive pole.

inductors (coils, choke coils) are incorporated within the circuit to smooth the current so that it simulates the ideal battery current.

We must always protect and isolate the patient from the power source. To do this isolation transformers must be incorporated in all electromedical apparatus operated from power lines. The isolation transformer prevents dangerous shocks when the patient or physician accidentally touches grounded objects, such as plumbing or electric fixtures.

Direct current flow is controlled by a simple rheostat or, better, by a potentiometer (Fig. 17-2). The rheostat (adjustable resistance) is placed in series with the patient. A potentiometer (resistance with adjustable tap) is placed across the voltage source in parallel with the patient. The potentiometer is preferred because output voltage is less affected by patient resistance and a smoother increase in current output is possible. A milliammeter is used to measure direct current and must be placed in series in the circuit. This is the only way one can measure direct current dosage and lessen the chance of burn with galvanic generators.

Every constant (galvanic, direct) current generator has a positive and a negative pole. Only direct current, never alternating current, is applied according to polarity. To be therapeutically effective, an electrode must be connected to the proper pole. Terminals must be clearly marked positive (+) or negative (−). However, when a power line is the source of direct current, the polarity of the terminals will change whenever the plug is inserted into the supply outlet in a different direction.

If there is any question regarding correct polarity, test by inserting the terminal tips, about 2 inches apart, into a weak salt solution. When current is turned on many small bubbles of hydrogen gas soon appear about the negative pole or cathode. Fewer and larger bubbles of oxygen gas appear about the other tip, the positive pole or anode (Fig. 17-3). In addition, a red spot will appear at the cathode tip if the terminals are touched to blotting paper moistened with dilute phenolphthalein solution (effect of alkaline NaOH).

Ion Transfer

In its pure state water does not conduct electricity. Aqueous solutions containing acids, bases, or salts are conductors of electricity known as electrolytes. When electrolytic substances (salts) dissolve in water, they dissociate into component-charged ions until an equilibrium is reached between the dissociated ions and the amount of salt dissolved. Metals, bases, and alkaloids are electropositive; acids and acid radicals are electronegative. The process of dissociation is called ionization (this does not imply that ions are driven into the body by electricity).

If a direct current is applied to an electrolytic solution it passes through the solution due to the migration of dissociated ions. Positively charged ions (cations) travel to the negative pole (cathode) while negatively charged ions (anions) migrate to the positive pole (anode). Movement of ions under electrical influence or "pressure" is called ion transfer. Iontophoresis (New Latin) refers to the introduction of drugs through normal (uninjured) skin by the transfer of ions effected by means of the application of a direct current. It is the medical term used to

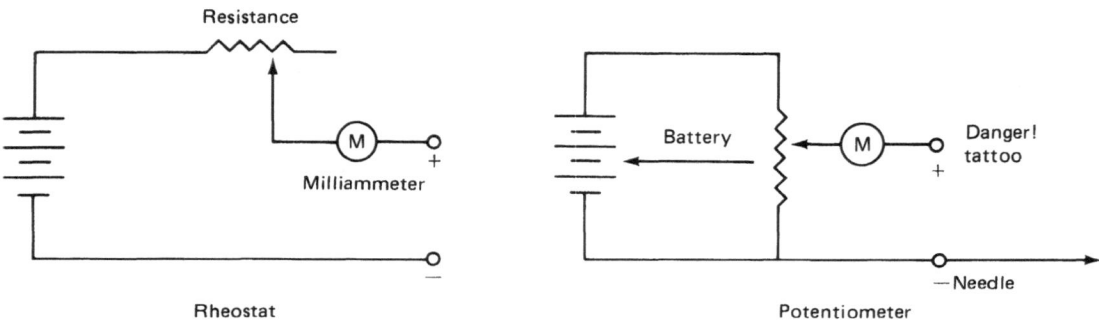

Figure 17-2. Diagrams of rheostat and potentiometer—devices used to control direct current applications. In galvanic surgery, including electrolysis, the negative electrode is used for destruction to prevent metallic tattoo of tissue.

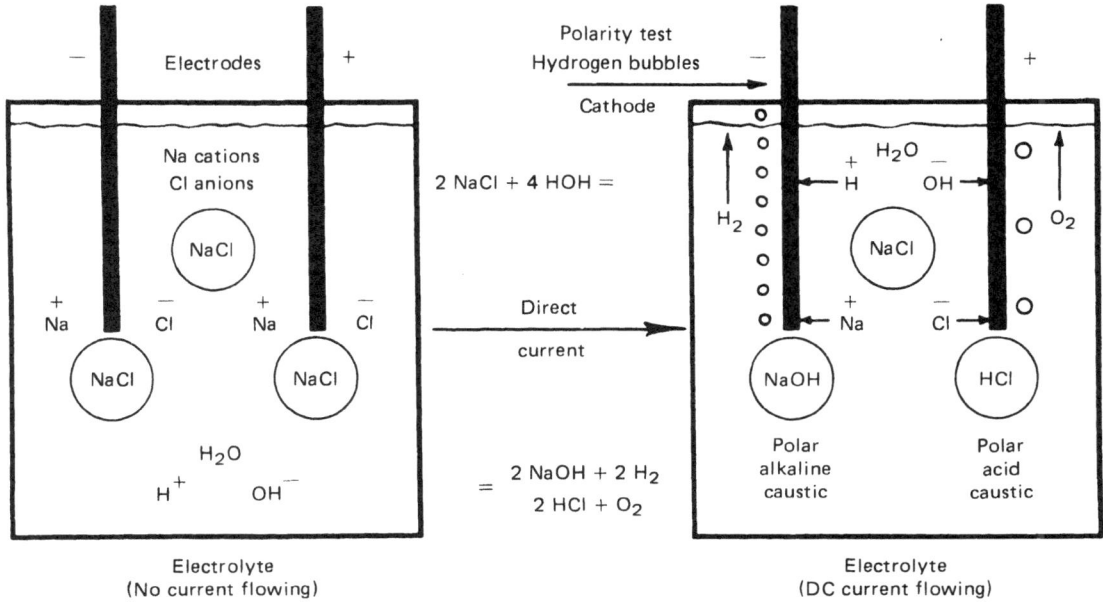

Figure 17-3. Dissociation of ions (ionization) and effect of direct current application (ion transfer) in electrolytes. The principle of ion transfer is used to test for polarity, to force ions into the body (iontophoresis), and for galvanic surgery (including electrolysis). Note that secondary chemical reactions cause polar alkaline and acid caustic effects in saline solutions, including those in body tissues.

indicate therapeutic transfer of ions into the body.

Whenever a direct electric current is impressed on an electrolyte such as sodium chloride ($NaCl$) solution ionization results. Charged sodium and chlorine atoms are attracted by and migrate to the pole with an opposite charge. Sodium cations ($Na+$) travel to the cathode ($-$Pole) while chlorine atoms move to the anode ($+$ Pole), and they lose their charges through chemical reactions when they arrive at their polar destinations. As unelectrified free atoms they cause secondary chemical reactions. An alkaline reaction occurs at the negative pole due to the formation of caustic sodium hydroxide ($NaOH$) and hydrogen (H). Hydrogen is liberated to rise to the surface of the solution in the form of gas bubbles, as in the polarity test. At the opposite positive pole a caustic acid reaction occurs as hydrochloric acid (HCl) and oxygen (O) are formed. Oxygen also escapes from the solution in the form of gas bubbles (Fig. 17-4). The intensity of the reactions is directly related to the strength and density of the electric current at each pole. Since acid and alkaline reactions in the electrolyte occur only in the vicinity of the poles (electrodes) they are described as polar effects. The same sequence of events occurs in the salt solution of body tissues. Formation of alkaline and acid caustics can result in destruction of tissue and is the basis of galvanic surgery. Precipitation of heavy metals such as copper, zinc, and silver may occur under electrodes applied to the surface of the skin; formation of such insoluble proteinates may hinder penetration of ions into the body during iontophoresis.

Colloidal molecules, fat droplets, and other body cells may be charged electrically by absorption; electrophoresis or cataphoresis occurs when these substances move toward the negative pole under the influence of direct current. Electroosmosis results when the water content of tissue shifts physically through electrically charged membranes. Thermal effects also develop. The continuous passage of current in fluids of different ionic composition and conductivity, as well as across or around cell membranes of varying permeability, is a complicated biophysical process. The clinical effects of direct current in tissue are outlined in Table 17-2.

Although skin is relatively impervious to the passage of water, the epithelium acts as a porous membrane and the extracellular fluid of the corium acts as an electrolytic solution. An

Table 17-2   *Clinical Effects of Direct Current, from Positive and Negative Poles, on Tissue*

DC Effects	Anode (+ Pole)	Cathode (− Pole)
Feeling of heat	Mild	Mild
Vasomotor change	Stimulation	Stimulation
Type of ions repelled	Metal, alkaloid	Acid, acid radical
Pain (intensity)	Moderate to severe	Mild
Tissue change	Tissue hardened	Tissue softened
Effect on nerves	Nerves sedated	Nerves irritated

electric current may be used to repel medicinal ions with a like charge and push or drive them into the skin (iontophoresis), despite the fact that the body part will not absorb the electrolyte (Fig. 17-4). Again, it will be obvious that knowing the polarity will permit us to connect electrodes to the proper terminals.

During iontophoresis precipitation of heavy metals such as copper, zinc, and silver may occur beneath electrodes in contact with the skin or mucosae. These precipitates may combine with tissue protein to form a barrier of insoluble proteinates, which hinder penetration of ions into the body. Such alterations and "hardening" of tissue at the positive pole may cause metal electrodes to stick to mucous membranes. Since current from the negative pole softens tissue, reversal of current flow will loosen adherent applicators.

It has been noted that we also use galvanic current (DC) for medical and surgical galvanism, as well as for heating the electrocautery and creating the flame of the plasma torch. Medical galvanism occurs when direct current is impressed on substances such as distilled water [23] or tap water [2] to force "nonmedicinal" ions into the skin. Surgical galvanism refers to the destruction of tissue with the negative electrode due to the polar (localized) alkaline caustic effect, which follows ion transfer. Electrocautery is not related to ion transfer, since the operating tip (electrode) is heated to incandescence by ohmic resistance of metal to the passage of either direct or alternating current. Ionization as it develops in the plasma torch will be discussed in Chapter 24.

Moist pad electrodes are always used for medical galvanism and iontophoresis. Electrodes may be concentrating or dispersing as they are smaller or larger. Mistakenly, it has become the practice to call only the concentrating electrode "active." All electrodes are active to some degree. Since electrodes must be properly moistened at all times, foot or hand baths may serve as both wet pad electrodes for medical galvanism and iontophoresis, and as the dispersing electrode in surgical galvanism. Electrodes should be of equal size whenever localized polarity effects are not important, as in medical galvanism.

In iontophoresis we want to drive electrically charged ions into the skin. After polarity is determined, electrodes are connected to the proper terminals. Ions with a positive charge will be pushed into the skin by a positive charge, while negatively charged ions will be impelled by a negative charge. The so-called active, driving, or concentrating electrode may be smaller than the dispersing electrode. It is improper to refer to the latter as inactive.

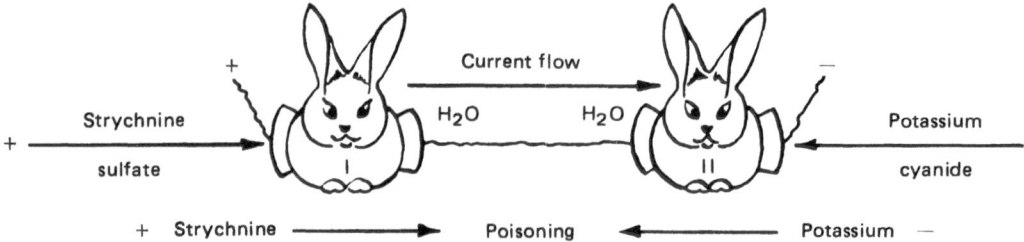

Figure 17-4.   Iontophoresis (Leduc's experiment). Direct current is passed through two rabbits connected in series. Electrodes are soaked in strychnine sulfate, water, and potassium cyanide as indicated. When DC flows the positive strychnine ion is repelled by the positive pole while the negative cyanide ion is repelled by the negative pole. The ions are forced into their respective rabbits so that both rabbits die, one of strychnine poisoning and one of cyanide poisoning. If current flow is reversed the ions are not repelled and the rabbits are unharmed. Modified from Watkins AL: A Manual of Electrotherapy. Philadelphia, Lea & Febiger, 1958.

Electrodes are best placed in contact with only unbroken, normally sensitive skin. To prevent shock gradually increase current from zero to the desired level. A current reversing switch is desirable; in medical galvanism this permits treatment of two extremities without changing electrodes. After completing iontophoresis current should be reduced slowly, and then reversed for a short time. Reversal may be necessary to loosen an electrode following the application of some metals to mucosal surfaces. Initially treatment should last 15 or 20 minutes; as tolerance develops time may be doubled.

There should be no undue patient discomfort if iontophoretic applications are correct. Initial mild tingling or prickly sensations, followed by a feeling of pleasant warmth, are to be expected. Painful or burning sensations, such as "hot spots," mean that the current is too intense or improperly concentrated. Remove, inspect, and reapply electrodes! Take special precautions if there is any disturbance of sensation (disease or scar), or if the skin is broken (abrasion or ulcer). Petrolatum, cold cream, collodion, adhesive plaster, and sheet rubber should protect inflamed, fissured, and denuded skin.

Epilation by electric current is presently considered the only safe and cosmetically acceptable method to permanently remove hair. Hair may be removed either by direct current of low voltage and amperage or by alternating current of higher voltage and amperage. Electrolysis implies only direct current destruction of the hair root by localized polar chemical cautery; heat results from the formation of alkaline caustic sodium hydroxide at the tip of the negative electrode (Fig. 17-5). Epilation by alternating current is possible after the hair root is destroyed by conversive heat: high frequency electric oscillations are converted into heat as the tissues resist passage of the waves. Both types of epilation will be discussed together because techniques and results are similar.

The rheostat or potentiometer used to control direct current for ion transfer is also used for electrolysis. High frequency spark gap, vacuum tube, or solid-state machines, to be discussed in Chapter 18 are used for hair removal by alternating current. Inserting a proper resistance to reduce current into the biterminal coagulation circuit of a spark gap

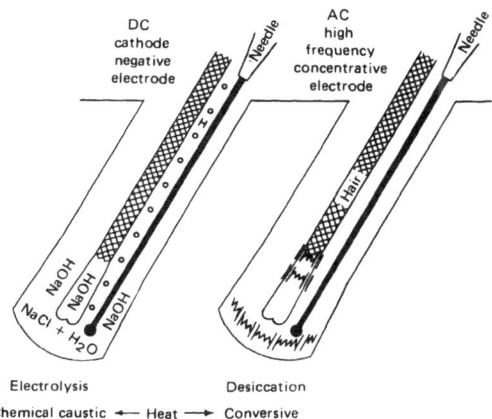

Figure 17-5. Epilation by electric currents (diagrammatic). In electrolysis direct current from the negative electrode causes formation of destructive caustic alkaline chemicals and liberation of hydrogen gas. High frequency alternating current destroys the hair because tissue resistance causes conversion of electrical energy into destructive heat.

machine, eg, the "Bovie," makes the reduced current satisfactory for epilation.

Before attempting electrolysis, attach the needle to the negative electrode! Surgical galvanism or negative galvanism results in ion transfer, formation of caustic sodium hydroxide, and release of hydrogen. Tissues are softened or liquefied by alkaline (caustic) cautery and the hair root is destroyed. The needle does not stick in the follicle. Pain is largely due to caustic, not to galvanic current. Since positively charged metallic ions (cations) are attracted to the negative pole they are retained as part of the needle. This prevents deposit of metallic ions in tissue, and tattoo is impossible.

If the needle is incorrectly attached to the positive electrode ion transfer will lead to the formation of acid caustic (hydrochloric acid) and oxygen. Tissue is destroyed, but hardened, so that the needle tends to stick. Metallic ions are repelled from the anode and deposited in tissue, causing tattoo. In any application, the dispersing electrode of gauze, fabric or sponge with a metal backing or core is is saturated with salt solution and pressed on by, or held in, the patient's hand.

Many more or less therapeutically active substances can be forced into the body by ion transfer. Substances may become fixed in the skin, they may penetrate and be circulated by the blood stream, or they may act as counterirritants (Table 17-2). We must be aware that when potent chemicals such as histamine and methacholine are introduced into the skin dramatic and undesirable systemic reactions can occur, duplicating those that follow injections. In addition, the patient may be burned. Although some dermatologists continue to use direct current for hair removal, today most prefer alternating current.

Iontophoresis has been in use for many years. There is little doubt that at present it has much theoretical and limited practical value. Some investigators foresee a brighter future for this modality. However, misinterpretation, overenthusiasm, and differences of opinion have created much criticism. With few exceptions controlled clinical studies with iontophoresis are lacking, and it is hard to compare the results with those obtained by other methods. Harris [12] discusses iontophoresis in detail.

Medical Galvanism

Medical galvanism is an effective, slow way to treat hyperhidrosis, or produce experimental anhidrosis, of the palms and soles. The method of treatment is the same as that with iontophoresis, but medicinal ions are not added to the electrolyte. Large, equal-size electrodes are attached to the anode and cathode. The electrodes are placed in nonconducting containers filled with enough tap water (as satisfactory as any other electrolyte and less expensive) to cover the treatment area and are covered with cloth pads. An extremity is placed on each pad. Direct current is applied to the comfortable limit of patient tolerance. Because the positive anode current is more effective than is the negative cathode current, it is wise to reverse polarity halfway through treatment periods, which last 20 to 30 minutes every other day.

Five to 10 treatments are usually necessary to stop sweating and large treatment areas may require up to 50 or 75 mA of current [2]. Relief may last 6 weeks and retreatment courses are shorter than the original series.

Surgical Galvanism

Galvanic current may be used to remove small benign tumors (surgical galvanism). Cosmetic results are good, but the process is somewhat time consuming. Skin tags, selected fleshy nevi, fibromata, spider nevi, and telangiectasias may be chemically destroyed by transfixation. A needle attached to the negative pole is repeatedly inserted into the mass following a pattern like the spokes of a wheel or a piece of graph paper. As in epilation, a current of up to 2 mA is impressed with each insertion for 30 to 60 sec. The growth is not removed, but involutes in a couple of weeks. However safe the procedure may be, pigmented cellular nevi should not be removed in this fashion when biopsy examination is anticipated. In treating spider nevi the needle is inserted into the center to destroy the central vessel. Current reduction will probably be necessary to avoid too much pain. In the same manner surrounding capillaries or any telangiectatic vessels may be destroyed by repeated applications along their course.

At present, one can only recommend the use of direct current for experimentation, galvanic surgery (including electrolysis), treatment of hyperhidrosis, electrocautery, and operating the plasma torch. Procedures are reasonably safe, but the patient should be told that burns may develop with any application of direct current. Some skin damage, not always minimal or avoidable, sooner or later will follow hair removal.

18

Epilation

Hugh M. Crumay

Epilation with high frequency alternating current apparently is replacing hair removal by direct current (electrolysis). Removal of hair by galvanic current is safer, less likely to cause scars, probably less painful, and slower than is removal by diathermy. For these reasons, epilation by direct current should be recommended to lay persons. Removal with high frequency machines requires greater concentration and skill than does electrolysis, since diathermy current destroys hair more quickly and there is less time to correct mistakes. Technique, on the other hand, is simpler and time is saved. Both methods have staunch advocates. Dermatologists will almost certainly prefer high frequency current generators and probably will choose more sophisticated, automatically timed epilators if planning extensive hair removal.

Peereboom-Wynia [19] studied the effects of high frequency and galvanic currents on hair roots by epilating the beards of hirsute women. Some regrowth of hairs followed applications of either current, necessitating retreatment. Comparatively speaking, those hairs regrowing after use of alternating current had decreased diameters and a greater percentage were of the "dysplastic/dystrophic" variety. Both methods were effective. Hair density in the test sites was decreased more rapidly by diathermy current, but there was no difference in the time required for complete destruction.

A unique hand-held galvanic epilator has been designed for self-epilation by the patient. It has been used effectively by physicians to remove a few hairs. The device incorporates a "spring-loaded round-headed needle" that should lessen the chance of damage to the hair follicle. The outer metal case, while held in the hand, acts as a dispersing electrode. The power source is a 7-V battery with current flow varying from 0.5 to 1.3 mA, depending on skin moisture and firmness of grip. Investigation led Sternberg [24] to conclude that "the 'Perma Tweez' is an acceptable electrolysis instrument for permanent removal of hair by the lay person." In most cases determination, longanimity, and practice are prerequisites for success. Once mastered this technique can save the patient much money. A larger, greatly improved model, recently introduced, may interest some dermatologists as an accessory unit.

High frequency epilating instruments are either of the spark gap or vacuum tube type. Tissue is destroyed by conversive heat resulting from tissue resistance to the passage of rapidly oscillating alternating current. The wave form is respectively damped or undamped (Chapter 20).

The majority of dermatologists are familiar with spark gap machines such as the Bovies or the Hyfrecator types. The 0-3 type Bovie or

197

the Bantam Bovie, for instance, uses a current-limiting resistor in the coagulation circuit to reduce current. Using too little current to destroy hair quickly is a common error. The most widely recommended application is biterminal (never "bipolar"). The epilating needle is attached to the concentrating terminal (to form the "active" electrode) while the patient's hand, or other bare skin area, is placed on the dispersing electrode. Monoterminal (incorrectly called "monopolar") epilation is possible. Robinson [21] did this with a spark gap machine. It is standard procedure with "high frequency" valve tube epilators, to be discussed below.

Familiarity with one's machine, whatever the type of application, is essential as characteristics vary. When using spark gap units it is wise to determine the setting that will produce a minimal spark when the needle is almost touching the operator's wet thumbnail or a palmar callus. A machine that produces a large spark at minimum (near zero) setting should not be used for epilation because destruction and scarring would be too great. Current flows only when the hand or foot switch is closed. Hence, control, as with direct current, is always manual. The 0-3 Bovie unit has been a good, though painful, reasonably satisfactory epilating machine.

Much better units are the valve tube–type higher frequency (shorter wavelength) machines designed especially for electrolysis, such as the Fischer, Hoffman, Instantron, and Kree models [16]. These epilators are sophisticated units with automatic power and time controls. When the switch is closed a definite predetermined amount of current is applied for a short interval. More intense current applied for a shorter time usually hurts less than milder current applied for a longer period. The application is reproduced each time the switch is closed. Removing the foot quickly may result in a shorter burst of current. Most of these machines can be set for manual operation.

One of these shorter wavelength epilators, for example, operates at a frequency of about 13 megahertz. The application is monoterminal (not monopolar): a single electrode, which is the needle, is used. Operation is manual or automatic. Automatic settings may be more or less than a common average of 0.5 sec. With this particular unit hair can also be removed by electrolysis. In this case, however,

use of direct current requires two electrodes, one the concentrating needle attached to the negative pole, and one a wet dispersing electrode attached to the positive pole. Intensity of current is measured by a milliammeter.

It is possible to remove hair by a combination of direct current and alternating current. First, a short application of direct current is made to "open the follicle"; next, alternating current is applied to destroy the hair root; finally, direct current is again impressed to "soften the follicle" and facilitate removal of the hair. It is unlikely that dermatologists will be interested in this "combined" approach.

In 1975 and 1976, a high frequency epilator, operating at a frequency of about 25 megahertz, was widely promoted to the laity by beauticians with the promise that it would painlessly and permanently remove hair. The concentrating electrode is not the usual "needle" type to be inserted into the hair follicle, but a small "forceps" type used to grasp and gently manipulate the hair protruding from the skin. One might say that the hair is "teased" while the current flows until the hair becomes loose. Deductively, it seems unlikely, or even impossible, that an electric current could safely destroy hair roots in this fashion; intuitively then one must suspect a hoax. We have been unable to unearth any scientific evidence to the contrary. Until proven otherwise, it may suffice to say that Kligman [14] could find no evidence of postepilation destruction in biopsy specimens. Caveat emptor!

Clean skin and comfortable positions for patient and physician are prerequisites for epilation. Light should be good and the operator may wish to wear a magnifying lens. A fine needle, preferably with a rounded or bulbous tip, is attached to the negative electrode for electrolysis or to the concentrating electrode for high frequency epilation. A bulbous tip decreases the chance of escape from the follicle and damage to the skin. The needle is slipped into the pore and advanced into the follicle parallel to and touching the hair; the slant of the follicle is followed until resistance is encountered when the bottom of the follicle is reached, 3 or 4 mm below the surface. Additional slight introduction (up to 0.5 mm) may increase the percentage of hair root destruction. Needle insertion should be easy, smooth, and relatively painless. Pain, with or without bleeding, usually indicates untoward penetration of the lateral wall of the follicle.

The foot or hand switch should be closed (current turned on) after the needle reaches the bottom of the follicle, and opened (current turned off manually or automatically) before removal. Current flowing during entry or exit will cause unpleasant pain and "shock." Skin may be destroyed and undesirable scarring may result, especially if high frequency current is being used. The amount and duration of current application may vary because of patient characteristics, anatomic variations, hair coarseness, multiple sites of germination, stage of the growth cycle, contact with the dispersive electrode, needle placement, and the machine. Failure to destroy the papilla (and permanently remove the hair) may result for the same reasons.

Additional current is usually necessary to remove coarse hair. When a papilla is destroyed the hair is easily removed. Removal by fingertips is evidence of destruction, but "forceps delivery" is more satisfactory. One or more additional short current applications (bursts) are necessary if a hair remains fast, the need for each being determined by repeated gentle tugs, with or without removal of the needle.

The potentiometer controlling the galvanic epilator should be adjusted to deliver 0.5 to 1.0 mA (rarely as much as 2.0 mA). In galvanic generators only the milliammeter will indicate the actual current flowing to the patient. Usually after 15 to 20 sec, sometimes longer, a small bubble of hydrogen will appear at the ostium. A few more seconds of current flow are allowed before gently tugging on the hair to see if the papilla is destroyed. Longer current flow may be needed, depending on the milliammeter setting, but more than 60 sec of flow is seldom necessary. A few hair removals should determine the average duration and milliammeter setting for each patient. The procedure is somewhat painful and definitely time consuming. Experience is necessary to best control the high frequency diathermy epilator, though the manufacturer will suggest a setting. In shortwave units, the milliammeter does not register the amount of energy passing to the patient, but simply reflects the fact that current is flowing. In the absence of a recommended trial setting, the dermatologist can estimate if

current is "safe" by using his or her own skin. Initial settings are carefully modified as needed. Manually controlled longwave diathermy current should be applied in short bursts, lasting less than 1 sec; 3 to 6 such bursts will usually suffice. Interruption of current occurs at set intervals with the automatic shorterwave diathermy machine. Even so, some will prefer repeated shorter untimed bursts. Repeated shorter bursts are less painful than are more sustained applications.

It is important that the highest concentration of current occurs at the point of the needle where destruction is desired. Excess current flow causes a cone or cylinder of destruction to extend peripherally around the shaft of the needle, resulting in unwanted damage. Short bursts of current should tend to limit destruction to the papilla. Sometimes, during epilation, small bits of coagulated or desiccated tissue stick to the shaft of the needle. Current concentrates about such accumulations and subsequent "shorting" causes superficial (but not papillary) destruction. Needles must be kept clean.

To lessen the chance of scarring, contiguous hairs should not be removed unless they are 3 or 4 mm apart. How many may be epilated at one sitting will depend largely on the skill of the operator, but also on the location and type of hair (the chin is preferred to the lip or neck). Seventy-five to 100 hairs can be removed in 15 to 20 min with the 0-3 Bovie unit. Under ideal conditions, skillful operators using sophisticated epilators have claimed removal of 40 to 50 hairs in little more than 5 min.

Sorely afflicted patients should be advised that epilation is a lengthy process. They should be informed that they have more hairs than anyone can count on any given day, and that new hairs can "grow" during the period of treatment. Following diathermy epilation 20 to 30% of hairs may regrow and require removal. With more time-consuming galvanic epilation (electrolysis), the percentage of regrowth should be less. It is estimated that, overall, one type of removal is as efficient as is the other. Usually the patient will be happier with high frequency epilation because immediate results are more impressive than are delayed results; as Cervantes wrote, "a bird in hand is worth two in the bush."

19

Electrocautery

Hugh M. Crumay

Heated metal, such as a soldering iron, a soldier's sword, or even a whaler's lance has been used for centuries as a "cleansing" cautery. Cautery is derived from the Greek word *kautérion* (branding iron); this, in turn, comes from *kaiein* (to burn). When tissue is cauterized microorganisms are destroyed and bleeding is controlled. Fine cautery tips, in the form of wire loops or blades, may be used for cutting. In the past the metal tip of the cautery was heated by fire. Electrocautery simply involves heating the metal tip by electricity. Heat develops due to ohmic resistance to the passage of electric current. Electrocautery should not be considered a form of electrosurgery; the latter term refers only to surgery accomplished by the application of high frequency current with a cold electrode.

Comparatively inexpensive cauteries are available to destroy and remove tumors. Common commercial alternating current (60 cycles, 110 V) is usually reduced by a step-down transformer to heat a metal tip, often composed of silver or platinum (Fig. 19-1). The resulting current is of low frequency (60 hertz), low voltage (5 V), and high amperage (± 15 A). It is controlled by a rheostat so that the operating cautery tip can be heated to the necessary degree. Small galvanocauteries, such as those made by Concept, Inc., contain a battery to produce direct current and heat the cautery tip. Use is limited, but portability is a valuable

asset. They can be carried like a fountain pen to be used for office and bedside minor surgery.

Destruction of tissue is due to heat conducted from a hot body to a colder body. The cautery tip should be dull to bright cherry red, depending on the judgment of the operator, to produce respectively lesser or greater destruction. Increased experience leads to better decisions, but brighter cherry red means greater heat and more destruction.

Electrocautery tips are made in various shapes and sizes. Small wire loops and flat blades, in various shapes, are usually preferred for dermatologic surgery. Extensive cautery excision, practiced today by few surgeons, requires special considerations. It is adequately discussed by a staunch advocate, Ervin Epstein, in his book *Skin Surgery* [10]. Burdick capably discusses the removal of minor skin lesions by electrocautery in the same text [4].

Little preoperative preparation is required. It may be sufficient to acquaint the patient with details of what is to follow, stressing that one may be repulsed by the odor of burning flesh and disturbed by a feeling of heat conducted beyond the area of anesthesia. Most surgeons prefer to use an anesthetic, though some may consider it superfluous. Unless anesthesia precedes surgery stoicism is required of the patient. Proper heating, however, is said to lessen pain. Apparently, James Percy, inventor of the cautery bearing his name, did extensive

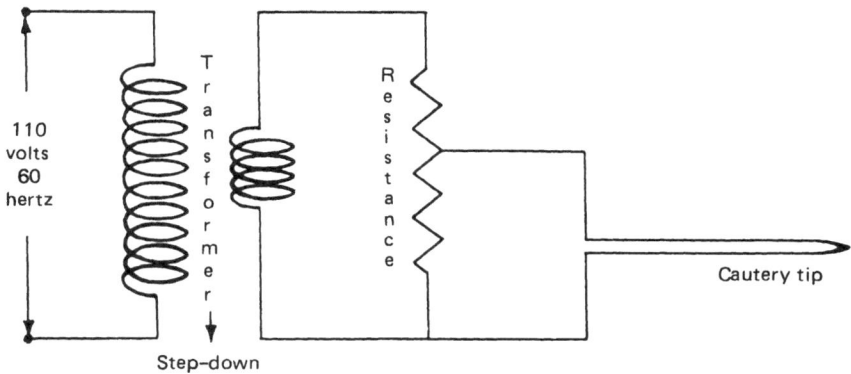

Figure 19-1. Electrocautery: diagram of basic circuitry. The operating cautery tip becomes red-hot due to ohmic resistance to the passage of low frequency, low voltage, high amperage current.

surgery without anesthetization. Since the cautery sterilizes as it burns, skin cleansing is not absolutely necessary unless injections are contemplated. The operator should take care not to ignite alcohol, unnecessary drapes, gauze pads, or clothing.

Actual surgery may be immediately heroic or accomplished in a more leisurely fashion, depending on the inclination and disposition of the surgeon. Burning can be ''layered'' with alternate curettement or even cold-steel cutting, so that the final goal may be reached in easy stages. This is an inherent advantage of both electrocautery and electrosurgery. A major asset of electrocautery is that hemostasis is usually adequate, even in a wet field. By exercising great care it is possible to remove a tumor from blood vessel walls due to the cooling, and hence protective, effects of circulating blood [10].

The amount of heat, visually determined by the experienced operator, and duration of application determine the amount of tissue destruction. Destruction is minimal if the tip is heated to a dull cherry red and lightly applied to tissue. Electrocautery proponents may argue that tissue damage is more easily controlled than it is with electrosurgery. Electrosurgeons will disagree; most, perhaps only because of experience, will find it easier, and more practical, to vary the degree of tissue destruction with high frequency current. Either type of application can be regulated to a fine degree.

Primary closure is impossible after electrocautery. Several days after being burned tissue begins to slough out. It will somewhat resemble pus for 7 to 10 days, or longer if large amounts of tissue have been destroyed (eg, third degree burn). Most patients, and even inexperienced physicians, will confuse the resulting appearance with infection. Forewarn the patient and point out that large wounds may not heal for more than a month. Usually crusts separate spontaneously after 10 to 14 days. Healing may be even slower in certain areas, such as the hands and feet, the scalp, and the intertriginous surfaces. Healing has been speeded by grafting on clean granulation tissue.

Electrocautery burns heal more quickly if they are kept clean and dry, terms that may be synonymous. It is advisable to remove excess burned or carbonized tissue with the curette. Alternate cauterization and curettement, destroying or ''biting off'' the desired amount of tissue with each step, allows gradual safe removal of superficial and deep tumors. Since the techniques of removal are much the same as in electrosurgery, they are discussed in Chapter 20.

Scars following electrocautery or cautery excision eventually have a better appearance than the inexperienced physician or layman might expect; usually they are cosmetically acceptable. After extensive excision, when healing may be prolonged for months, cosmetic results are less predictable. The wary physician will guarantee nothing. The patient's welfare must be given first consideration, but unavoidable risks exist and some patients are unreasonable. If one does excellent work and promises little, the average patient will be pleasantly surprised, happy, and often grateful; it is hard, on the other hand, to justify unwarranted optimism that leads to patient depression.

If hypertrophic scars are expected it may be wise to apply steroids to depress fibroblastic proliferation, though healing may be somewhat prolonged. Aerosol steroids (with antibiotics added only when necessary) may be easier to apply, promote dryness, and may be more effective. Intralesional steroids frequently flatten scars and relieve itch or other discomfort.

Electrocautery may be used wherever electrosurgery is effective. Most dermatologic surgeons prefer to use high frequency current. Electrocautery may be chosen to remove any wart; nevi without junctional activity; vascular tumors including large ectasias and granuloma pyogenicum, but not those of the telangiectatic variety; seborrheic keratoses; actinic kera-

toses; and skin cancers. Numerous operators consider the electrocautery tip ideal for incising abscesses and infected or noninfected cysts, especially if they are tender. The sac or cavity should be probed and explored with a hot tip to promote drainage and resolution. Proper technique often results in extrusion of the entire cyst sac through the cautery incision, with subsequent permanent disappearance and minimal scarring.

The virtues of electrocautery are much the same as those of electrosurgery (Chapter 20). Only personal experience can determine when and how often each will be preferred. Superior hemostasis in a wet field is a distinct advantage when using the electrocautery. Contrarily, slow healing is probably the chief handicap.

20

Alternating Current: Electrosurgery

Hugh M. Crumay

Electrosurgery should only refer to the removal or destruction of tissue by conversion of electric energy into heat through tissue resistance to the passage of high frequency alternating current. The terms cautery or electrocautery should not be used to describe such surgery. Electrosurgery results from surgical diathermy. Diathermy, in turn, involves the use of rapidly oscillating electric current to heat tissue; the word is derived from the Greek words *dia* and *therme* ("through heat"). Electrosurgical energy is so intense that the concentrating electrode will fulgurate, desiccate, coagulate, or cut integument and flesh. The degree of destruction depends on the wave form of the oscillations and the power of the electric current. Characteristics and uses of alternating current employed in medicine are summarized in Table 20-1.

A fully damped wave form causes marked tissue destrution and good hemostasis, but it does not cut. A completely undamped wave form causes minimal tissue damage and does not stop bleeding, but cuts dramatically. Either wave form can be modified to resemble the other and tends to mimic the other's effects. When two dispersing electrodes are used intervening tissue is medically heated (gently and uniformly). However, if one electrode is concentrating surgical heating and destruction (more or less intense and limited) occurs wherever it is applied (Fig. 20-1).

Increasing the voltage of the usual household or commercial current will provide sufficient power for surgery. The available current is impressed on the primary coil of a step-up transformer, which is a device for increasing the voltage of alternating current. Through electromagnetic induction current then flows in the secondary coil of the transformer. The secondary coil of a step-up transformer has more turns of wire than does the primary coil and the voltage will be raised in direct proportion to the increase in number of turns; eg, if the secondary coil has 20 times as many turns the voltage will be 20 times greater. Conversely, whenever the secondary coil has fewer turns of wire than does the primary the voltage decreases proportionately (a step-down transformer).

It is not sufficient to simply increase voltage, but rather the frequency must also be greatly increased. Why can't this be done mechanically? A generator producing 60-cycle "household" current rotates 3600 times every minute (3600 rpm). To produce 1,000,000 hertz a generator would have to operate at 60,000,000 rpm (a mechanical impossibility). Fortunately we can easily solve this problem because an electric oscillating circuit consisting of condensers, a coil of wire (solenoid), and a small air gap (spark gap or thermionic tube) can produce electric current that oscillates millions of times each second. Mirable dictu! Thus, low voltage, low frequency commercial current is

Table 20-1   *Types, Characteristics, and Uses of Alternating Current (AC) Employed in Medicine*

| | Type of Alternating Current | | |
	LOW FREQUENCY	HIGH FREQUENCY	ULTRAHIGH FREQUENCY
Frequency			
Cycles/sec	<10,000	>100,000	>10,000,000
Kilohertz	<10	>100–10.000	>10,000–3,000,000
Megahertz	<0.01	1 (commonly)	>10–3,000
Wavelength	Long	Short	Ultrashort
Meters	>30,000	<3,000–30	<30–3
Diathermy		Longwave	Shortwave
Usual Current	Faradic or induced	Damped	Undamped
Sensation	Shock	Heat (conversive)	Heat (conversive)
Uses			
Major	Tetanize	Surgical	Medical
Minor		Medical	
Associated terms	Ruhmkorff coil	Currents:	Electromagnetic field
		D'Arsonval (solenoid)	Electric Field
		Oudin (resonator)	

converted into high voltage, high frequency current for electrosurgery (Fig. 20-2).

Spark gaps, thermionic tubes (diodes or triodes), and solid-state substitutes produce oscillations. In the spark gap generator condensers (capacitors) are charged by high voltage current from the secondary coil of the high tension transformer. After a condenser is filled to capacity it will empty itself across properly adjusted contact points of a spark gap. The discharge is always oscillatory. Varying spark gap resistance will cause oscillations to die down more or less rapidly: the resulting wave form is more or less damped. If any air gap is too large no discharge can occur. Oscillations are sustained by the solenoid (inductance); hence, it is the most important element in the

oscillating circuit. Each turn of the solenoid (wire coil) acts as an impedance (inductive resistance) to the flow of current so that it oscillates animatedly with subsequent production of wave trains. Frequencies of resonator (oscillating) circuits are altered by varying the values of capacitance and inductance; this is accomplished by respectively changing the size of the condensers and the coil.

Oscillations are either damped or undamped. Spark gap generator waves are damped because the resistance offered by the gap causes successive wave amplitudes to gradually decrease to zero, just as the excursions of a pendulum are finally stopped by frictional resistance. Both widening the gap and increasing the resistance will result in longer

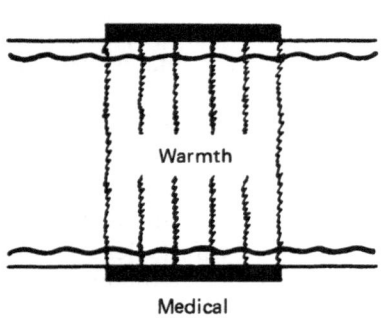

Warmth

Medical

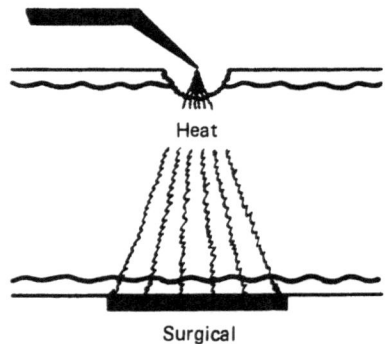

Heat

Surgical

Figure 20-1.   The effect of electrodes on current concentration. Two dispersing electrodes (left) permit "gentle" uniform heating (warmth). A concentrating electrode (right), on the other hand, concentrates the same amount of heat in a small area so that it becomes destructive.

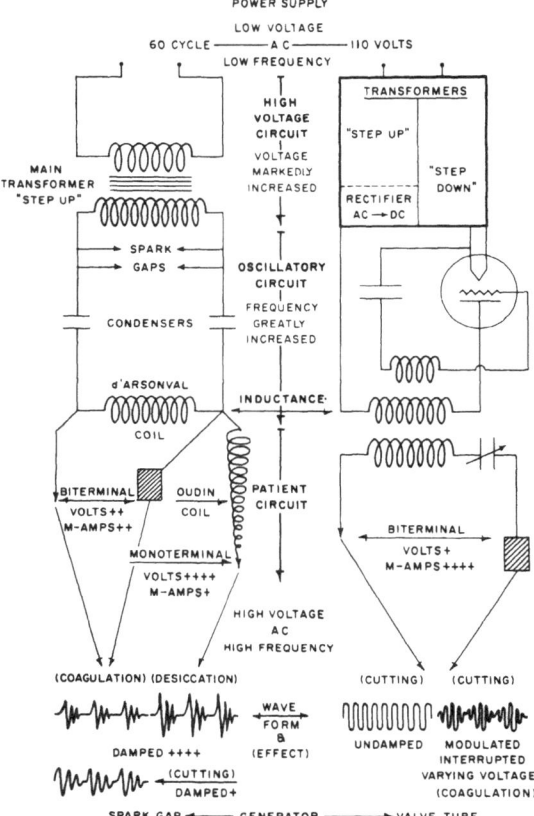

Figure 20-2. Schematic diagram of simplified diathermy circuits (spark gap and valve tube) and wave forms (damped and undamped) produced. Each circuit has a "high voltage circuit" (to increase voltage) and an "oscillatory circuit" (to greatly increase frequency). Basic wave forms may then be modified to produce varied effects. Modified from Moschella SL, Pillsbury DM, Hurley HJ: Dermatology, Vol. 2. Philadelphia, Saunders, 1975. Courtesy of W. B. Saunders Co.

rest periods between wave trains, and, consequently, greater damping. In contrast, overcoming internal resistance in the valve tube circuit permits the amplitude of each wave to continue unchanged (Fig. 20-3). The oscillator circuit is composed of a pair of oscillator tubes,

a plate circuit, and a grid circuit. Both circuits contain coils and condensers with fixed values of inductance and capacitance. The two circuits mutually energize each other because they are resonant to the same frequency: each oscillation receives a slight boost through a feedback mechanism and "perpetual" oscillations are sustained.

Wave forms may be modified by changing the characteristics of the oscillating circuit. Damping decreases in the spark gap generator as the voltage is slowly returned to zero. As damping decreases wave trains get closer together and eventually approach the undamped form. If a triode (a tube containing filament, grid, and plate) is used in the valve tube circuit the wave form will be completely undamped: a continuous sine wave. If a single or double diode (containing only filament and plate) replaces the triode, respective half-wave or full-wave rectification results, and the undamped waves will somewhat resemble moderately or slightly damped wave forms (Fig. 20-4).

Maximum destruction, synonymous with maximum coagulation and maximum hemostasis, results when a highly damped wave from a spark gap oscillator, with a frequency of 0.5 to 1 megahertz, is applied with two terminals (Table 20-2). These effects are somewhat decreased, but remain emphatic, when the wave form is moderately damped. Raising voltage adequately permits monoterminal application causing electrodesiccation and excellent, though more superficial, hemostasis. When the wave form is only slightly damped, however, so that it closely resembles an undamped wave train, tissue can be cut easily, while decreased coagulation is still sufficient to provide appreciable hemostasis. Voltage drops and optimum results demand the use of two (concentrating and dispersing) electrodes.

The vacuum tube oscillator, with an approximate frequency of 1 to 3 megahertz, produces undamped waves (continuous sine

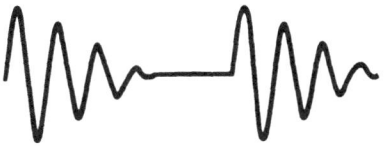

Spark gap—Damped wave

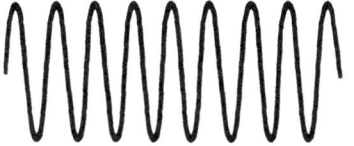

Tube—Undamped wave

Figure 20-3. Basic wave forms of currents from spark gap and valve tube generators.

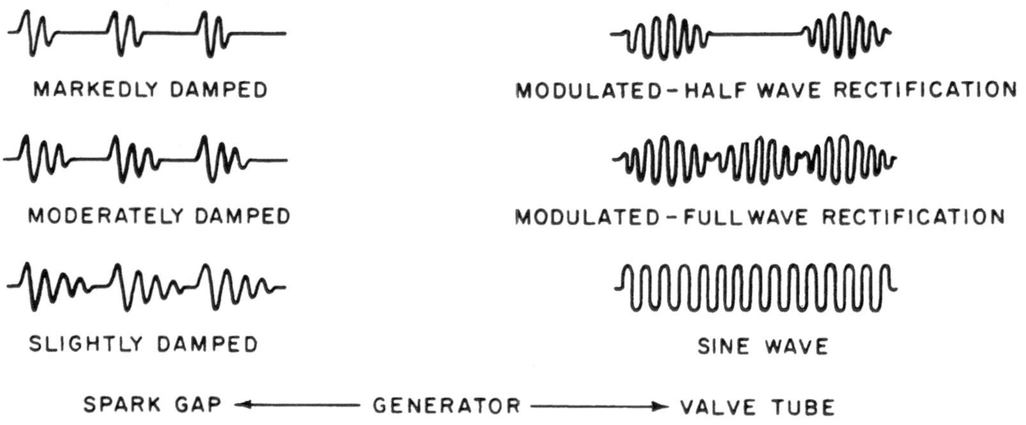

MARKEDLY DAMPED   MODULATED-HALF WAVE RECTIFICATION

MODERATELY DAMPED   MODULATED-FULLWAVE RECTIFICATION

SLIGHTLY DAMPED   SINE WAVE

SPARK GAP ◄──────── GENERATOR ────────► VALVE TUBE

Figure 20-4. Modifications of high frequency wave forms from spark gap and valve tube generators.

waves); coagulation is minimal, hemostasis is practically nil, and cutting is maximal—permitting healing by first intention under ideal conditions. According to Martin [17], if the wave form of the tube-type oscillator is modulated by varying the voltage so that amplitude of oscillations increases and decreases in each wave train, the output will resemble a damped wave and limited coagulation with hemostasis will result. Furthermore, these effects can be obtained with less destruction and charring than may be associated with moderately damped waves. This is true whenever maximum voltage decreases, as in the vacuum tube oscillator compared to the spark gap generator. Some dermatologists prefer such a tube-type machine for certain surgical procedures.

Effects of High Frequency Current on Tissue

When frequency is sufficiently high, current passing through tissue causes heat but has no other effect. Probably not all the factors responsible for heating tissue have been fully explained. Bovie [3] wrote that "the conduction of an electric current through tissue is in general like the conduction through solutions. It is electrolytic rather than metallic. . . . But the transfer of charged matter, and therefore

Table 20-2 *Dermatologic Applications (Spark Gap Apparatus)*

	Electrodesiccation	*Electrocoagulation*	*Cutting*
Wave form	Damped (markedly)	Damped (moderately)	Damped (slightly)
High tension transformer	Secondary (Oudin)	Primary (d'Arsonval)	Primary
Electrodes	Monoterminals (concentrative)	Biterminal (concentrative and dispersive)	
Application	In tissue	In tissue	In tissue
Modifications	Fulguration (no contact)	Resistance added to remove hair	
Volts	2000–10,000	300–500 (underload)	100–500
Milliamperage	150	200–500	3000
Advantages	Superficial	Penetrating	Minimal damage
	Easy control	Greater destruction	Seal small vessels
	Less destruction	Danger of secondary	? First intention healing
	Good hemostasis	hemorrhage after	
	Little danger of	heavy coagulation	
	bleeding		

From Moschella SL, Pillsbury DM, Hurley HJ: Dermatology, Vol 2, Philadelphia, Saunders, 1975. Courtesy of W. B. Saunders Co.

the current, is a more complicated process than that which occurs in simple solutions." We have seen that recognizable ion transfer and polarization are impossible with high frequency current; hence, no chemical heat is formed as with direct current. Huntoon [13] stated that "the cell behaves with respect to the high frequency current as if it were a small bit of salt solution surrounded by a good, but very thin insulator, the whole immersed in another conducting fluid. This makes the electrical equivalent of the cells immersed in body fluid a circuit of small condensers, shunted by, and in series with, small resistances." It follows that the body becomes a capacitor. High frequency current passes through tissues both as a capacitive current and a conductive current (Fig. 20-5).

High frequency electromagnetic fields may cause heat in any dielectric medium, including the body, as the result of dielectric polarization. Direct current and low frequency alternating current, to a lesser degree, cause slight relative shifts of electrons in atoms and molecules under the influence of an electric field (polarization). Oscillations may become so rapid that there is no chance for "obvious" shifting. Nevertheless, an electric field properly applied always causes infinitesimal "to-and-fro" movements of atoms and molecules. Such polarization dissipates energy, which is transformed into heat. As Elliott [9] pointed out, "the alternating electric field set up in the tissue between electrodes displaces or stresses the molecules, first in one direction and then in the other, as the polarity of the field is reversed. Since the electric elasticity of dielectrics is not perfect, friction results from molecular motion in the tissue and heat is generated irrespective

of tissue conductivity. This phenomenon is called dielectric hysteresis or dielectric loss." Furthermore, an electromagnetic field induces eddy currents in conductive substances and, if of sufficient strength, they generate heat in soft tissues of the body. Consequently, high frequency alternating currents cause heat in tissues due to conductive resistance, capacitive resistance (the most important factor), and eddy currents.

We have noted that high frequency current causes more or less tissue destruction and more or less hemostasis, in direct relation to the degree of damping or separation of successive wave trains. How rapidly the voltage dies down to zero in each wave train determines the amount of damping. A faster drop of voltage to zero widens the distance between bursts of discharge and increases the damping effect. Changing the characteristics of the oscillation circuit, such as widening or narrowing the spark gap, respectively raises or lowers the voltage and decreases or increases frequency. Billin [1] explained that in older equipment, the spark gap was used in this manner to control power. In the early 1930s electrosurgical units contained two spark gap structures in one machine—one closely spaced for cutting and the other widely spaced for coagulation. Improved techniques led to modern units that function with one fixed spark gap setting. By changing parameters of inductance and capacitance the entire function of the electrosurgical unit can be controlled. Blending currents is not necessary.

No one is certain why a pure sine wave current (completely undamped) cuts best. McClean's investigations [3,18] demonstrated

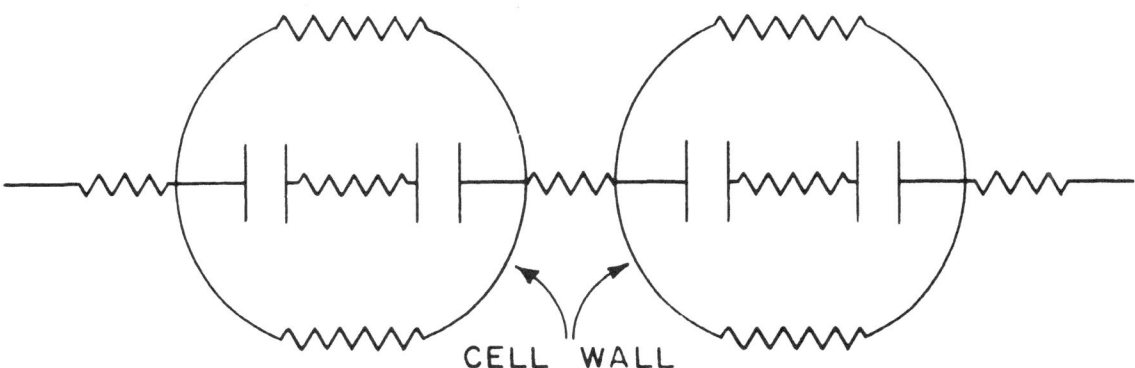

Figure 20-5. Schematic diagram: the electric equivalent of cells.

that "electrosurgical incision is shown to be independent of frequency or wave form, and to depend on current density." Due to high current density the arcing discharge of a cutting current was seen in a revolving mirror as a "compact tight pencil," sharply concentrated so that heat distribution was sharply limited. Contrarily, the discharge of a noncutting (coagulation or desiccation) current is wide like a brush or a diffuse spray, concentration is poor, and heat is distributed over a relatively large area. McClean [18] adds that "persistence of ionization, requiring high current density, of the gap between the electrodes and the tissue" apparently accounts for arc concentration. He concludes, "Rationally then, either damped or undamped oscillations can produce either cutting or deep heating effects, provided that for cutting there is maintained a high current density and an adequate electrode-gap ionization, and for deep heating a relatively low current density and no persistent ionization of the electrode gap (through more sluggish interruptions of oscillating trains, either damped or undamped)." Billin [1] agrees that "cutting action seems to depend on the formation of a minute arc between the electrode and tissue"; and that "the more easily this arc can be formed and maintained, the more easily the electrode will cut." As a matter of fact, cutting can be done with direct current, but it is incompatible with life.

Histopathologic changes from all types of electrosurgical applications tend to be similar. Burdick [5] carried out experiments on freshly excised breasts, using "minimal currents and time" as well as "a special modification of Verhoeff's stain to demonstrate more adequately the extent of tissue destruction." Changes "after fulguration, desiccation, and coagulation" were remarkably alike. He observed more damage than expected after cutting with a pure sine wave. Comparing damage to that following electrocautery, he notes that radiofrequency currents may cause extensive damage. This warning is simply a reminder to exercise care and judgment. We agree that "the speed, simplicity, and safety of these techniques justify even more popular use of electrosurgical procedures."

Classically, monoterminal applicatons of current cause dehydration, so that cells look "mummified." Though cells are shriveled, outlines and nuclei are preserved; Clark [6] termed this desiccation. Current applied biterminally, with concentrating and dispersing electrodes, causes greater heat and cell outline is entirely lost. An amorphous mass of coagulated tissue remains, as though it had been "boiled in its own juice"; this has been loosely called hyalinization. The majority of the blood vessels are thrombosed. Round cell infiltrates appear peripherally in a few days after both desiccation and coagulation. When biterminal cutting current is used, coagulation is more or less reduced depending on current density and cutting speed. Tissue seems to separate ahead of the cutting arc and perhaps explosive vacuolization occurs as the result of intercellular steam pressure. Effects of longwave diathermy are reviewed in Table 20-3.

As one might expect, stronger desiccating currents can cause some coagulation, and weaker coagulation currents may cause only desiccation. Charring and carbonization are due to excess voltage—penetration is a function of the amperage. The extent of scarring after electrosurgery is related to the amount of tissue destruction, the anatomic location, and individual responsiveness. As noted, scars in general tend to be surprisingly good and are often superior. On those few occasions when a dissatisfied electrosurgeon recommends corrective plastic surgery postoperatively, the patient is apt to consider it unnecessary. Keloid incidence is no greater after electrosurgery than following cold-steel surgery. On the other hand, there is a slight increase in hypertrophic scarring if coagulation has been extensive, especially in areas such as the back and shoulders. Injecting depot-type steroids intralesionally (and sublesionally) can hasten and even improve the amelioration due to time. The electrosurgeon (or surgeon) should make every reasonable effort to avoid extensive cancer surgery that may result in scarring that could cause contractions of the inner canthus or localized retractions of the upper lip.

Precautions in the Use of Electrosurgical Applications

Techniques of surgical diathermy are so easy to imitate that safety is often taken for granted. However, certain precautions are necessary. Advice to read and follow the manufacturers'

Table 20-3 *Effects of Longwave Diathermy Currents*

	Long Wave Diathermy	
Spark Gap ——————	Generator —————	Vacuum Tube
	EFFECT ON TISSUE	
	(heat according to Joule's law: I^2RT)	
	CHARACTERISTICS	
	(high frequency, shortwave)	
	ELECTRODES	
Heat (medical)	Dispersing/Dispersing	Heat (medical)
Destruction (surgical)	Concentrating/Dispersing	Destruction (surgical)
	DERMATOLOGIC APPLICATIONS (PATHOLOGY)	
Fulguration (dehydration)		Cutting
Desiccation (dehydration)		(explosive vacuolization)
("mummification")		(slight coagulation)
Coagulation (hyalinization)		(disintegration)
Epilation (dehydration)		
Cutting (mimics Tube effect)		
	ADVANTAGES	
Controlled destruction		Destruction minimal
Excellent hemostatis		? First intention healing

From Moschella SL, Pillsbury DM, Hurley HJ: Dermatology, Vol 2, Philadelphia, Saunders, 1975. Courtesy of W. B. Saunders Co.

instructions seems superfluous, but it is surprising how many operators fail to do this. Perhaps this is especially true of those who have acquired expertise in the use of "similar" units. As power increases more care is required. Modern equipment has many built-in safety features, such as isolation transformers, plate isolation adapters, and capacitors in the output (therapeutic or patient) circuit. One can guarantee safe operation within tolerable limits; no one can assure mistake-free applications. The unit must be properly grounded and all external wires and connections must be in good repair. Spark gaps, tubes, and terminal wires may need to be replaced at long intervals, but good electrosurgical equipment needs surprisingly little maintenance.

Pillsbury [20] cautions that "deaths have resulted from deficiencies in such units and their use in the presence of volatile explosive gases." The increasing use of nonexplosive anesthetics reduces a risk understood by everyone, but explosions have also resulted from ignition of flammable gas in the intestines or of hydrogen gas generated in the bladder. Probably the most frequent injury is a burn, resulting from improper grounding of the patient. Aerosols and alcohol on the skin, or in gauze, have been set ablaze. Distorted physiologic signals and disturbed monitoring devices can cause concern. High frequency electric currents (ra-

diofrequency waves) can have adverse effects on cardiac pacemakers. Demand pacemakers of the "triggered" ventricular-inhibited type, especially if they are "external" and not implanted, are much more easily disturbed than are the "untriggered" fixed-rate types. The medical literature indicates that electric signals from the following generators may deactivate pacemakers: "electrocauteries" (an unfortunate incorrect term, because all references to electrocautery actually incriminate cutting and electrocoagulation with high frequency alternating current), radiotelemetry apparatus, certain ultraviolet light (UVL) units, medical diathermy machines, another pacemaker, microwave ovens, radar warning devices, neon lights, electric shavers, and spark plugs. Bradycardia (sometimes injurious) and, less frequently, asystole and ventricular fibrillation, have resulted from such interference.

Adverse effects during surgery have usually been reported in the urologic literature, and cutting current, rather than coagulation current, seems to be the dangerous modality. To our knowledge, accidents have not occurred during dermatologic electrocoagulation, but caution is advisable. Greene and Merideth [11] advise the following precautions: placing a well-lubricated ground plate (dispersing electrode) under the buttocks ("far" away from the heart) during urologic surgery to keep the radiofrequency field small; arranging electrode and ground plate (concentrating and dispersing electrodes) wires perpendicular to pacemaker electrode wires, because parallel wires form a better receiving antenna; using grounded (3-prong) plugs; and removing external battery pacemaker packs as far as possible from the radiofrequency field. Greene and Merideth add, however, that newer modifications of pacemakers should make interference by high frequency currents unlikely: incorporation of radiofrequency filters; provision for automatic reversion of unfixed demand-type pulsing to fixed-rate pacing if there is external interference; and, most recently, covering pacemakers with titanium to make them impervious to outside electric influence.

Krull [15] suggests the following recommendations: "(1) Use another method of treatment if possible. (2) If not, discuss the patient, the kind of procedure, and the specific pacemaker carefully with the cardiologist, realizing that he may not be knowledgeable about your electrosurgical unit or its affect on pacemakers. (3) It is highly desirable to perform electrosurgery in a hospital environment with appropriate assistance and monitoring, fixed-rate conversions, and resuscitation facilities available. (4) Complete the circuit with the inactive electrode as far from the heart as possible. (5) Use short (5 seconds or less) bursts of energy. (6) Have all circuits well grounded."

In our experience, electrodesiccation and electrocoagulation, intelligently used, have not interfered with pacemaker function, but everyone should be aware of the possibility. Luckily for dermatologists, most, if not all, serious mishaps have occurred in the hospital and not during office surgery. *Safe Use of High Frequency Electrical Equipment in Hospitals,* a manual published by the National Fire Protection Association [18a], is recommended reading for all electrosurgeons, especially those who contemplate hospital surgery. Incidentally and importantly, during electrocautery, if the term is properly used, no current passes through tissue.

It also pays to remember that electric currents flow through a complete circuit. This is not always evident. The dispersive electrode provides a safe, controlled, desirable path for high frequency current, introduced by the concentrating electrode, to return to the machine.

If there is relatively poor contact, or a poor connection, the current will favor the path of least impedance (resistance). This is most likely to be any type of metal on, or in contact with, the operating table and the patient. Indeed the unwary surgeon who touches patient and machine or other grounded object may become the return part of the circuit. Burns develop along such devious pathways. If the dispersive plate is forgotten, or if monoterminal application is premeditated, the high frequency current returns to ground in any possible way. Electrons are shed to the immediate environment. Current simply spills over the table edge (like water over a dam) and seeks the "easiest" course to ground. Such action requires adequate voltage and makes monoterminal electrodesiccation possible.

Use of excessive electrosurgical current leads to unnecessary tissue destruction. Current intensity is a function of output power plus time. Gentle current applied for a "long" time often does a better job than "blasting" with a harsh current for a short period—the former also leads to better cosmetic results. Maintaining a dry field (by stretching, pinching, using pressure rings, or any other effective maneuver) will permit hemostasis by less current applied for a longer period—and less tissue destruction will reduce scarring. It is always wise to use the smallest, "coolest" effective spark. Electrode tips should be kept clean and bright (by scraping, by emery papering, or by rubbing a gently sparking electrode across metal edges on the electrosurgical unit). The proper current for surgery must be carefully selected; the surgeon is more surprised than is the patient if epilation with intense coagulation current is unwittingly attempted. Unnecessary carbonization and charring, two hallmarks of the poor electrosurgeon, should be avoided. The electrosurgeon should be careful not leave excess burned tissue and "dead spaces," thus helping to prevent infection and speed healing. Depressed removal sites should be converted into a "shallow saucer," whenever possible, to avoid precipitous sides and overhanging edges.

We should consider trying various operative techniques on fresh moist flesh (eg, a large piece of veal, a beef heart, or a freshly excised breast) before approaching the living subject. If there is any question about the effect of a less powerful current application, such as that used in epilation or for destruction of telangiectasias, on the patient, it is wise to use one's own arm for testing. As Pillsbury [20] suggests, the patient may be reassured, and the unit tested at the same time, by "sparking" a palmar callus (or a fingernail). In removing benign lesions this caveat should never be violated: the smallest amount of current that will do the job should be used, even if operating time is prolonged. The cosmetic result is the electrosurgeon's first, and often only, concern. When dealing with cancers, on the other hand, it pays to be determined and overenthusiasm is commendable. Here, total removal of the tumor at any reasonable cost must be the goal.

Clinical Applications

Electrosurgery results only from the controlled application of high frequency alternating current to living tissue, in such a fashion that living tissue is destroyed to a desired degree. Also, for best results some form of cold-steel cutting is essential to most applications. A necessarily complete electric circuit requires a clearly visible concentrative (focusing) electrode and a dispersing (diffusive) electrode, which may or may not be evident.

Electrosurgery may be accomplished by means of fulguration, desiccation, coagulation, or cutting. All these techniques act in the same fundamental manner and effects often vary only in degree. Similarities and disparities become apparent when we consider each technique separately. Types of current employed and their effects on tissues are understandable only when each one is compared to all the others (Table 20-4).

Electrofulguration

Electrofulguration (from the Latin, *fulgur,* or lightning) is actually a form of electrodesiccation; the currents employed and the means of conduction are identical. However, the technique of using the electrode is different. While the electrode (commonly shaped like a ball or needle) must contact the body during electrodesiccation, it does not contact the body during electrofulguration—the electrode is simply held close enough so that a spray of sparks can be played over the tissue being treated. The resultant heat, developing within tissue, dries out cells and superficial desiccation results. The amount of damage varies with the power of the applied current, but fulguration never de-

Table 20-4 *Electrosurgical Applications in Dermatology*

	Modalities				
	ELECTRODESICCATION	ELECTROCOAGULATION		ELECTROSECTION	
Oscillator	Spark gap	Spark gap	Tube	Spark gap	Tube
Inductance	Secondary (Oudin)	Primary (d'Arsonval)	Primary	Primary	Primary
Wave form	Damped	Damped	Undamped (M)	Damped (close spaced)	Undamped (sine or M)
Electrodes	MT	Biterminal		Biterminal	
Modifications	Fulguration No contact	Epilation R added	Mild MT		Epilation MT
V	2000–5000	100–500 (under load)		100–500 (under load)	
mA	150	200–500		100–2000	
Frequency	0.5–1 mh	0.5–3 mh		1–3 mh	
Wavelength	600–300 m	300–100 m		300–100 m	
Advantages	"Superficial"	"penetrating"		? First intention healing	
Hemostasis	3 plus	4 plus	2 plus	2 plus	0 or 1 plus
Destruction	3 plus	4 plus	2 plus	1 plus	½ or 1 plus

M, modulated; MT, monoterminal; R, resistance; m, meter; mh, megahertz.

stroys deeper tissue because superficial carbonization forms an insulating barrier that protects underlying structures. As the electrode is moved about during electrodesiccation (and even during electrocoagulation or improper cutting) some sparking, off the tip or sides of the electrode, can occur. For this reason inadvertent fulguration (not harmful except possibly when cutting) may accompany all electrosurgical applications.

Electrodesiccation

Electrodesiccation (from the Latin, *desiccare,* to dry up) results when highly or moderately damped current is radiated through a monoterminal (concentrating) electrode as it touches, or is inserted into, tissue. A single electrode is connected to the secondary coil in the oscillator circuit of the high frequency generator. This secondary coil (Oudin coil) is added to the primary coil (d'Arsonval coil) or solenoid of the oscillator circuit. The high frequency transformer formed by the combination of these two coils further increases the voltage so that only one electrode is required to destroy tissue. This high frequency transformer must not be confused with the low frequency, high tension main transformer that initially raises the voltage. As expected, amperage is lowered as voltage is raised, penetration is less, and damage is more superficial than it would be if current from the d'Arsonval (primary) coil was used.

Desiccation (and fulguration) current is produced by a spark gap generator. Typical characteristics of the relatively high voltage, low amperage current include marked to moderate damping, 0.5 to 1 megahertz frequency, 2000 to 5000 V (peak value), and 150 mA. Minimal power causes only epidermal damage and no scarring. Maximal power, on the other hand, may cause coagulation and subsequent increased scarring, in addition to desiccation.

Electrocoagulation

Electrocoagulation (from the Latin, *coagulare,* to curdle) occurs when moderately damped or modulated undamped current is applied biterminally, with both concentrating and dispersing electrodes. A variation where two closely spaced, combined concentrating electrodes are inserted into tissue to cause "in-between" lo-

calized coagulation probably is not being used in dermatology. The concentrating electrode may either contact or enter the tissue to be destroyed; the dispersing electrode is usually a metal plate large enough to contact comparatively large skin areas, eg, the palm. To avoid interference with monitoring devices, should they be present, the dispersing electrode must be placed so that the current path between the two surgical electrodes does not include or coincide with the position of the monitoring unit electrodes. In addition, electrocautery may be safely substituted for electrosurgery if there is any threat of interference.

While spark gap units are most often used for coagulation in dermatology, valve tube generators may be preferred by some surgeons since they produce so-called "white coagulation" (without charring) and less tissue damage. However, the chance of inadequate hemostasis is greater than with a spark gap machine. To be effective coagulators, valve tube machines must produce modulated interrupted undamped current with increasing and decreasing voltage in each wave train. Typical characteristics of these lower voltage, higher amperage (compared to desiccation) currents are 1 to 3 megahertz frequency, 100 to 500 V (under load), and 200 to 500 mA (depending on technique).

Coagulation, with either moderately damped or modulated undamped wave forms, can cause extensive destruction and there is some chance of delayed secondary hemorrhage due to unmeasurable depth of penetration and associated unknown damage to hidden blood vessels. In many areas it is possible to elevate full thicknesses of skin by pinching and lifting it between fingers, so that the chance of damage to nerves and blood vessels is markedly diminished. In actual practice such bleeding is rare following dermatologic surgery; in any event, the expert electrosurgeon will know when to anticipate untoward reactions and take steps to avoid trouble.

Electrosection

Electrosection (cutting) results when slightly damped, modulated undamped, or undamped (sine wave) currents are properly applied. Two electrodes are necessary: the application is always biterminal. The concentrating electrode must not be heavy or coarse as bulk will slow cutting and cause unnecessary tissue destruction. The "delicate knife" electrode should be activated as it enters tissue (not beforehand) and deactivated as it comes out (not afterward). Undesirable destruction will follow if current flows during entry or exit. Skillful cutting requires courage and precision. A rapidly moving electric knife cuts cleanly (like a hot knife through butter) and inflicts little damage on incisional margins. Proper placement of the dispersive electrode is even more important here than it is during coagulation.

The slightly damped current of a spark gap apparatus cuts easily, destroys little tissue, and controls bleeding quite well. It is the type of current Bovie developed to make much of Cushing's brain surgery practical. A modulated undamped valve tube current with closely spaced wave trains cuts a bit better, damages somewhat less tissue, and retains fair hemostatic properties. The true undamped current (pure sine wave) cuts best, destroys almost no tissue, and has no appreciable ability to prevent bleeding. Under ideal conditions all three wave forms produce incisions that can heal by first intention. Obviously, the greatest success in this respect is achieved with the sine wave current.

In dermatology there is little or no need for current that only cuts; we prefer a modality that also provides adequate hemostasis. Comparatively low voltage, high amperage cutting current is characterized by 1 to 3 megahertz frequency, 100 to 500 V (under load), and 100 to 2000 mA.

Certain principles, to some degree, apply to all electrosurgical procedures. Most dermatologists may never use cutting current because rapid movements are required and this makes control difficult. Nevertheless, a cutting current with good hemostatic properties, like that from a spark gap, is a good modality for excision of tumors and for removing acceptable biopsy specimens from soft or vascular tumors. A quick swoop with a wire loop electrode, for example, may be used to gouge tissue for biopsy from a granuloma inguinale mass. It is also true that everything we can do with cutting current can be done by cutting with cold steel plus desiccation or coagulation. Furthermore, mechanical cuts can be made relatively slowly; hence, there is less chance of making errors,

especially those involving too much tissue removal.

General Procedures

Electrodesiccation and electrocoagulation are ideal modalities that are employed frequently by many dermatologists. Usually they are more effective tools when used in conjunction with some form of cutting, most often with the curette, scissors, or knife, in that order. Competent electrosurgeons do not simply "burn things off," unless they are removing tiny superficial lesions with very light current; eg, the desiccation needle with the current control set at, or near, zero may be used as an "electric eraser" to wipe off verrucae planae with little or no subsequent scarring. When lesions are larger and especially thicker, it is more difficult to determine the amount of current necessary to adequately remove undesirable tissue without damaging adjacent or underlying normal structures. It should be evident that burning off lesions is an inaccurate, inelegant, inept, and entirely unsatisfactory method of removal. Results are far better if the bulk of a tumor is removed by cutting, either in layers (bit by bit) or in toto, with each removal followed by application of the "exact" amount of electric current that will control bleeding and destroy only the desired amount of tissue (Fig. 20-6). With few exceptions, this is the type of electrosurgery referred to throughout this chapter.

Patients should be prepared for the smell of burning flesh (not always noticeable), for the possibility of heat transfer from the "hot" anesthetized operative area to surrounding tissue (not by conversion, but by conduction), and for comparatively slow healing. The convalescent period may be one of anxiety as the patient and the patient's family ponder over postoperative "scabs." They should be informed that the eventual cosmetic results, barring contractures, are always far better than can be expected from simply contemplating the wound.

As indicated previously, a surgical implement (mechanical or electric) should be used to "saucerize" the removal site, when practical, so that the resulting scar margins will gradually blend into the surrounding skin. Relatively large superficial tumors may be safely removed from the eyelids since there is no need of deep excision, but only experience will warn when

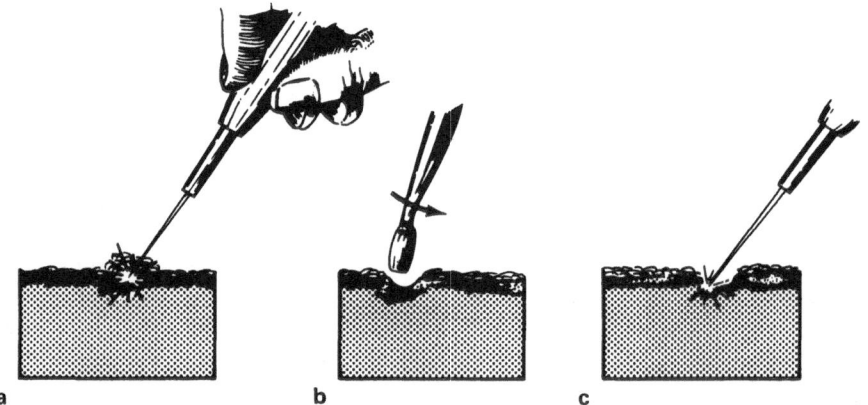

Figure 20-6.   Removal of superficial benign, or very early malignant, lesions (seborrheic keratoses, warts, solar keratoses). *a.* Initial electrodesiccation: often omitted, especially with tumors other than warts. May be repeated after curettage. *b.* Superficial curettage, before or after desiccation; may be repeated, alternating with electrodesiccation. (Scissors or scalpel may be substituted for, or alternated with, the curette.) *c.* Final electrodesiccation of base, using only enough current to produce desired result, and thus avoiding needless tissue destruction. From Pillsbury et al [20]. Courtesy of W. B. Saunders Co.

undesirable reactions such as ectropion are apt to follow. Judicious removal by electric and mechanical means can save patients from skin grafting and hospitalization. Excision of large, especially deep, lesions may lead to contracture of the upper lip and ala nasi, depression of the center nose (especially the tip), and notching of the rim of the ear.

Nonetheless, it is true that scars are usually cosmetically acceptable, often surprisingly good. A large round surgical defect often heals in a linear fashion, simulating the scar seen following excision and suture. Even cold-steel disk excisions of cancers and peripheral normal skin down to the fat, followed by electrodesiccation on electrocoagulation, often heal with surprisingly good results. Indeed, the scar following electrosurgery may be more attractive than is the appearance of a skin graft. If a superficial tumor can be wholly or partially removed by surgical shaving or planing and the base contoured so as to mimic the normal skin curvatures, little or no appreciable scarring will follow the use of light desiccation current to control bleeding.

Scarring will be less, as a rule, than the inexperienced physician or patient will expect from observations during the period of healing. It is wise to reassure the patient and to explain that healing will take from 1 to several weeks.

Necrotic tissue under the postoperative crust will suggest pus and infection to the uninitiated observer. Removal of large, loose crusts during convalescence will speed healing and improve appearance. Crusts that are soggy due to underlying "pus" should also be removed. The same is true of thick, yellowish, more or less greasy crusts that develop in oily skin areas, eg, around the nose. On the other hand, tightly adherent dry crusts are good protective covers and should be left undisturbed.

Dryness of the electrosurgical postoperative site is desirable and may be promoted by exposing the wound to air and by frequently applying 70% alcohol. Sometimes, especially if postoperative wounds are large, it is preferable to avoid dry thick crusts. If so, hydrogen peroxide may be applied so as to mechanically cleanse the removal site four times daily; residual liquid is removed each time by blotting prior to applying a thin film of a nonsensitizing antibiotic ointment. Wounds should be covered by dressings only for protection or cosmetic purposes. Short periods of "masking" do little, if any, harm and are good for morale.

Delayed bleeding postoperatively always alarms the patient who is not prepared for that possibility. The wise physician will explain beforehand that direct pressure with a few folds of cloth, such as gauze or a handkerchief, will control bleeding just as it did during surgery; he will make it clear that appreciable blood loss occurs only when fear interferes with rational behavior.

Extensive preoperative preparation is seldom necessary with electrosurgery. Rarely do patients require sedation. To save patients needless worry surgery should be performed, if possible, immediately after it is recommended. Patients, including an occasional physician, are pleasantly surprised when they realize how little discomfort accompanies electrosurgical procedures. It is advisable to tell subjects how much pain they should feel. If procedures are minor and the surgeon believes that no anesthetic is necessary, he should demonstrate the fact by testing on his own skin. Sterile drapes and gloves are not needed, since electrosurgical procedures are inherently antiseptic applications. Skin is thoroughly washed and then scrubbed with 70% alcohol before operation. A 3-min (or more) alcohol scrub is advisable before injecting an anesthetic under the skin of the hands or feet.

All patients are grateful for anesthesia unless minimal current can be used to remove small superficial lesions. It is hard to understand the callousness that prompts a surgeon to avoid anesthesia whenever possible. In fact, many people will ask for a "freezing" spray ethyl chloride) prior to injection, once they have experienced the slight numbing sensation that follows its use. A 1 to 2% local anesthetic (eg, Carbocaine or Xylocaine) is usually adequate for dermatologic surgery. Epinephrine is seldom required; it should never be injected into fingers! Finger tourniquets are rarely needed; if deemed necessary they should be applied for short periods. Skin tension and finger pressure are adequate to produce a reasonably dry field most of the time. A dry field permits use of a weaker current; bleeding is more easily controlled while tissue damage and charring may be decreased.

The needle electrode should be kept clean when operating. Wipe or scrape off charred and dehydrated bits of tissue with gauze, a fingernail, or a sharp metal edge. Keep in mind that the amount of destruction is directly related to both time and power. A clean, as well as a slim, electrode results in better concentration and more precise application. In this writer's experience, however, delicate, very sharp needle electrodes are generally unsatisfactory for desiccation and coagulation; when moved rapidly they tend to catch and make tiny superficial cuts in tissue. A moderately sharp needle of medium thickness is ideal for nearly all applications. Power should be increased when the needle is constantly kept in motion; to produce the same results with a relatively stationary needle, current should be reduced.

Inexpensive, thin, easily broken razor blades (not those made of hardened or stainless steel) make superior cutting instruments to use in conjunction with electrosurgery. They may be reduced to any manageable size and many shapes with a "blade breaker," an instrument similar to a small hemostat with flat, smooth jaws, which subsequently serves as a handle for these custom-made scalpels. These blades are very sharp and very thin, characteristics that permit fine, delicate, exquisite cutting. They are ideally suited for "shave excision" because they make it relatively easy, when compared with standard scalpels, to follow body (skin) contours. Blades can be made sufficiently small to work in depressed areas such as the nasolabial folds. If a razor blade is held between the fingers and bent (curved) so that the convexity is directed toward the skin, some tumors may be completely excised (sliced out) with the wound being saucerized at the same time.

Thin shave biopsy specimens, often including the entire tumor and certainly better than curettings, may be obtained from many lesions, eg, flat warts, seborrheic keratoses, and actinic keratoses. A narrow strip biopsy can also be removed from large lesions with the razor scalpel in order to further minimize scarring. The electrodesiccation needle is brushed lightly over the wound surface to control minimal bleeding.

Pinpoint electrodesiccation, and sometimes electrocoagulation, can be used to stop bleeding from larger superficial blood vessels. If such tiny desiccated, or small coagulated, areas are not close together, little or no scarring should result. After such spotty desiccation Monsel's solution may be widely applied to immediately stop minor oozing. This does not cause permanent pigmentation due to iron deposits, contrary to established doctrine, if surgery is superficial, as in removal of seborrheic keratoses. A temporary elegant hemostatic nonocclusive dressing can be made by covering the wound wih Gelfoam powder before applying flesh-tinted Micropore tape.

It is advisable to try various operative techniques on fresh moist flesh, eg, a piece of veal, before approaching the living subject.

Electrosurgical Treatment of Specific Lesions

Papillomatous, Filiform, and Digitate Tumors

Tumors such as skin tags, papillomas, and filiform warts are cut off by snipping the narrow trunk with small scissors. Bleeding is controlled with light electrodesiccation current. If tumors are tiny, local anesthesia may not be necessary. When tumors are sessile, or large enough to have a thick stalk, anesthesia is advisable and shave excision with a razor blade scalpel followed by electrodesiccation is recommended.

Vascular Tumors

Vascular tumors, if not too large, are easily treated by electrosurgery, with or without cutting. What constitutes suitable size must be determined by the experience of the surgeon. Telangiectasias and spider angiomas are sclerosed (destroyed) by repeatedly touching or puncturing the epidermis (every few millimeters) over the course of the dilated vessels or over the central punctum of angiomas with the desiccation or coagulation needle. A fine needle may be actually inserted into larger vessels. When using a spark gap generator, one will probably prefer the epilating (weak coagulation) current. A modulated undamped cutting current from a tube-type generator, applied monoterminally, is also effective, takes a little more time, causes more bleeding, and hurts less. Local anesthesia may be desirable, but telangiectasias scattered over a large area and the tendency of injected fluid to obliterate small vessels may make infiltration impractical. When spider angiomas are distinct and localized, anesthetics can be injected circumferentially or even sublesionally. A short waiting period gives lesions obliterated by injection a chance to reappear while adequate analgesia is retained.

Local anesthetics are always indicated, if there are no contraindications to their use, before removal of larger lesions, such as senile angiomas, angiomas of the mucous membranes (including the lip), and small mature hemangiomas of any type. Excellent results follow scalpel or scissors excision, or preferably shave excision when it is adequate, and subsequent electrodesiccation. As always, experience teaches each operator what size limits are to be observed.

With rare exceptions, hemangiomas should not be treated electrosurgically or by excision before a patient is 10 years of age. Watchful waiting will almost always permit mature development and coincident spontaneous resolution. Indeed, one should attempt to remove vascular birthmarks, especially port-wine stains, at any age by electrosurgery and/or cryogenic surgery, only after cautious applications to a limited area. Judicious trials should satisfy the patient that the result of such surgery will be preferred to the original appearance.

Verrucae

Verrucae are so common that every busy dermatologist will sometimes hope never to see a wart again. Treatment problems challenge every aspect of the art and the science of medicine. Warts are contemplated too casually by uninformed patients and physicians. Usually patients seek help from the dermatologist after their warts have been present for many months, or even many years, growing and increasing in number with or without treatment. In our experience it is unwise to "let warts alone," hoping that they may disappear eventually. If many warts follow in the wake of viral autoinoculation, a more difficult treatment problem ensues.

It is far better to remove one or two warts unnecessarily than to cultivate difficult treatment problems. It is wise to always point out that unseen, apparently "hibernating" wart virions may produce warts in other areas, or cause recurrences (especially in younger children). The patient must understand that we have no way of determining how capriciously the wart virus may act in any given individual. After long practical experience, many frustrations, and review of the literature it is difficult to be scientific about wart management. One can promise that treatment will be successful only when every virus particle is destroyed or removed, and the sufferer is not exposed to reinfection.

Warts can be removed in many ways. The method that is least traumatic for the particular patient is always selected. If scars did not follow electrosurgery, it would be the method of choice for removal of verrucae (Fig. 20-7). At the same time, it is true that very few patients complain about such scars as long as the face is spared. We agree with Shelley [22] that "the single most reliable method" of removing ugly, large, deforming warts (especially of the hands) is to cut them out prior to thorough electrodesiccation of the base (Fig. 20-6). Strangely enough, such proper electrosurgical removal of subungual and periungual warts, a procedure shunned by many surgeons, results in remarka-

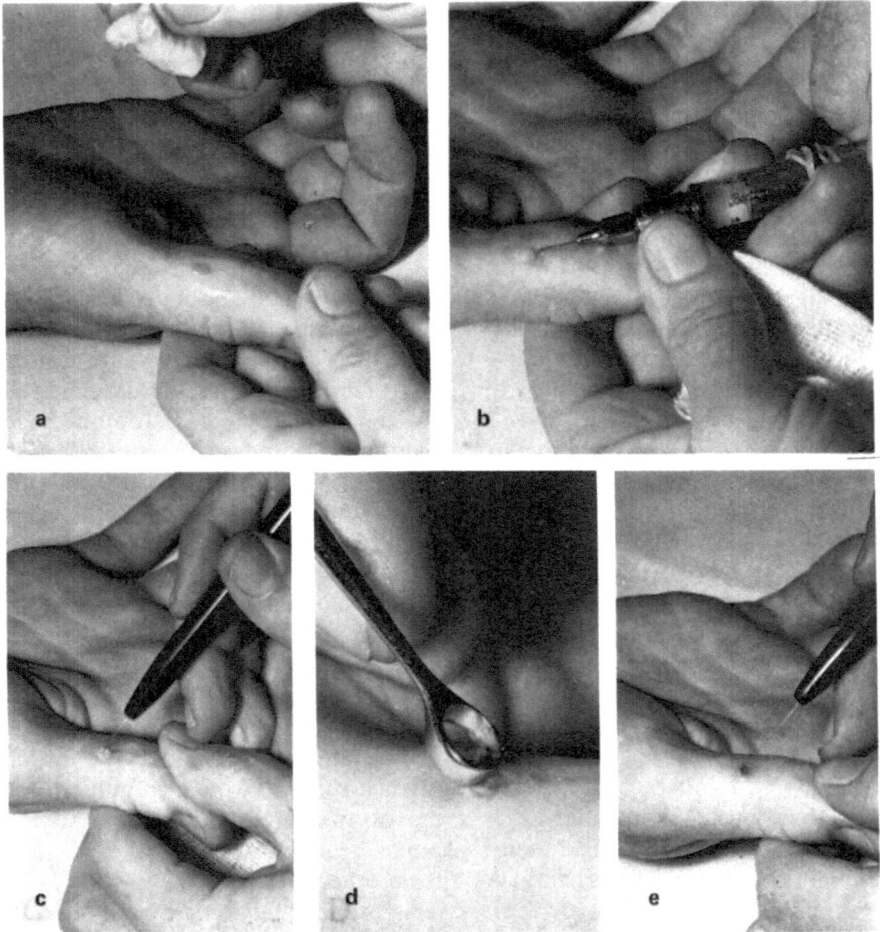

Figure 20-7. Technique of wart removal. Removal may be much more extensive than is pictured here, especially if tumors are periungual. Remove overlying nail if warts are subungual. *a.* Preparation of operative site: scrub with 70% alcohol for 3 min; use sterile instruments. *b.* Infiltration of local anesthetic around and under wart. Avoid needling infected tissue. Do not inject epinephrine into digits. Some surgeons will prefer nerve block. *c.* Electrodesiccation around, and in, wart; this step may be omitted. *d.* Removal of wart tissue before or after desiccation with curette. Often it is desirable to trim periphery of wound with small curved scissors. *e.* Electrodesiccation of entire removal site, lightly but thoroughly, to destroy residual virions. No viable cells should remain on the surface. Control of bleeding is a planned bonus. From Pillsbury et al [20]. Courtesy of W. B. Saunders Co.

bly little scarring or deformity. The finger may be somewhat more tapered after extensive surgery.

One should avoid being lulled into a sense of false security. Poor wart surgery is too often the rule rather than the exception. No doubt this results from the foolish, disdainful attitude that wart surgery is extremely simple—anyone can do it. As a result, incomplete removal or excessive destruction, or both, are frequently encountered. This is to be expected when tumors are simply "burned off."

Local anesthesia is mandatory before electrosurgical removal of any but the smallest warts; for extensive involvement of a finger, some surgeons prefer digital nerve block. It is wise to keep the anesthetic needle out of the wart to prevent reflux and seeding of viable virus into surrounding uninvolved tissue. It may be best to desiccate a ring of apparently normal skin immediately adjoining the wart in order to destroy any inapparent advancing infection. Some prefer to desiccate the wart itself to the point of beginning incandescence by multiple insertions of the operating needle before excision. However, total destruction of all virions without risking excessive damage to uninfected tissue is not possible and should not be attempted. Rather, every bit of visible wart is removed by repeated curettement, so that at worst only a very thin layer of infected cells can remain. It is then easy to destroy any remaining virus, and at the same time control bleeding, with a light desiccating current that is unlikely to damage excessive normal tissue. The wound is left uncovered as much as is practical.

If the technique of removing warts from the hand is mastered, one should have little difficulty in other areas. When treating subungual warts it is important to cut off enough nail to expose the entire tumor and a narrow peripheral margin of normal tissue before attempting removal. The patient should be informed that permanent nail dystrophy is always a possibility when a wart overlies the matrix or involves much of the nail bed. Actually, despite this possibility, objectionable deformity is rarely a prominent sequel of good surgery.

Since it is difficult for patients to protect their hands and feet adequately, secondary infection is always a threat; but it is usually easy to control with warm soaks and systemic antibiotics. Healing is frequently delayed in areas subjected to moisture, in creases, and over knuckles. Scars from previous wart surgery (or x-ray therapy), abutting on or admixed with newly infected tissue, may complicate surgical procedures, but are not a contraindication to further excision.

Many dermatologists avoid removing plantar warts electrosurgically, although such surgery is usually successful and without subsequent painful scarring. Apparently a minority of dermatologists routinely manage all but the largest plantar warts, including those of the mosaic variety, in this manner. The clue to success is probably meticulous blunt dissection, followed by very light but thorough desiccation in a dry field. An uninfected epidermal collarette is made by cutting with small curved scissors or scalpel into the normal skin, often thickened (callused), around the plantar wart. The wart is then dissected from the surrounding base with a blunt curette; it may be scooped out with a spoon curette. If surgery is properly performed, the pattern of dermatoglyphics can be seen in the dry field before the base is lightly electrodesiccated. Unfortunately, the recurrence rate is higher if desiccation does not follow curettement. An irrational (the histologic picture having been disregarded) and reprehensible procedure is full thickness excision of the skin containing the wart followed by suture repair. Not only is the recurrence rate high, but satellite warts often develop around excision scars, including those that are deemed "perfect," so that therapy is needlessly complicated and prolonged. The possibility of painful scarring, however infrequent, makes removal of verrucae plantares over pressure points fraught with more risk than removal from other areas.

Venereal warts are easily removed by desiccation or coagulation, with or without excision, after podophyllin chemotherapy fails. Vaginal and rectal mucosal warts should be suspected in every case, and removed to prevent recurrence in the skin. Following any type of wart removal, the patient is urged to return as soon as there is any suspicion of recurrence. Careful, thorough surgery by competent dermatologic surgeons is more successful than a review of the literature suggests.

Nevi

Nevi, more or less pigmented, are ubiquitous in the skin; it has been estimated that the average adult has 40 moles at 30 years of age. Many of these tumors are objectionable because they are irritated or cut, as in shaving, or are cosmetically offensive. Cosmetically speaking, no form of removal can improve on the results that follow expert shave excision and subsequent electrosurgery. If and when pigmented nevi should be removed by electrosurgery is debatable, however, because they may be the foci for malignant melanomas. Some authorities insist that pigmented nevi should be excised in toto or left untouched. Many dermatologists, including this writer, believe it is safe to remove any biopsy-proven benign nevus electrosurgically. Probably the majority of dermatologists approve of the electrosurgical removal of elevated nevi, followed by wide excision if ominous junctional activity is observed under the microscope. Obviously, flat nevi cannot be removed by shave excision. They should not be destroyed by any type of electric current, since no specimen is available for biopsy and scarring can be excessive. Flat nevi should be excised and subjected to microscopic examination; small lesions may be excised with a punch.

Actually it may be safe to remove unchanging elevated nevi, judged benign by competent dermatologists, without subsequent histologic examination. This has been the daily routine for many years in some quarters, but such practice cannot be recommended. Histologic examination should be undertaken, not so much because malignant melanoma may be present, but to avoid potential malpractice actions.

High frequency electric currents are not carcinogenic. No one has proven, to our knowledge, that electrosurgery of any type, let alone light electrodesiccation, has ever been responsible for a malignant melanoma. This is a remarkable and most significant fact, because thousands of nevi are partially removed by good and bad electrosurgery every day. Daily trauma repeated for years is probably more dangerous than gentle partial excision. Decrying all electrosurgery in management of nevi is hard to justify. Large numbers of people have benefited from such surgery; to deprive patients of this aid is inconsistent with our goal of helping as many people as possible at reasonable cost.

Cosmetic removal of nevi, particularly those on the face, requires commendably precise technique. Following local anesthesia the razor-blade scalpel (or conventional scalpel) is used for shave excision of the protruding portion of the tumor, following the normal contours of the involved area. Any concavity that will result in a slight depression should be avoided. The least intense effective electrodesiccation current is sharply localized to control points of comparatively marked bleeding. The operating needle may then be moved rapidly back and forth over the excision site to stop minor oozing. The electrode can also be used as an electrosurgical curette or electrosurgical eraser to further contour any irregularities. A monoterminal diamond-shaped wire-loop electrode, activated by a mild modulated undamped cutting current, may be lightly brushed to and fro over the wound to accomplish similar results. Monsel's solution may be safely used to stop minimal bleeding.

No dressing is required, but there is no objection to a temporary Gelfoam–Micropore cover (previously described). The excised nevus is examined under the microscope to rule out any possibility of premalignant or malignant malanoma. If there is any suggestion that the residual nevus left in the skin will threaten the patient's future welfare, it is widely excised. Appearance of a small melanotic freckle after complete healing is no cause for concern in the light of favorable biopsy findings; melanocytes are carried up out of a follicle during epithelization.

Seborrheic Keratoses

Seborrheic keratoses (basal cell papillomas), though benign, frequently annoy and disfigure the senior citizen. They grow on some skins by the dozens, or even hundreds, and it is not uncommon to find tumors that measure more than 25 mm in diameter. Generally speaking, these warty, pigmented, plaquelike tumors tend to get larger, thicker, darker, crustier, and uglier with the passage of time. Frequently they itch, and moisture causes maceration: they can cause considerable discomfort under an overhanging breast. It is our belief that seborrheic keratoses should be removed as soon as they become objectionable for any reason, and before increase in size and numbers makes them a plague.

Commonly, seborrheic keratoses are easily excised from (scraped off) the skin by a curette, which need not be razor sharp. Occasionally, despite the histologic picture, they become quite adherent as they grow older, are much harder to remove, and the base is rough rather than smooth. After the bulk of a lesion is removed the base is smoothed by further curettement. The most active bleeding points are controlled by the desiccation current. Minimal, more generalized bleeding (slight oozing) of the surface can be controlled by rubbing the area rapidly with the desiccation current needle, by applying Monsel's solution, or by covering with a Gelfoam–Micropore dressing. As a matter of fact, all these methods are used in some cases. The Gelfoam–Micropore dressing is preferred on the face because Monsel's solution makes a darker crust that adheres for a longer time. This method of postoperative management is less messy than that of watchful waiting and pressure dressings. Minimal scarring, or frequently no scarring, follows the artistic removal of seborrheic keratoses.

Actinic Keratoses

Actinic keratoses (solar keratoses, senile keratoses) are precancerous tumors and should be removed soon after they are discovered. They are often considered as squamous cell cancers, grade $\frac{1}{2}$. Probably, malignant degeneration would eventually occur in every one if the patient lived long enough. Fortunately, however, such secondary (to damage by sunlight) cancers are much less likely to metastasize than are those that arise de novo. Once actinic keratoses have started to develop, it is a wise policy to reexamine the patient every 6 months, or sooner if tumors erupt frequently.

Topical 5-fluorouracil (5-FU) will eradicate, more or less permanently, actinic keratoses. If the patient agrees this chemical should be employed before surgery, especially when there are many lesions. Surgery may be avoided or postponed in this manner. Numerous patients will refuse the chemical when acquainted with its inflammatory effects and alternate methods of treatment. It is also true, in our experience, that a majority of those who have used 5-FU one or two times elect to have recurrences or new lesions removed surgically (by electrosurgery or cryosurgery).

Actinic keratoses are removed much like seborrheic keratoses, but the curette should be sharp because they are adherent and harder to excise. Painstaking, complete electrodesiccation of the entire tumor base, after thorough curettement, is necessary because of their cancerous predisposition. If biopsy is desirable, adequate tissue should be removed by curettement or shave excision. The latter may provide a more satisfactory specimen. After obtaining material for histologic examination, one may immediately remove the entire tumor or postpone definitive surgery (Fig. 20-8). Some scarring always follows electrosurgical removal of actinic keratoses. Usually it is not marked, but it may be objectionable because of hypopigmentation. A cutaneous horn (cornu cutaneum) can be a hyperkeratotic hypertrophic solar keratosis and is excised in the same manner.

Epitheliomas

Epitheliomas (skin cancers) are eradicated by proper electrosurgery more than 95% of the time. Crissey [7] states that "the 5-year cure rate for this technique compares favorably with the 5-year cure rate for other methods of treatment. He points out that the 5-year cure rate for Mohs' series, removed by his chemosurgical technique, is 99.1%" and that this percentage is remarkable when one considers that many of Mohs' cases may be described as "cutaneous disasters." Unfortunately, it is impractical and impossible to treat every skin cancer in this fashion. Fortunately, on the other hand, it is not necessary. From a practical standpoint, electrosurgical removal (cutting/curettement followed by electrocoagulation) of skin cancers is enthusiastically recommended (Fig. 20-9). It may be well to recall that electrosurgical procedures are rapid, safe, effective, aseptic, painless, and frequently save the patient considerable time and expense. Several studies suggest that breakdown products of tumor cells partially destroyed by electrocoagulation may act as antigens and stimulate an immune mechanism that destroys

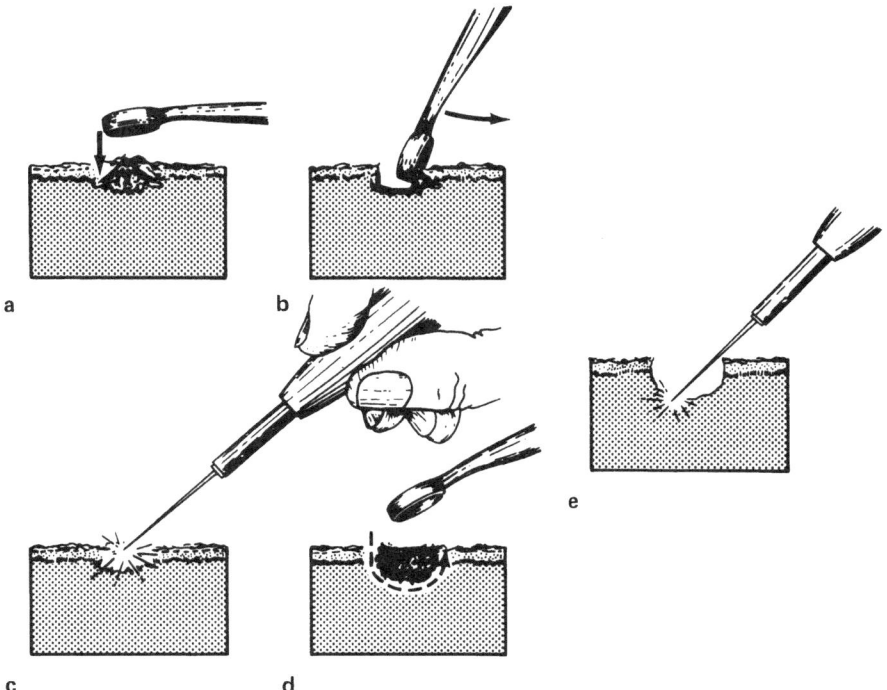

Figure 20-8. Technique of biopsy and electrosurgical (excision and electro-dessiccation or electrocoagulation) removal of skin tumors. For elevated nevi, substitute scalpel shave for curettement, thus avoiding any concavity. *a* and *b*. Removal of material for biopsy. Sharp curette, firm downstroke to base of lesion (a); removal of adequate specimen (b). Scissors or scalpel may often be substituted for the curette. Infiltrate local anesthetic around and under lesion before cutting.
c. Biterminal (not bipolar) coagulation (monoterminal desiccation may be preferred).
d. Thorough, firm, meticulous curettage to, or into, surrounding normal tissue to remove and saucerize wound. Demarcation is often sharp and distinct, but search for malignant pseudopods with small curette. *e*. Biterminal coagulation of periphery. Curettage and coagulation may be repeated several times. From Pillsbury et al [20]. Courtesy of W. B. Saunders Co.

residual cancer tissue; at present this theory cannot be proven.

All skin cancers, except malignant melanomas, can be removed electrosurgically. It is, nevertheless, safe to biopsy malignant melanomas electrosurgically if total, en bloc excision of the tumor follows within the week. The technique of biopsy of any cancer is the same as the technique of removal, but only representative tissue is removed and eradication of the tumor is postponed. As a matter of fact, the expert dermatologist usually recognizes the nature of the lesion beforehand, and one excision can serve both purposes. Older and larger cancers are, naturally, more difficult to remove, and, as expected, have a slightly lower cure rate. Malignant cells may extend as pseudopods and

escape detection by the searching curette, to be subsequently unearthed by Mohs's chemosurgical technique. Luckily, the extent of most cancers can be determined by the curette and complete removal, in expert hands, is the rule rather than the exception. As Pillsbury [20] has pointed out, "there is possibly no aspect of dermatologic therapy more satisfying than the early recognition of basal cell epithelioma and its removal as an office procedure." Figure I-1 demonstrates that cosmetic results may be superior.

Probably no one should attempt to make hard and fast rules about the sizes of tumors that are suitable for electrosurgical removal. Both the type and location of a cancer are important. In the past a majority of dermatolo-

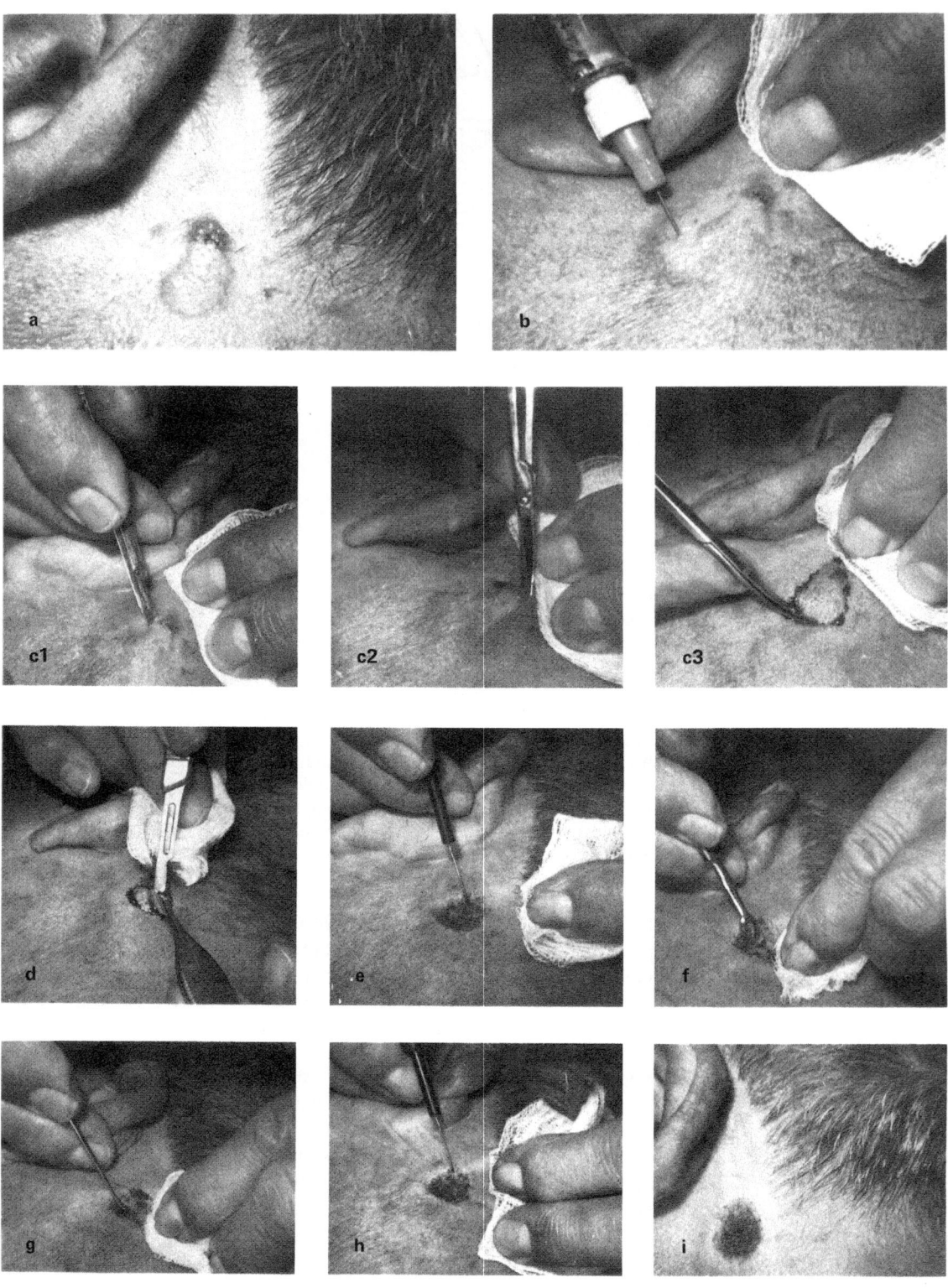

gists have been too conservative, but Crissey [7] has wisely suggested the following sizes: "4 cm in any area" and "1 cm on the tip of the nose or ala nasa" unless the lesion is superficial. These are, we agree, reasonable rules of thumb, especially for the beginner, meant to be violated as one gains experience and the situation demands. We have, as have Whelan [27] and Whelan and Deckers [28], often successfully exceeded such limitations.

Sclerosing basal cell cancers usually respond to audacious electrosurgery, and recurrences, normally recurring superficially in the scar and readily observed, are easy to remove. On occasion it may be better to treat these recurrences chemosurgically, cryosurgically, with x rays, or by wide excision with subsequent grafting. The same is true when bone is involved. Cartilage, on the other hand, even when stripped of all overlying tissue over a wide area, withstands the onslaught of high frequency current surprisingly well. The eventual result will seem almost miraculous to the inexperienced observer. There is no need to worry about painful chondritis or necrosis. Selected cancers of the eyelid margins and the vermillion borders of the lips can be removed electrosurgically with very good to excellent results. The fact that electrosurgery spares tissue around the eyes, nose, mouth, and ears may be of great importance.

Too many dermatologists, as well as most nondermatologic surgeons, refuse to remove any prickle cell epithelioma (squamous cell carcinoma) by excision and electrocoagulation. However, like a growing number of dermatologists and nondermatologists, it is our belief that a majority of squamous cell skin cancers can safely, and should, be removed by cutting, curettement, and electrocoagulation. It has already been mentioned that squamous cell cancers, arising in actinic (solar) keratoses, compared to those arising de novo, are not agressive carcinomas and have almost no metastatic potential. This new biologic concept proposed by Graham et al in 1969 [10b] strengthened our belief in the efficacy of such surgery and helped explain successes that had been questioned by others. The technique of removal is exactly like that described for extirpation of basal cell cancers. It has been my experience that wide excision of sequelae (wounds or scars) following thorough electrosurgery— prompted because of doubt, fear, histologic observation, or skepticism—has usually failed to reveal residual cancer.

Freeman et al [10a], as well as Williamson and Jackson [29], reported the results of studies that justified the use of curettement combined with electrodesiccation to treat squamous cell cancer. Honeycutt and Jansen [12a] cured 98.9% of 281 squamous cell carcinomas by electrodesiccation and curettage. This impressive cure rate is greater if only lesions not exceeding 2 cm in size are considered; there was only one recurrence after 264 excisions. They believe that such therapy, which we consider proper electrosurgery, is the treatment of choice in selected cases because of excellent to superior results, good cosmetic effect, and reduction in medical expense.

Preceding removal of any cancer, uninvolved skin surrounding the tumor is infiltrated with local anesthetic. It seems best to avoid needling the lesion itself, lest cancerous cells be carried into uninvolved tissue. The entire cancer can be removed, usually piecemeal, by vigorous curettement with a sharp instrument. Cancer tissue is often soft, with a consistency somewhat like that of a firm melon, so that it is easily separated from harder normal tissue. Smaller curettes are used to search every nook

---

← ———

Figure 20-9. Removal of skin cancer by electrosurgery (cutting and electrocoagulation). *a.* Basal cell cancer. Lower portion resembles a seborrheic keratosis. *b.* Infiltration of local anesthetic around and under cancer after scrubbing skin with 70% alcohol. Avoid needling malignant tissue. *c*1, 2, 3. Incision into peripheral uninvolved skin with scalpel or scissors preparatory to undercutting tumor. A sharp curette is often preferred to scalpel or scissors. In any event, it is often wise to incline the cutting instrument to saucerize the wound. *d.* Undercutting tumor to remove malignant tissue en bloc. *e.* Electrocoagulation of major bleeding points. This step may be omitted or repeated as needed. *f.* Curettement to ensure complete removal. This step is not necessary if one is certain all cancer tissue has been removed. *g.* Searching for pockets (pseudopods) of malignant tissue. *h.* Final electrocoagulation of base and periphery of wound. This step not only controls bleeding, but also destroys superficial residuals of cancer that may have escaped detection. *i.* Final appearance after electrosurgery.

and cranny of the resulting depression or cavity for pockets and pseudopods of cancer cells. The entire exposed area of the cavity (surgical defect) is then electrocoagulated, or heavily desiccated, so that an additional 2 or 3 mm of tissue is destroyed. Coagulated or charred tissue is curetted away, and the entire process of curettement, search, and electrocoagulation is repeated once or twice. Since peripheral margins are potential sites of recurrence and gently sloping edges make a more cosmetic depression, a scalpel or curved scissors is used to further saucerize the wound; the chance of cure is increased and the somewhat larger scar will look better than does a smaller chasm with precipitous sides.

The described technique may be modified, more or less frequently, to produce better results. Cutting current or a cold knife may be used in conjunction with curettement and electrocoagulation. Electrosurgery also includes the use of cutting current with good hemostatic properties to excise the entire cancer, with or without subsequent closure, and hopefully with healing by first intention if sutures are used. For years it has been my practice to excise and destroy cancers by a modified technique of curettement, cutting, and electrocoagulation. As expected the second and third curettements remove decreasing amounts of tissue. There is always some chance that marginal small foci of cancer cells were missed by the curette and the coagulating current. For this reason, in the majority of cases the entire process of curettement and electrocoagulation has been repeated 7 to 10 days later, after histologic evaluation, to

enhance the chance of complete removal (Fig. 20-10). Considerably more tissue is removed and experience indicates that the final cosmetic result is prejudiced very little, if at all, by this epilogue surgery.

Treatment of cancer is wisely followed by conscientious and determined efforts to have the patient return for routine regular check-ups no less than every six months for at least 5 years. Not only can recurrences be treated at an early date, but many precancers and numerous new cancers, unrecognized by the untrained eye, will be discovered.

Precancerous Lesions and Carcinomas in Situ

Precancerous lesions, generally comparable to actinic or senile keratoses, and carcinomas in situ should also be treated by curettement (and/or cutting) and electrodesiccation (and/or electrocoagulation). Erythroplasia of Queyrat occurring in mucous membranes (usually on the glans penis; sometimes on the prepuce, vulva, or oral mucosa) is an intraepithelial squamous cell cancer: it is the equivalent of Bowen's disease, which is an intraepidermal squamous cell cancer (cancer in situ). Paget's disease is carcinoma in situ, classically involving the female nipple; now and then the male nipple is attacked. It is external evidence of deeper ductal cancer of the breast and the entire organ should be removed despite its normal appearance. Extramammary Paget's disease of the axillae, genital area, and anal region also heralds probable or possible underlying carcinoma. The apocrine glands (cousins of the

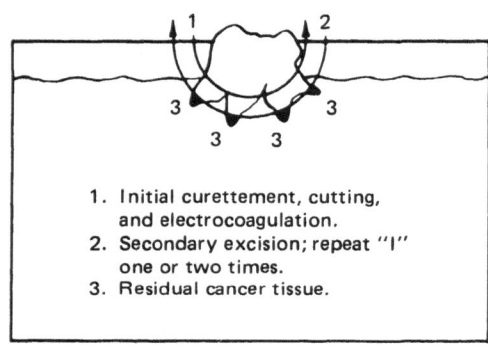

1. Initial curettement, cutting, and electrocoagulation.
2. Secondary excision; repeat "l" one or two times.
3. Residual cancer tissue.

a

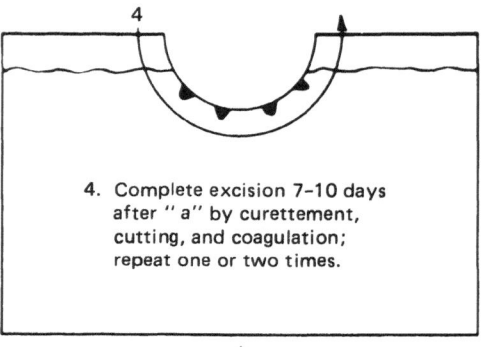

4. Complete excision 7–10 days after " a" by curettement, cutting, and coagulation; repeat one or two times.

b

Figure 20-10. "Epilogue" removal of epithelioma. *a.* Classical removal of epithelioma by curettement, cutting, and electrocoagulation, as in Fig. 20-8. *b.* "Epilogue" removal 7 to 10 days after initial procedure. This removal is made easy due to previous electrocoagulation, and increases chance of cure.

mammary gland) are involved in the axillae and genital area; the mucus-secreting goblet cells are involved in the anal region.

Leukoplakia is the mucosal counterpart of senile keratosis in the skin; it may affect the lips, the oral mucous membranes, or the vulva. Arsenical keratoses may histologically resemble either senile keratosis or Bowen's disease.

Areas of x-ray atrophy, fortunately seen with decreasing frequency during our lifetime, are prone to develop radiation keratoses (akin to actinic keratoses) and cancers (often manifested by ulceration). These scarred sites of excessive radiation should be carefully examined at least every 6 months; at such times degenerative lesions can be annihilated.

Cysts

Cysts (wens), usually keratinous, seldom sebaceous, may be removed electrosurgically by Danna's method [8]. He used a diathermy needle (usually monoterminal) to create an opening, about 5 mm in diameter, in the thinnest part or center of the cyst top. The amount of tissue slough, depending on how much current was applied, determined the size of the opening. Following this procedure Danna allowed the contents of the cyst to be naturally extruded over a period of weeks with eventual excellent cosmetic results. The method is particularly valuable if the cyst is inflamed or infected; the opening can be made without benefit of anesthesia.

An alternate method of removal, requiring local anesthesia, is usually preferable. An opening is made in the cyst, with cold knife or electrosurgery needle, and the contents are evacuated. The walls of the cyst cavity are then curetted (scraped) and desiccated, prior to removal of the cyst wall (sac) by small forceps and manipulation. Burdick [5] recognizes the efficacy of this technique, but he prefers burning the inside of the sac with a hot cautery tip to desiccating the walls with a cold high frequency needle. On other occasions some will prefer to make a small scalpel incision through the top of the cyst. After evacuation of contents the use of curette, forceps, and pressure manipulation (often quite forceful) results in extrusion of the entire sac. The incision is closed by suture when desired. If removal appears incomplete one may elect to desiccate (or cauterize) the margins of the incision and the remaining sac, proceeding as though the scalpel had not been employed.

Miscellaneous Lesions

Miscellaneous lesions are more or less amenable to the electrosurgical procedures that have been described. An incomplete list includes pyogenic granuloma, molluscum contagiosum, mucus retention cyst, rhinophyma, xanthelasma, hidradenitis suppurativa, trichoepithelioma, adenoma sebaceum, sebaceous adenoma, senile sebaceous nevus, sebaceous nevus of Jadassohn, syringoma, hidrocystoma, and small circumscribed lymphangioma.

Removal or destruction is necessarily followed by relative scarring. Benign tumor surgery is advised only when the scar is expected to be preferable to the tumor. In many instances the advisability and choice of electrosurgical removal will be determined by the number and the location of lesions. If in doubt, or in the presence of many tumors, one or a few may be removed as a test procedure, as a prelude to contemplated additional surgery weeks to months later.

Cutting and curettement followed by desiccation may be the treatment of choice for pyogenic granuloma, mucus retention cyst, trichoepithelioma, and certain stages of hidradenitis suppurativa. Lesions of hidradenitis suppurativa are "marsupialized" (in lieu of excision and graft) by excising the skin overlying cavities and sinus tracts. The exteriorized bases and sides are completely curetted and electrocoagulated. Such wounds heal slowly.

Few surgeons will find office removal of massive rhinophyma a practical procedure; less severe involvement is another matter. The nose is artistically reshaped by shave excision of excess tissue with a damped or modulated undamped cutting current scalpel. Switching to electrocoagulation current may be required to stop localized, more profuse bleeding. Electrosection is far better than traditional scalpel surgery in such cases. There is evidence that electrosurgical shave followed by cryogenic surgery may prove to be the treatment method of choice.

A nevus of Jadassohn is a precancerous tumor. Basal cell cancer may develop in more than half of them. Most dermatologists will probably recommend complete excision about the time of puberty; smaller tumors of the scalp can be destroyed by electrocoagulation if a depressed scar will not be objectionable.

There can be no doubt that proper electrosurgery is a most valuable modality that can be employed many times each day to cure disease, to correct deformity, to provide great relief, to give much pleasure, to promote happiness, to conserve precious time, to prevent loss of work, and to reduce the cost of medical care.

Unfortunately, electrosurgery is often misused because the techniques of application are deceptively simple. The dermatologist is less likely than are other physicians to make such mistakes. His familiarity with all the vagaries of skin morphology makes the competent dermatologic surgeon the physician of choice to apply electric current advantageously for skin surgery. Electrosurgery is too often avoided, to the patient's detriment.

References

1. Billin AG: Personal communication, 1971
2. Bouman HD, Lentzer EMG: The treatment of hyperhidrosis of hands and feet with constant current. Am J Phys Med 31:158, 1952
3. Bovie WT: Cited in McClean AJ: Characteristics of adequate electrosurgical current. Am J Surg 18:417, 1932
4. Burdick KH: Electrocautery of minor skin lesions. In Epstein E (ed): Skin Surgery. Springfield, Ill, Thomas, 1970
5. Burdick KH: Electrosurgical Apparatus and Their Application in Dermatology. Springfield, Ill, Thomas, 1966
6. Clark WL, Morgan JD, Asnis EJ: Electrothermic methods in treatment of neoplasms and other lesions, with clinical and histological observations. Radiology 2:233, 1924
7. Crissey JT: Curettage and electrodesiccation as a method of treatment for epitheliomas of the skin. J Surg Oncol 3:287, 1971
8. Danna JA: A simple treatment for sebaceous cyst. New Orleans Med Surg J 98:5, 1945
9. Elliott JA Jr: Electrosurgery. Its use in dermatology, with a review of its development and technologic aspects. Arch. Dermatol 94:340, 1966
10. Epstein E: Cautery excision. In Epstein E (ed): Skin Surgery (3rd Ed). Springfield, Ill, Thomas, 1970
10a. Freeman PG, Knox JM, Heaton CL: The treatment of skin cancer: a statistical study of 1,341 skin tumors comparing results obtained with irradiation, surgery, and curretage followed by electrodesiccation. *Cancer* 17:535, 1964
10b. Graham JH, Bendl BJ, Johnson WC: Solar keratosis with squamous cell carcinoma: a new biologic concept. *Am. J. Pathol* 55:26A, 1969
11. Greene, LF, Merideth J: Transurethral operations employing high frequency electrical currents on patients with demand cardiac pacemakers. J Urol 108:446, 1972
12. Harris R: Iontophoresis. In Licht S (ed): Therapeutic Electricity and Ultraviolet Radiation. Waverly Press, Inc. Baltimore, MD. 1967
12a. Honeycutt W M , Jansen G T : Treatment of squamous cell carcinoma of the skin. *Arch. Dermatol.* 108:670, 1973
13. Huntoon RD: Tissue heating accompanying electrosurgery. An experimental investigation. Ann Surg 105:270, 1937
14. Kligman AM: Personal communication, 1976
15. Krull EA: Pacemakers. Cutaneous Surgery Course. Annual Meeting of the American Academy of Dermatology, 1974
16. Lincoln CS Jr: Epilation. In Epstein E (ed): Skin Surgery. Springfield, Ill, Thomas, 1970
17. Martin JW: Personal communication, 1972
18. McClean AJ: Characteristics of adequate electrosurgical current. Am J Surg 18:417, 1932
18a. National Fire Protection Association: Manual for the Safe Use of High Frequency Electrical Equipment in Hospitals. Boston. NFPA No. 76CM, 1976
19. Peereboom-Wynia JDR: The effect of electrical epilation on the beard hair of women with idiopathic hirsutism. Arch Dermatol Res 254:15, 1975
20. Pillsbury DM, Shelley WB, Kligman AM: Dermatology. Philadelphia, Saunders, 1956
21. Robinson MM: Removal of superfluous hair by monopolar coagulation. Med Ann DC 15:531, 1946
22. Shelley WB: Consultations in Dermatology with Walter B. Shelley. Philadelphia, Saunders, 1972
23. Shelley WB, Horvath PM, Weidman FD, et al: Experimental militaria in man, production of sweat retention anidrosis and vesicles by means of iontophoresis. J Invest Dermatol 11:275, 1948
24. Sternberg TH: Clinical Study of Perma Tweez Self-Use Electrolysis. Los Angeles, General Medical, 1972
25. Watkins AL: A Manual of Electrotherapy. Philadelphia, Lea & Febiger, 1958

26. Watkins AL: A Manual of Electrotherapy, 3rd ed. Philadelphia, Lea & Febiger, 1968

27. Whelan CS: Electrocoagulation in the treatment of skin cancers about the head and face. Surgery 62:1017, 1967

28. Whelan CS, Deckers PJ: Electrocoagulation and currettage for carcinoma involving the skin of the face, nose, eyelids, and ears. Cancer 31(1):159, 1973

29. Williamson GS, Jackson R: Treatment of squamous cell carcinoma of the skin by electrodesiccation and currettage. *Canad Med Assoc J* 90:408, 1964.

21

Phototherapy: Light Sources

Isaac Willis

The resolution of certain skin diseases following exposure to sunlight was recognized as early as two centuries ago, and this recognition has had a significant impact on the manner in which succeeding generations of practitioners manage many of their dermatologic patients. However, because sunlight is so capricious in its nature it soon became necessary for more modern clinicians to attempt to determine the particular wavelengths of sunlight that were of greatest therapeutic importance, and to equip themselves with some type of artificial light source(s) that could produce these wavelengths and the desired effects within both a predictable and reasonable period of time. Herein we will describe the major light sources that are currently available for this purpose, their advantages and disadvantages in therapy, and the skin diseases that are most responsive to phototherapy.

Light Sources

Types of Artificial Light Sources

It is just as important to know the appropriate light source to use in the treatment of a disease as it is to know that the disease can be effectively treated by light. It is therefore necessary to have knowledge of (1) the spectral and energy output of one's lamp source, and (2) the specific wavelength requirement (action spectrum) for obtaining resolution of the disease.

Advances in the field of dermatologic photobiology can be used to help resolve some of the diversities of opinion concerning the ideal type of lamp source. Thus, it must be realized that direct cutaneous effects resulting from light exposure may be mechanistically and pathologically different when caused by different wavelengths from different lamp sources (eg, 254 nm versus 290 to 320 nm versus > 320 nm erythema responses) [2,3]. Thus, one's therapeutic objectives will be influenced by the types of radiation in use. Also, precise action spectrum data that are now known for specific phototherapeutic chemicals will dictate the wavelength requirements and lamp source that are required for a particular desired photochemotherapeutic effect.

Artificial light sources can be divided into two basic types: incandescent and arc. Incandescent light sources emit mainly visible and infrared radiation, and are therefore used mainly for visible lighting and in some cases to produce heat. Since certain chemicals useful in skin diseases (eg, neutral red in herpes simplex infections) are activated by visible wavelengths, these lamps do have some limited phototherapeutic value. Arc light sources are the type most commonly used in phototherapy. Although they are best known for their emissions in the ultraviolet (UV) spectrum, many of these lamps are also capable of emitting tremendous amounts of visible and infrared radiation.

Types of Arc Light Sources

Arc light sources are of two types: open and enclosed. The carbon arc lamp is prototypical of the open arc lamp. It was popularized by Finsen who employed its UV emissions for the treatment of cutaneous tuberculosis. However, in spite of its nearly ideal solar-simulating (sunlight) spectrum of radiation, its practical, technical, and economic disadvantages have led to its disuse and to the need for the enclosed type of arc sources. The enclosed arc light sources are of numerous types, the most common of which include the mercury, xenon, and quartz–iodine arcs currently in use in dermatology practices in this country [7]. These will receive more detailed description below.

Choosing a Light Source

The ultimate decision as to which lamp(s) to use in one's practice should be based upon two factors: (1) the type(s) of photobiologic response(s) which must be elicited in order to achieve phototherapeutic success, and (2) the technical, economic, practical, and medical advantages and disadvantages of a chosen source.

The first point requires a basic knowledge of the effects of different wavelength ranges of light on skin and also the effects of the wavelengths on photosensitizing chemicals used in phototherapy [4,6,8]. It is helpful to divide wavelengths into the UVB (290 to 320 nm), UVA (320 to 400 nm), visible (VIS) (400 to 700 nm), and infrared (IR) (> 700 nm) ranges for this purpose (Fig. 21-1). Light sources that emit radiation mainly in the UVB range will cause sunburn, desquamation, some pigment darkening, and melanogenesis with delayed pigmentation. However, this type of source is not as useful for eliciting certain photochemically dependent phototherapeutic responses as are those sources that simultaneously emit not only UVB but also UVA and VIS radiation. Although high doses of UVA are capable of causing direct effects on skin that are similar to those caused by UVB, UVA's primary effects include enhancement of UVB effects and inducing certain important photochemical phototherapeutic reactions (eg, Oxsoralen phototoxicity) in skin [4,5,9]. The effects of VIS radiation are in some respects similar to those of UVB but to a lesser extent. In addition, VIS

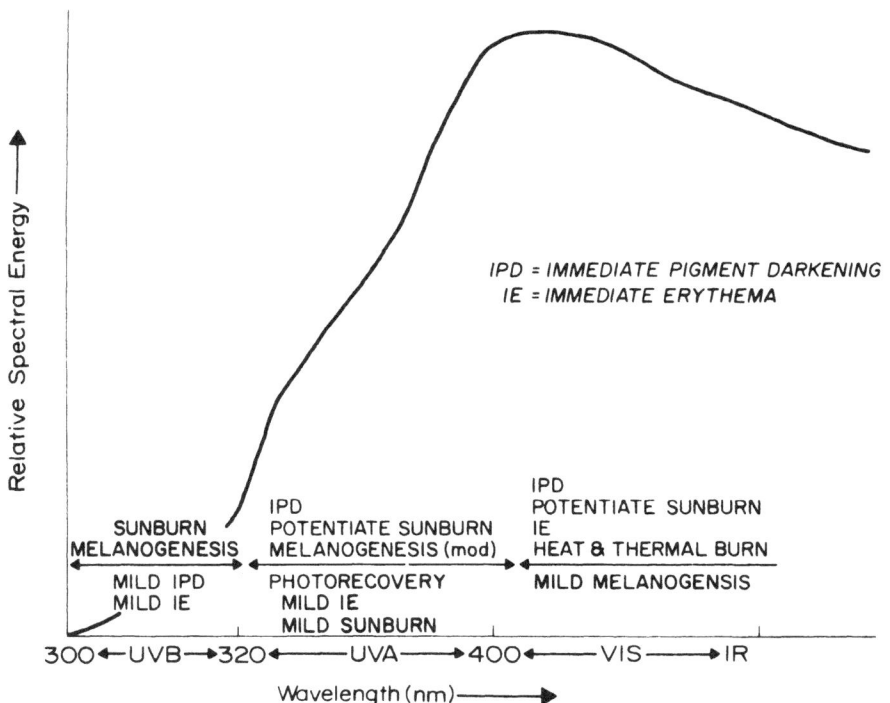

Figure 21-1. The potential effects of different portions of the ultraviolet and visible spectrum of global radiation on human skin.

wavelengths, like IR wavelengths, may cause a thermal burn [8].

A desirable light source should possess at least the following features.

1. A continuous (solar-simulating) and reproducible spectrum and intensity of radiation
2. An operating life span in excess of 200 hr
3. An intensity of energy sufficient to obtain the desired photobiologic or photochemotherapeutic response over a reasonable-sized field within a short period of exposure (ie, at least within 3 to 5 min)
4. Reasonable initial and replacement costs
5. Simplicity in operation and maintenance
6. Rugged construction
7. Mobility if required or desired

With the above features in mind, and one's ideas as to the desired photobiologic responses, the dermatologist may then choose to equip himself with one or more of the types of lamp sources as outlined in Table 21-1. The spectral characteristics for these sources in comparison to global radiation (ie, sunlight at the earth's surface) are outlined in Figs. 21-2–21-8. From the data in Table 21-1 and the figures, it becomes apparent that each lamp has its unique advantages as well as disadvantages. However, for the average practitioner, fluorescent sunlamps and/or blacklight (BL) lamps will allow him to treat practically all of the diseases for which phototherapy has been recommended (Table 21-2). Together, these sources emit a continuous solar-simulating spectrum of UVB, UVA, and near-visible light. Their only possible disadvantage lies in the moderately low intensity of energy emitted by the regular-type blacklight tubes. In an attempt to overcome this disadvantage, the author recommends that either a bank or cabinet unit of tubes be employed. The regular blacklight tubes (ie, 48-inch, 40-W or 24-inch, 20-W BL fluorescent tubes) can be mounted in the standard 4-channel fixtures with reflecting aluminum backing surfaces, or the number of tubes can be increased to 8 per bank, spaced at 0.5-inch intervals. This type of bank arrangement can then be mounted in a cabinet or suspended from an adjustable overbed serving table for patient exposure. A bank of the BL tubes at 12 inches will elicit a phototoxic reaction to topically applied 1% 8-methoxypsoralen (when applied 0.5 hr prior to irradiation) within a 2- to 5-min period. An average minimal erythema dose for FS-20 bulbs, arranged similarly to the above and located at a patient-to-lamp distance of 12 inches, will be less than 60 sec. Obviously, in each and every distance, one should establish the desired response by initial testing of small (ie, 1 to 2 cm) skin sites before exposing larger or entire body surfaces. High intensity blacklights will soon be available to overcome the problem of low intensity. It should be clear that the eyes of both the patient and clinician should be thoroughly protected when ultraviolet light sources are employed.

Clinical Use

The following describes the manner in which lamp sources may be employed for the treatment of photoresponsive diseases (Table 21-2).

Fluorescent Sunlamp

The fluorescent sunlamp may consist of a bank of 4 to 8 bulbs of either the FS-20 or FS-40 type mounted at 0.5- to 1-inch intervals in parallel series. It should be used only for the treatment of UVB-responsive diseases. The minimal erythema dose (MED) requirement for each patient should be established prior to therapy by exposing 1 cm² squares of normal skin to increasing doses (25 to 50% increments) of radiation at a lamp-to-skin target distance of 12 inches. The initial MED test exposures in untanned white skin should range from 30 to 90 sec, while those in black or darkly pigmented skin should range from 60 to 180 sec. Greater or lesser exposures may be given depending upon the results observed at the above test sites 24 hr postexposure. Having established the MED, the initial phototherapeutic exposure may be given at the 1-MED dose level. Subsequent exposures at 1- to 2-week intervals may be increased by 25% of the previous exposure. Care should be taken not to exceed the exposure required to induce a brisk 24-hr erythema. In addition, the patient should be cautioned regarding the potential hazards of using or taking photosensitizing chemicals and of further exposure to UV from sunlight or high intensity artificial light during the course of phototherapy.

Table 21-1 *Common Lamp Sources*

Types	Characteristics	Advantages	Disadvantages
Xenon arc	High intensity; continous spectral emission; constant output; long life span; may be filtered to emit solar-simulating radiation in all important wavelength ranges	All light effects can be accomplished using short exposure times	High initial and moderately high maintenance costs; small radiation field; not portable
Quartz–Iodine	Same as above except for a lack of high intensity UVB (290–320 nm) radiation	UVA (320–400 nm) and visible (400–700 nm) light effects can be accomplished using short exposure times; portable	Is not an adequate source for testing in the UVB range; high costs; small radiation field
Carbon arc	High intensity; continuous but irregular spectral emission; variable output; short life span varies with carbons; may be filtered to emit radiation in all important wavelengths ranges	Light effects can be accomplished using short exposure times; low costs; moderately large radiation field; may be portable	Too much variability in energy intensity and spectral emission; carbons are too short lived
Hot quartz (high pressure mercury arc lamp)	High intensity; linear spectral emissions in all wavelength ranges; constant output; long life span	Many light effects can be accomplished with short exposure times if the desired action spectrum corresponds to emissions from the lamp; large radiation field; portable	Many important photoactivating wavelengths are not emitted
Cold quartz (low pressure mercury arc lamp)	Linear spectral emission, approximately 90% of which is at 253.7 nm; constant output; moderate intensity; long life span	None for routine phototesting	Most important photoactivating wavelengths are not emitted
Black ray lamp (100 W)	Low to moderate intensity; continuous spectral emission of 320–420 nm radiation with peak emission at about 360 nm	UVA effects can be accomplished if only short exposure times are required; low cost; reasonable size for radiation field	High operating temperature; should be operated only intermittently; operating time should not exceed 5 min before cooling for twice as long
Fluorescent sun lamp (FS20T12 or FS40T12)	Moderate intensity; continuous spectral emission of 280–350 nm radiation with a peak emission at 320 nm; constant output; long life span	UVB effects can be accomplished with moderately short exposure times; a reflecting bank containing several lamps may be used; low costs; large radiation field; portable	Is not an adequate UVA and visible light source
Blacklight fluorescent lamp (24-inch, 20-W or 48-inch, 40-W)	Low to moderate intensity; continuous spectral emission of 320–420 nm radiation with peak emission at about 360 nm; constant output; long life span	UVA effects can be accomplished; a reflecting bank containing several lamps may be used; low costs; large radiation field; portable	Moderately long exposure times are required for effects; is not an adequate UVB and visible light source
High output blacklight fluorescent lamp: Ultralite (Voltare) and Westinghouse 72-inch H-O BL	High intensity; continuous spectral emission of 320–420 nm radiation with peak emission at 350 nm; constant output; long life span	UVA effects with or without photoactive chemical can be accomplished using relatively short exposure times when a bank or cabinet arrangement is employed; large radiation field; may be portable; low cost is possible	Somewhat high cost depending upon accessories employed; is not useful for UVB effects

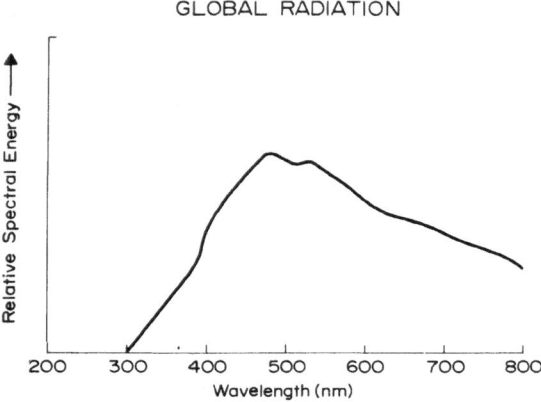

Figure 21-2. Global radiation is a continuous spectrum of energy.

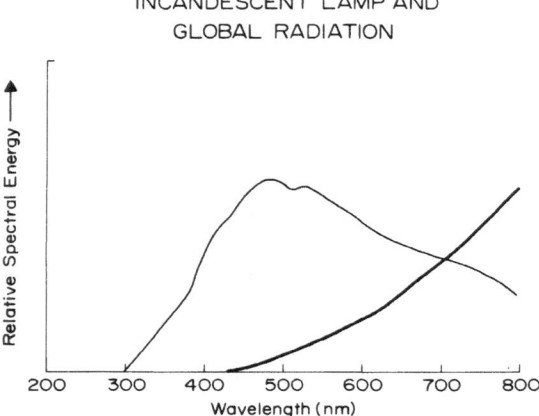

Figure 21-3. Incandescent lamp and global radiation.

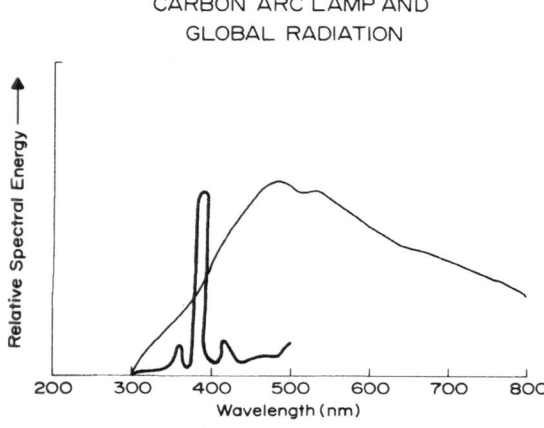

Figure 21-4. Carbon arc lamp and global radiation.

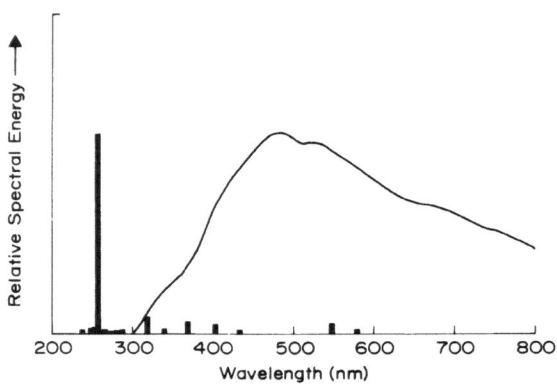

Figure 21-5. Low pressure mercury lamp and global radiation.

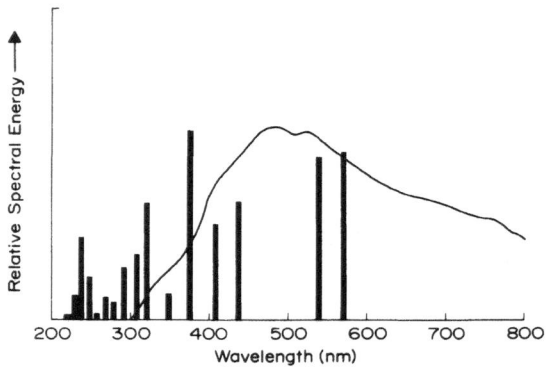

Figure 21-6. High pressure mercury lamp and global radiation.

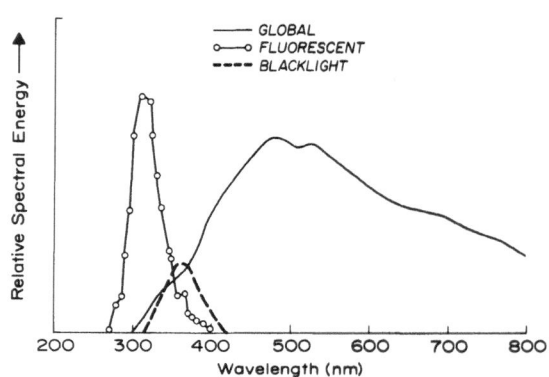

Figure 21-7. Fluorescent sunlamp, blacklight lamp, and global radiation.

XENON ARC LAMP AND GLOBAL RADIATION

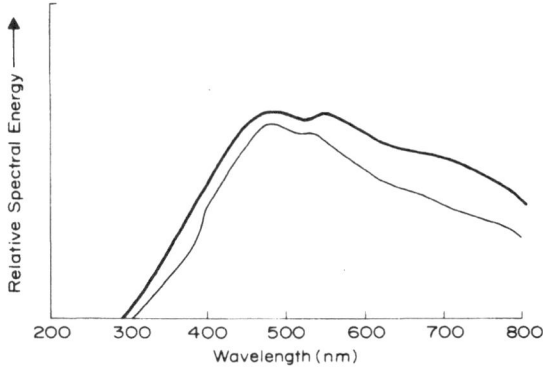

Figure 21-8. Xenon arc lamp and global radiation.

Table 21-2 *Effective Wavelengths for Specific Diseases*

Disease	Effective Wavelengths
Acne vulgaris	UVB ± drug or UVA + drug
Alopecia areata	UVB or UVA + drug
Atopic dermatitis	UVB or UVA + drug
Bacterial (cutaneous) infections	UVB and/or UVA
Congenital jaundice	VIS (blue light)
Erythrocyanosis	UVB
Herpes simplex infections	VIS–UVA + dye
Lupus vulgaris	UVB
Mycosis fungoides (erythrodermic and early plaque stages)	UVB or UVA + drug
Neurodermatitis	UVB or UVA + drug
Parapsoriasis (chronic types)	UVB or UVA + drug
Pityriasis rosea	UVB or UVA + drug
Psoriasis	UVB or UVA + drug
Rickets	UVB
Seborrheic dermatitis	UVB
Stasis ulcers	UVB
Vitiligo	UVA + drug

Blacklight

The blacklight source should consist of a bank of 4 to 8 bulbs of the 20-W or 40-W BL type, mounted at 0.5- to 1-inch intervals in parallel series. It should be used mainly for the treatment of those disorders that are responsive to UVA-dependent photochemical reactions, but may be useful if the disorder responds to UVA alone. Its main use has been for the activation of the psoralen chemicals in the treatment of vitiligo and psoriasis.

It is helpful to initially determine the minimum dose of UVA that is required to induce a mild to moderate phototoxic response, since more intense reactions over large body areas are undesirable. A series of 1-cm² test sites should be exposed to increasing doses of UVA at a skin-to-lamp distance of 10 inches at a specific time following the administration of psoralen. In the case of orally administered psoralen, the UVA dose requirement depends upon a host or variables that have not been fully elucidated; however, oral doses of greater than 10 mg of 8-methoxypsoralen generally require exposures in excess of 10 min to induce a clinical response. In contrast, the phototoxic response to topically administered 8-methoxypsoralen is quite predictable. At 30 min postapplication, test sites should receive exposures ranging from 45 to 180 sec. Observations should be made at 48 to 72 hr postexposure since peak phototoxicity does not occur until then.

The initial phototherapeutic exposure should be equal to that dose of UVA required to induce a mild to moderate 72-hr erythema response at the test site within the area to be treated. Subsequent exposures may be given as often as every 7 days. However, these should not be increased by more than 25% of the previous exposure until the patient is clearly unresponsive to a preceding exposure.

Blacklight (high output)

High output blacklight sources emit essentially the same continuous spectrum of energy as that emitted by regular lower intensity blacklight sources (ie, 320 to 400 nm). These 6-foot tubes are generally arranged 1 to 2 inches apart in parallel when installed in some type of unit design such as a square, ellipse, or circle.

This source can be used in the same manner and for the same disorders as described for regular blacklight. The major advantage is that less time will be required to obtain a desired therapeutic response. While a bank of blacklights as described above will emit only between 1 and 3 mW/cm² at a target distance of 8 to 10 inches, high intensity blacklight units will emit anywhere from 7 to 15 mW/cm² at the same target distance. Output will vary depending upon construction and design of the unit (ie, with or without grid covering, handles, etc, between the patient and the light tubes) and the operating age of the bulbs.

High intensity blacklight, which may be used for total body or large area exposure, has added a significant new dimension to dermatologic therapy, most notably in the case of psoriasis. Although its use at this time is still in the investigational stage to determine optimal dosages and potential adverse cutaneous, ophthalmologic, and hematologic effects, it has proven to be practical in terms of time required for treatment when systemic psoralens are administered. At present, if a dose of 0.6 mg/kg of 8-methoxypsoralen is given by mouth 2 hr prior to exposure, an optimal starting dose may be accurately determined by exposing a series of 1- to 2-cm² test sites to increasing doses of UVA and making observations of the test responses at 72 hr as described above. Subsequent doses may be increased by 25% of the preceding dose unless erythema is present at the time therapy is to be given. An alternate approach to this precise dose determination is to use the standard suggested dosages based upon skin types (ie, responses of different types of skin to 30 min of midday temperate zone summer sunlight). These are shown in Table 21-3.

For a particular light source the equation to use for determining the exposure time in minutes is as follows:

$$\text{Time (min)} = 16.67 \times \frac{\text{prescribed UVA dose (J/cm}^2)}{\text{Energy output of the particular light source (mW/cm}^2)}$$

For example, if the output of a light unit is 10 mW/cm² and a dose of 5 J/cm² is desired, the exposure time would be 8.3 min as calculated by the above equation ($16.67 \times 5/10 = 8.3$).

Treatments should not be repeated more often than every third day since the maximum phototoxic response will not occur until 48 to 72 hr post–psoralen-UVA (PUVA) therapy.

For patients who will receive photochemotherapy of the type described above, it is essential to warn them against the concomitant use of topical, oral, or parenteral photosensitizing drugs and agents. They should be instructed to wear UVA-filtering eyeglasses for at least the entire day of therapy and to avoid sunbathing for at least 24 hr prior to treatment and 72 hr posttreatment.

Hot Quartz

A hot quartz source such as the Alpine lamp should be employed so that a large surface area can be treated. The Krohmayer Lamp is unsuitable because of its small field of irradiation. Hot quartz radiation is used mainly for the treatment of UVB-responsive disorders, but it may be used for disorders that require UVA in their treatment. In the latter cases a Schott WG 345 (2 mm) or window glass (3 mm) filter must be used to eliminate exposure to sunburn rays.

Exposure times should be predetermined for each patient as outlined for the previously described lamp sources. At a lamp-to-skin distance of 18 inches, the average MED range is 30 to 60 sec.

Cold Quartz

The cold quartz type of lamp is recognized for its effectiveness in the treatment of disorders (eg, acne) that respond to superficial desqua-

Table 21-3 *Standard Suggested Dosages Based on Skin Type*

Skin Type	History	Exposure Dosage (J/cm²)
I	Always sunburn, never tan	1.5 to 3.0
II	Always sunburn, but sometimes tan	2.5 to 5.0
III	Sometimes sunburn, but always tan	3.5 to 7.0
IV	Never sunburn, always tan	4.5 to 9.0
V	Moderately pigmented persons (Indians, Asiatics, Mexicans, Puerto Ricans, Mongoloids)	5.5 to 11.0
VI	Blacks	6.5 to 13.0

mation following an acute erythema induced by 254 nm radiation. An average MED is 30 sec when the lamp is held at a distance of 12 inches from the subject.

Other Sources

Other sources such as the xenon arc and quartz–iodine lamps were not primarily designed for phototherapy. In both instances, their fields of irradiation are too small for practical clinical use.

References

1. Arnold HL, Rees RB: Report: American Academy of Dermatology: Herpes simplex (by John M. Knox). Cutis 13:472, 1974
2. Bachem A: Time factors of erythema and pigmentation produced by ultraviolet rays of different wavelengths. J Invest Dermatol 25:215, 1955
3. Breit R, and Kligman AM: Measurement of erythemal and pigmentary responses to ultraviolet radiation of different spectral qualities. In Urbach F (ed): The Biologic Effects of Ultraviolet Radiation. Oxford, Pergamon, 1969, p 267
4. Buck HW, Magnus IA, Porter AD: The action spectrum of 8-methoxypsoralen for erythema in human skin. Preliminary studies with a monochromator, Br J Dermatol 72:249, 1960
5. Fitzpatrick TB, Arndt KA, Mofty AM, et al: Hydroquinone and psoralen in the therapy of hypermelanosis and vitiligo. Arch Dermatol 93:589, 1966
6. Pathak, MA, Stratton K: Effects of ultraviolet and visible radiation and the production of free radicals in skin. In Urbach F (ed): The Biologic Effects of Ultraviolet Radiation. Oxford, Pergamon, 1969, p 207
7. Task Force on Photobiology of the National Program for Dermatology: Report on ultraviolet light sources. Arch Dermatol 109:833, 1974
8. Willis I: Sunlight and the skin. JAMA 217:1088, 1971
9. Willis I, Kligman AM: Effects of long ultraviolet rays on human skin. Photoprotective or photoaugmentative? J Invest Dermatol 59:416, 1972

22

Light Therapy

Farrington Daniels, Jr.

Every winter many thousands, perhaps millions, of Europeans and North Americans fly south and bask in the sun of the Mediterranean, Caribbean, or Gulf of Mexico. Many of them become sunburned and a number of them develop skin cancer in later years, but most seem to find something enjoyable about the experience. On their return to work they are the subject of envy and admiration of their less-tanned Caucasian fellow-workers. In a survey [30] in Queensland where the incidence of skin cancer in the white population is the highest in the world, 42% said that they would "do anything" to get a good tan. It is hard to believe that all these people flying south and taking pride in their tans are not receiving some health benefits, but what are these benefits? Importantly, does the ability to obtain sunshine in the winter have anything to do with the better health of the upper and upper-middle economic classes compared to that of the poorer classes? If there are beneficial effects from sunlight, and if they are due to certain wavelengths in the ultraviolet (UV) spectrum, then these benefits can be brought indoors by the illuminating engineers.

Ultraviolet irradiation of city children, if deemed beneficial, would involve not only the white population that seeks a tan, but also the dark-skinned populations that are most prone to develop overt signs of ultraviolet-ray deficiency, ie, rickets. This was found to be a problem among the dark-skinned immigrants to Britain from India and Pakistan [1,3,9].

Fresh air and sunlight have long been considered healthful. However, the "air vitamin" has never been discovered and, aside from the synthesis of vitamin D, now supplied as a nutritional supplement, the beneficial effects of sunlight have also not been explained in terms of physiologic mechanisms. Some of the psychologic benefits of an acquired tan are plausible. The winter vacation in the Caribbean indicates a certain degree of financial success. Becker [2] has written of the inversion of values: in years past the aristocracy avoided the sun so that they would not look like the workers in the field. In contemporary society, the workers in the offices and factories are pale and success and status can be demonstrated by a tan rather than by pallor.

Basking behavior is seen in many animals and its biologic functions are not fully known; presumably there is synthesis of vitamin D and some sparing of metabolic heat requirements. Once, at a meeting at the Oregon Primate Center, I observed that rhesus monkeys inside a cage were stretched out in the sun in a similar manner to that of humans stretched out on the lawn, with arms extended overhead and axillae warmed by the sun. One of the special adaptations provided man by his upright posture is maximal reception of the warming, but not sun-burning, rays of the early morning and late afternoon sun, while in the middle of the day only a small fraction of his body is exposed to the noon sunlight with its heat load and risks of sunburn [33].

The history of sun worship by man must be quite ancient. Stonehenge and other megalithic structures in Europe were apparently astronomic devices to keep track of the seasons. The sun was deified in many religions [18]. The ancient Greeks employed heliosis, ie, exposure of the body to the sun, for health purposes.[16] Vitiligo was treated in ancient India [10] with photosensitizing psoralens which would have required light for their action.

Herodotus is quoted thusly: ''Exposure to the sun is highly necessary in persons whose health needs restoring and who have need of putting on weight. In winter, spring, and autumn, the patient should permit the rays of the sun to strike full upon him, but in summer, because of the excessive heat, this method should not be employed in treating weak patients. . . . At all times the head must be protected by some kind of covering.''

With the advent of Christianity, sun worship and sun bathing were considered pagan practices; thus, there is scarce reference to the beneficial effects of sunlight from the early centuries A.D. until the 18th century [18].

Artificial Sources of UV Radiation

Hot Quartz Lamps

The most commonly used therapeutic sunlamp has been the medium pressure mercury lamp with maximum biological activity at 297 nm (Fig. 22-1). These lamps are known as hot

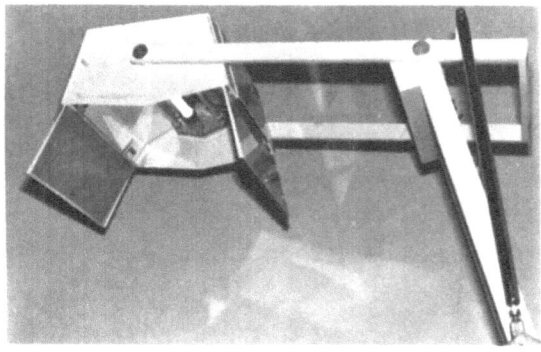

Figure 22-1. Medium pressure mercury arc lamp.

quartz lamps because of the temperature of the surface of the tubes and the fact that quartz envelopes are necessary to transmit the 297-nm radiation. These lamps may also produce considerable ozone from the 1810-nm wavelength that is emitted through the quartz. These units must be warmed up to reach a stable output, and when turned off cannot be turned back on until cooled. This makes them intrinsically more hazardous than either cold quartz or fluorescent lamps because they cannot be used with automatic timers but require constant nursing, physician, or technical supervision. On the other hand, they more closely simulate sunlight than do cold quartz lamps and have a much greater intensity than can be obtained with fluorescent sunlamps. It is usually possible to produce an erythema dose in approximately 30 sec with these lamps, depending upon distance. The erythema is more intense than with 254-nm radiation and there is more tanning. When the term sunlamp is used without qualification it will usually refer to this type of unit.

Eye protection is most important and the admonition to close the eyes cannot be relied upon for complete eye safety because there is always some blinking. The small-diameter dark glasses sold for use with sunlamps are best so that there is not an untanned, white area surrounding the eye (Fig. 22-2). A cotton ball placed under the small glasses is even better for protection from photophthalmia.

Lamps of this type are apparently widely used in gymnasiums and other health establishments, where the only safety features appear to be a posted list of instructions. Dermatologists see a number of patients with severe sunburn received at these installations.

In general, the high temperature implies that these units operate as relatively fixed pieces of equipment. However, one unit having greater mobility is the air-cooled Kromayer or Aerokromayer lamp (Fig. 22-3), shown in closer detail (Fig. 22-5). This is useful for treating such local lesions as plaques of psoriasis, but finds its greatest current application in light testing patients for clinical photosensitivity diseases. With our unit a 1-sec exposure normally produces a very faint pink response at 24 hr, a 3-sec exposure produces a 2+ erythema on the scale we use, and a 10-sec exposure produces a slightly painful 3+ or 4+ sunburn, on previ-

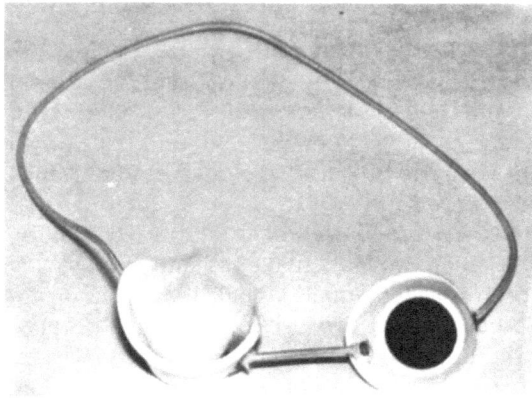

Figure 22-2. Dark glasses for eye protection.

ously untanned white skin. The same lamp can be used with various filters to determine whether the patient is reacting to longer wavelengths that do not ordinarily produce skin reactions. Surprisingly, some apparently light-sensitive patients have a high rather than a low erythema threshold. The great advantage of the

Aerokromayer lamp is its pistollike nature which aims a small beam. The patient and the doctor, nurse, or technician do not need to be heavily goggled and draped.

All hot quartz lamps gradually become somewhat fogged and unless they are replaced one moves gradually from effective to placebo therapy, and is then rudely confronted with severe sunburn when a new lamp is put in.

Cold Quartz Lamps

Low pressure mercury arc lamps, also called cold quartz lamps due to their low surface temperature, emit radiation principally at 254 nm (Fig. 22-4). Fluorescent lamps are low pressure mercury lamps incorporating phosphors that fluoresce at various longer wavelengths. Although 254-nm radiation does not traverse the ozone layer of the stratosphere and is not part of our natural environment, it has been extensively studied in photobiology because the lamps emit a large part of their energy at 254 nm, making it the cheapest way to obtain mon-

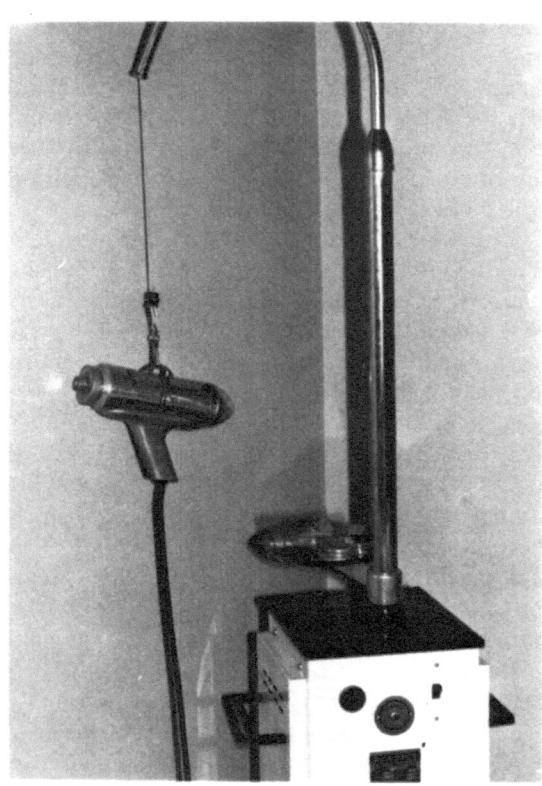

Figure 22-3. Aerokromayer lamp.

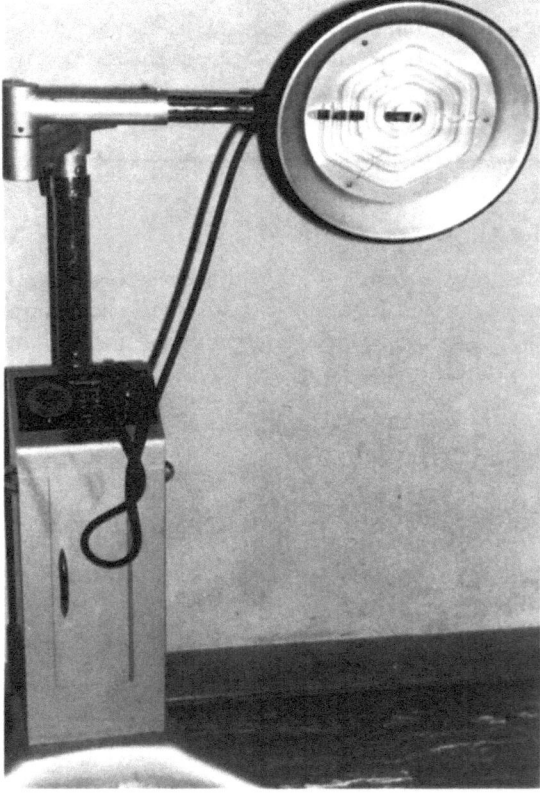

Figure 22-4. Cold quartz unit.

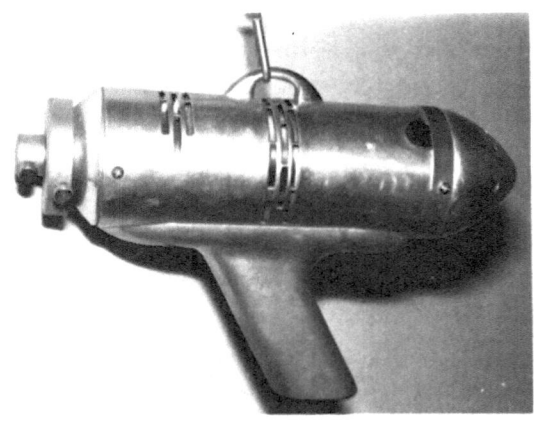

Figure 22-5. Close-up of Aerokromayer lamp.

ochromatic untraviolet radiation. The low pressure mercury arc lamp is also commonly called a germicidal lamp, not because other wavelengths do not kill bacteria and viruses, but because the peak action for this effect is near 254 nm. As germicidal lamps they have been used for water purification and in hospitals to reduce airborne infections. While the hospital installations are near the ceiling and are supposed to irradiate only air, there have been instances of eye irritation and of exacerbation of systemic lupus erythematosus. Germicidal lamps have also been used in some operating theaters for many years. Any quartz–mercury vapor lamp may produce some ozone at 185 nm.

Cold quartz lamps produce a paler erythema which appears earlier than does the 290 to 310 nm erythema. It can produce some peeling but relatively little tanning. The latter is an advantage in that the dose does not need to be increased as it does with the 290- to 310-nm radiation which causes tanning [40].

High Intensity Sources

Very high pressure mercury arcs have been used in a number of experimental therapeutic sources, particularly when the light is to be highly filtered or used as the source for a monochromator. They are also used for searchlights and other intense illuminators. In general, with all mercury arcs, at low pressures only the specific mercury lines are emitted; as the pressure is increased there is more broad background radiation between specific lines.

A more recent development in high inten-

sity sources is the xenon arc which provides a continuous spectral output most resembling that of daylight. It has been used experimentally in a number of solar simulators [4,17,34] and was used therapeutically [17] in centers giving a large amount of ultraviolet therapy. It is also the source of choice for the light in monochromators. Xenon arcs are probably the ideal light source for centers where photosensitivity diseases are studied and where a great deal of ultraviolet therapy is given, ie, a center large enough to support a physicist to supervise their use.

Fluorescent Lamps

Three types of fluorescent lamps are used in dermatologic therapy. One, the fluorescent sunlamp, emits a broad band in the sunburn range (290 to 320 nm) with lesser output in the longwave ultraviolet (UVA, 320 to 400 nm). The other two types are the blacklight fluorescent lamps. The phosphors selected for these lamps take the excitation energy of the 254-nm band of the low pressure mercury arc and convert it mostly into longwave ultraviolet radiation. When placed in nonfiltering glass (quartz is not needed because wavelengths shorter than 320 nm are not wanted) they also emit some visible light. These lamps are often added to banks of fluorescent sunlamps so that they will add a component of tanning as well as burning to the effects. They are also used with tar for the treatment of psoriasis, or with the psoralens (furanocoumarins) for the treatment of vitiligo [18] and psoriasis [27]. Fluorescent lamps in the longwave ultraviolet are supplied either unfiltered or with nickel oxide in the glass envelope to remove the visible light and convert the lamp into a blacklight unit, used principally to produce visible fluorescence for a wide range of effects. These lamps are used in the examination of patients with pigmentary disorders such as vitiligo, in mineralogy, to diagnose pseudomonas infections in burned patients, to detect porphyrins in the urine of patients with clinical porphyria and to produce special effects at iceshows.

Carbon Arc

For many years the most widely used artificial source of ultraviolet radiation was the carbon arc. In fact, the term, arc, derives from the curved beam of light emitted by the spark between two carbon rods. Pure carbon arcs do not produce a great deal of sunburn radiation (UVB), and various therapeutic carbons were developed with metals, particularly iron, added to provide their characteristic emissions. In general, carbon arcs became obsolete because there had to be a mechanical device to move the rods forward as they gradually burned up, and the arcs sputtered and produced a lot of oxidized iron. However, I personally believe they were abandoned unnecessarily. Starke [32] has recommended carbon arcs as continuous sources for evaluating light sensitivity. The more complete spectrum of the carbon arc, compared to the line spectra of low and medium pressure mercury arcs, probably did a better job of tanning as well as reddening the skin.

Ultraviolet Radiation and Vitamin D

As Loomis [19,20] and De Luca [8] have both emphasized and as I have previously reviewed [6] designation of vitamin D as a vitamin instead of a hormone is an accident: only a few foods contain a dietary sufficiency of vitamin D. Throughout most of human existence 7-dehydrocholesterol was converted in man's skin by ultraviolet radiation into vitamin D_3. Only in northerly climates and particularly with the advent of cities was the sun-produced vitamin D too little to prevent rickets in growing children and osteomalacia in adults. A recurrent theory is that Neanderthal man was not a separate species but rather Homo sapiens with rickets during a cloudy period of climatic change. In his review of rickets, Loomis [19] pointed out the particular cruelty to children of a tax on windows in many European cities. Of course, window glass transmits very little antirachitic radiation, and many of the windows may have been oiled paper, but to decrease light by taxation must be, in retrospect, a bizarre form of cruelty.

A recurrent and unanswered question, and one relevant to therapy with ultraviolet radiation, is whether it is possible to produce vitamin D poisoning by an excess of ultraviolet radiation. Loomis [20], in a widely quoted article, suggested that the Caucasian in the tropics should be vulnerable to vitamin D poisoning because of excess vitamin D production in the skin. However, this idea has been challenged by this author and others [7]. Ultraviolet irradiation of 7-dehydrocholesterol produces many photoproducts in vitro, although the conversion of the provitamin D to vitamin D_3 in skin is 100% efficient. Vitamin D_3 itself can be broken down by excess ultraviolet irradiation.

The Erythema Threshold with Ultraviolet Radiation

Ultraviolet therapy should be administered in relation to the patient's own baseline response. The minimal erythema dose (MED) was originally described as that UV radiation necessary to produce a minimal perceptible erythema on "normal untanned white" (Caucasian) skin. As with any test based on a threshold there has been considerable disagreement and confusion regarding the minimal perceptible erythema (MPE). The subject has been studied in depth by van der Leun [35–39]. Van der Leun did not depend upon a single reading but rather upon a series of 9 doses from a shutter device with windows approximately 2×7 mm in area. A series of doses through these windows appears in a semicircle on the skin because the shutter device is a circular shutter. He graded his steps to increase by a factor of $\sqrt{2}$ to obtain a geometric progression of the exposure times. The step dosage, therefore, increased approximately 40% for each step. The electrically controlled shutter used by van der Leun is not commercially available, but a shutter of cardboard with similar openings in a linear arrangement can be easily made. The crude use of 1-, 3-, and 10-sec exposures with the Aerokromayer as a screening technique for some light sensitivity and therapeutic situations has been discussed; this can be justified in a busy clinical situation but the more carefully graded shutter measurements are required for more thorough clinical or research uses. In spite of the theoretical and practical difficulties of the minimal erythema (whether defined as the MPE or the lightest erythema with a sharp margin, or as a + response on a scale of + to +++++ the method has been very useful. It should be remembered that different ultraviolet wavelengths produce different time–response curves, ie, 254-nm radiation has a quicker rise and fall of erythema than does 297-nm radiation, but that for convenience most clinical erythema baselines are based on a 24-hr observation following irradiation.

Use of Phototherapy in Various Diseases

Acne Vulgaris

To some, acne seems like a trivial and superficial disease. However, it can be devastating psychologically to the victim and to family relationships. Its maximum impact occurs at the time the adolescent boy or girl is trying to become independent and mature socially. One of the greatest satisfactions of a practicing dermatologist is seeing the troubled adolescent blossom and mature as his or her acne improves. Phototherapy is important. Most but not all patients with acne improve in the summertime. The role of ultraviolet radiation in this seasonal change is not better defined for acne than for other diseases, but ultraviolet radiation is believed to be involved. Hot quartz and cold quartz therapy are both used in the treatment of acne. The cold quartz produces less erythema and very little tan, but can produce peeling with removal of sebaceous gland plugs that are believed to play a role in acne pathogenesis. I personally prefer the small hand-held cold quartz (254 nm) lamp because it can be used by the physician or nurse while simultaneously discussing diet, family and academic pressures, amounts of sleep, and exercise with the patient. For home acne therapy the RS sunlamp, which is a combined tungsten and mercury lamp with a built-in reflecting surface and since it is used in a standard socket, it is useful, but is only supplemental to the office visit where more complete attention is available.

Pityriasis Rosea

Pityriasis rosea is a mild disease which alarms the patient because of the sudden appearance of a rash. Since the principal differential diagnosis is secondary syphilis, the disease must be taken seriously. Mild ultraviolet radiation is thought by some to shorten the duration of the rash; but possibly the ultraviolet erythema provides a less conspicuous background for the erythema and scaling of the lesions. Even if ineffective, phototherapy is a much safer treatment than are systemic steroids, which might

be an alternative treatment in a very apprehensive patient. The epidemiology of pityriasis rosea suggests a viral etiology, although this has not been established. There is therefore the remote theoretical rationale that the ultraviolet radiation may be viricidal.

Alopecia

Ultraviolet therapy has been used for many years to treat baldness of various kinds, particularly alopecia areata. This therapy also needs to be investigated, because there are background data that provide some support for a rationale.

Increased hair growth is characteristic of several photosensitive diseases, eg, porphyria cutanea tarda and erythropoietic porphyria (Günther's disease).

Some photosensitizing chemicals lead to increased hair growth. Acriflavine, used for treatment of gonorrhea in France in the early 1930s, led to photosensitization and increased hair growth as illustrated by Jausion and Pagès [13]. The technicians administering carbon arc radiation in the Finsen treatment for skin tuberculosis developed hypertrichosis on their arms.

Johnson [14,15] studied the effects of different wavelengths of ultraviolet radiation on hair growth and the hair cycle in mice. He irradiated the mouse skin both from above and below. Hair growth was inhibited during the telogen phase by 290- and 300-nm radiation, and during the early anagen phase by 280-, 290-, 300-, and 370-nm radiation. However, Johnson found, in contrast to the inhibition effects of the longer wavelengths in the UVB, that 250-, 260-, and 270-nm radiation given to mouse skin in the telogen hair phase initiated hair growth. At least two exposures were required. A cold quartz UV "comb" is illustrated in Fig. 22-6 for scalp treatments at 254 nm.

Mycosis Fungoides

Mycosis fungoides is initially, and often for many years, the mildest of cutaneous lymphomas. The disease is of interest for many reasons, including the fact that dermatologists can often detect its onset years before biopsy diagnosis can confirm the malignant nature of the disease. After years or decades the disease eventuates in a more serious lymphoma, such

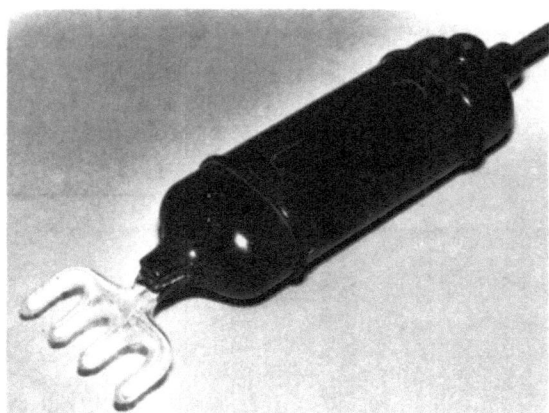

Figure 22-6. Cold quartz "comb" for scalp therapy.

as reticulum cell sarcoma. Mycosis fungoides is named for the mushroomlike appearance of the late lesions; no mycotic organisms are involved. In the early stages the disease is described as eczematous or infiltrative; during these stages the disease is often benefited by ultraviolet radiation. In the later nodular and ulcerated stages ionizing radiation or chemotherapy are required. The responsiveness of the early stages to ultraviolet therapy is often forgotten, and unnecessary ionizing radiation, electron beam therapy, or anticancer chemotherapy may be given because the diagnosis leads practitioners to think of the advanced rather than the early phases. Some cases are cured by contact sensitization immunotherapy. However, until it is shown that these more powerful agents actually "kill" the early malignant process, phototherapy should probably be given as long as it is effective. Some useful strategies include getting the patient a job in a fire-watch tower during the summer where it is socially possible to work naked in the sunlight all day, or having the family move to California or Florida where year-round sunbathing is possible. Mycosis fungoides has a polymorphous dermal infiltrate and intraepidermal abscesses, and the mechanism of the beneficial effects of UV radiation in the early stages is not known.

Neonatal Jaundice

Use of phototherapy in neonatal jaundice is important and widespread. The reader is referred to reviews in the pediatric literature [21,-29,31]. The procedure is apparently effective but also controversial because the hazards are not well defined. It is not usually supervised by dermatologists and hence is not reviewed in detail here. White or blue fluorescent lamps rather than ultraviolet lamps are used.

Psoriasis

The Goeckerman regimen [11,12] has gained wide acceptance as a standard therapy for psoriasis. This involves the application of crude coal tar preparations, removal of the tar (which is of course a good light filter), and ultraviolet radiation, usually from hot quartz lamps. The extensive experience of the Mayo Clinic is reviewed by Sams [28]. The therapy works best in the hands of those experienced in its use. We have been impressed with the number of patients with psoriasis who claim "they have had everything," but who have had neither ultraviolet therapy nor the Goeckerman regimen. In the absence of an organized dermatology center with nurses working full-time on the Goeckerman regimen, most dermatologists compromise by using a variety of "modified Goeckerman regimens." For example, the patient may apply tar himself, wipe it off with mineral oil, and present himself to the dermatology clinic to be exposed in a small room with aluminum reflecting walls and fluorescent sunlamps, sometimes supplemented with blacklight fluorescent lamps.

Crude coal tar is a pharmacologic nightmare, ie, an extremely heterogenous mixture. The active ingredients are presumed to be a variety of polycyclic hydrocarbons which are probably carcinogenic. This is mystifying initially, but most of the therapies that have had some beneficial effect on the nonmalignant proliferative disease of the skin, ie, psoriasis, have had carcinogenic potential: eg, inorganic arsenic as in Fowler's solution, ultraviolet radiation, antimitotic drugs such as methotrexate, and coal tar.

In spite of the carcinogenic nature of the tar and ultraviolet radiation, only a very few cases of skin cancer have occurred in patients treated with the Goeckerman regimen [26]. It is not known whether this is related to the nature of psoriatic skin, or to the fact that psoriasis tends to be located on unexposed skin and that the total Goeckerman exposure is only a small fraction of the lifetime exposure to UV radiation on the face and hands where skin cancers are most common. That natural sunlight may be a factor in the control of psoriasis is indicated by the findings of Miyaji [25]. He showed that in Japan psoriasis decreases from north to south, whereas skin cancers and lupus erythematosus increased from north to south.

Goeckerman [11] began his studies by recognizing the seasonal benefits of sunlight on psoriasis. He tried various known photosensitizing chemicals to potentiate the effect of ultraviolet light and rapidly identified coal tar as the most promising.

Before the advent of hydrocortisone and derivatives for topical use there were many claims regarding the benefit of the Goeckerman treatment, including its use in persistent pustular eruptions of the palms; this is probably a neglected treatment at present. Cole [5] described the beneficial effects in a variety of skin disorders, even though he readily admitted that the series was not strictly controlled. However, many of the diseases were chronic and rapid improvement in chronic diseases in a high percentage of cases does not automatically mean that a double-blind test is necessary, or even ethical.

In reviewing the Mayo Clinic experience with the Goeckerman regimen, Muller and Kierland [26] stated that they did not believe that photosensitization was a part of the unexplained benefits of the combination of tar and hot quartz lamp therapy. They report that 6 suspected, but not clear-cut, cases of skin cancer in the literature could be attributed to the Goeckerman regimen. Some of these cases were complicated by arsenic therapy or other confounding factors.

Goeckerman [12] observed that when the cutaneous lesions of psoriasis were improved by his regimen, concurrent psoriatic arthritis was also improved.

Sams [28] has also reviewed the experience with the Goeckerman regimen at the Mayo Clinic. Crude coal tar at a concentration of 2 to 5% in petrolatum is applied 2 to 3 times a day on the entire body from the neck down, but avoiding the axillae, antecubital fossae, and groin regions. The ointment is applied by hand and massaged in the direction in which the hairs point, in an effort to avoid the principal complication, ie, tar folliculitis. The patient is then placed in cotton pajamas and, if necessary, cotton gloves and socks. The next morning the tar is removed by wiping with a gauze pad saturated with cottonseed oil. The patient is then exposed to fluorescent sunlamps or to high pressure mercury vapor lamps; the latter usually become necessary during the 21 days of treatment because the patient tans and a lamp of greater intensity is needed. After the UV treatment the patient bathes with soap. The tar is then reapplied 2 to 3 times a day and UV irradiation is given each morning. Patients with exfoliative or pustular psoriasis should not be treated. The treatment can be given at home but the mess and odor of the tar ointment frequently make this objectionable.

At present, PUVA therapy (psoralens + UVA) (27) is under intensive study for the treatment of psoriasis, mycosis fungoides, and atopic dermatitis. However, further discussion is not given because FDA approval has not yet been forthcoming.

References

1. Arneil GC, Crosbie JC: Infantile rickets returns to Glasgow. Lancet II:423, 1963
2. Becker SW Jr: Deleterious effects of sunlight on the skin and their prevention. GP 21:82, 1960
3. Benson PF, Stroud CE, Mitchell NJ, et al: Rickets in immigrant children in London, Br Med J 23:1054, 1963
4. Berger D, Magnus I, Rottier, PB, et al: Design and construction of high-intensity monochromators. In Urbach F (ed): The Biologic Effects of Ultraviolet Radiation. Oxford, Pergamon, 1969
5. Cole HN: Goeckerman therapy in the management of common dermatoses. Arch Dermatol 80:788, 1959
6. Daniels F Jr: Physiological and pathological extracutaneous effects of light on man and mammals, not mediated by pineal or other neuroendocrine mechanisms. In Pathak MA, Harber LC, Seiji M, et al, (eds): Sunlight and Man. Tokyo, University of Tokyo Press, 1974, pp 247–258
7. Daniels F Jr, Post PW, Johnson BE: Theories of the role of pigment in the evolution of human races. In Riley V (ed): Pigmentation. Its Genesis and Biologic Control. New York, Appleton, 1972, pp 13–22
8. De Luca HF: Vitamin D. A new look at an old vitamin. Nutr Rev 29:179, 1971
9. Dunnigen MG, et al: Late rickets and osteoma-

lacia in the Pakistani community in Glasgow. Scott Med J 7:159, 1962

10. Fitzpatrick TB, Pathak MA: Historical aspects of methoxsalen and other furocoumarins. J Invest Dermatol 32:229, 1959

11. Goeckerman WH: The treatment of psoriasis. Northwest Med 24:229, 1925

12. Goeckerman WH: Treatment of psoriasis. Continued observations on the use of crude coal tar and ultraviolet light. Arch Dermatol Syph 24:446, 1931

13. Jausion H, Pagès F: Les maladies de lumière. Paris, Masson, 1933

14. Johnson BE: Potentiation of hair growth by ultraviolet light. Nature 187:159, 1960

15. Johnson BE: Action spectra for acute effects of monochromatic ultraviolet in mouse skin. In Urbach F (ed): The Biologic Effects of Ultraviolet Radiation. Oxford, Pergamon, 1969, pp 223–234

16. Johnson BE, Daniels F Jr, Magnus IA: Response of human skin to ultraviolet light. In Giese AC (ed): Photophysiology, Vol 4. New York, Academic Press, 1968, pp 139–202

17. Kimmig J, Wiskemann A: Lichtbiologie und Lichterapie. In Handbuch der Haut und Geschlechtskrankheiten, Suppl 5, pt 2. Berlin, Springer, 1959, pp 1021–1141

18. Licht S: History of ultraviolet therapy. In Licht S (ed): Therapeutic Electricity and Ultraviolet Radiation. New Haven, Licht, 1967, pp 191–211

19. Loomis WF: Rickets. Sci Am 223:7691, 1970

20. Loomis WF: Skin pigmentation regulation of vitamin-D biosynthesis in man. Science 157:501, 1967

21. Lucey JR, Ferreiro M, Hewitt J: Prevention of hyperbilirubinemia of prematurity by phototherapy. Pediatrics 41:1046, 1968

22. Luckiesh M: Applications of Germicidal, Erythemal, and Infrared Radiation. New York, Van Nostrand, 1946

23. Maughan GH, Smiley DF: Effect of general irradiation with ultraviolet light upon the frequence of colds. J Prevent Med 2:69, 1928

24. Mayer E: Clinical Application of Sunlight and Artificial Radiation. Including Their Physiological and Experimental Aspects with Special Deference to Tuberculosis. Baltimore, Williams and Wilkins, 1926

25. Miyaji T: Skin cancers in Japan. A nationwide 5-year survey, 1956–1960. Nat Cancer Inst Monogr 10:55, 1963

26. Muller SA, Kierland R: Crude coal tar in dermatologic therapy. Mayo Clin Proc 39:275, 1964

27. Parrish JA, Fitzpatrick TB, Tannebaum L, et al: Photochemotherapy of psoriasis with methoxsalen and UVA N Engl J Med 291:1207, 1974

28. Sams WM Jr: Phototherapy of psoriasis. In Pathak M, Harber LC, Seiji M, et al (eds): Sunlight and Man. Tokyo, University of Tokyo Press, 1974, pp 793–796

29. Schmid R: More light on neonatal hyperbilirubinemia? N Engl J Med 285:520, 1971

30. Scott, G: Some sociological observations on skin cancer in Australia. In McCarthy WH (ed): Melanoma and Skin Cancer. Cited Sydney, New South Wales Government Printer, 1972, pp. 15–22.

31. Sisson TRC: Visible light therapy of neonatal hyperbilirubinemia. In Smith K (ed): Photochem and Photobiol Rev 1. NY Plenum Press, 1976, pp 241–268

32. Starke JC, Jillson OF: Duplication of the sun spectrum with a modified carbon arc. Arch Dermatol 82:1012, 1960

33. Underwood CR, Ward EJ: The solar radiation area of man. Ergonomics 9:155, 1960

34. Urbach F: Solar simulation for phototesting of human skin. In Urbach F (ed): The Biologic Effects of Ultraviolet Radiation. Oxford, Pergamon, 1969, pp. 107–114

35. van der Leun JC: Theory of ultraviolet erythema. Photochem Photobiol 4:453, 1965

36. van der Leun JC: Delayed pigmentation and ultraviolet erythema. Photochem Photobiol 4:459, 1965

37. van der Leun JC: Ultraviolet erythema. A study on diffusion processes in human skin. Ph.D. Dissertation. University of Utrecht, Netherlands, 1966

38. van der Leun, JC: On the action-spectrum of ultraviolet erythema. In Gallo U, Santamaria L (eds): Research Progress in Organic, Biological, and Medicinal Chemistry, Vol 3, Pt 2. Amsterdam, North-Holland, 1972, pp 711–736 .

39. van der Leun JC: Observations on ultraviolet erythema. Photochem Photobiol 4:447, 1965

23

Laser Dermatologic Surgery
Research and Clinical Applications

Leon Goldman

The laser is a new physical modality of considerable interest to the dermatologist. The laser belongs to the group of so-called nonionizing radiation, ie, ultraviolet radiation, microwaves, modalities, and ultrasonics. The laser is essentially a strong light beam whose name is an acronym meaning *l*ight *a*mplification through *s*timulated *e*mission of *r*adiation. This powerful beam may be said, in brief, to be produced by raising molecules to a higher energy level by use of an external energy source and then causing all to return to their previous, lower energy state at the same time, emitting light (or other radiation). Einstein, in 1917, first proposed the concepts of stimulated emission, stimulated absorption, and spontaneous emission. But it was not until 1953 that Basov and Prokhorov, in Russia, and Townes, Weber, Schawlow, and Gould, in the United States, developed the concept of the laser. The first laser was shown to the public on July 7, 1960, by Maiman. Many references are available for a detailed review of laser physics [2,10].

The laser is a monochromatic, coherent light beam with tremendous high-energy and power densities. Some laser systems have differential color absorption. The laser range currently extends from near the x-ray region to the far infrared region. The laser systems may be solid, gas, chemical, or semiconductor types. The duration of the laser pulse may either be continuous wave (CW) or pulsed with the dura-

tion varying from milliseconds (msec) through nanoseconds (nsec) into picoseconds (psec). Table 23-1 reviews the laser systems of current interest to the dermatologist.

Since a laser is a beam of light, various optical instruments are used to transmit this beam of light from the optical bench to the operator. These include lenses; prisms; mirrors; curved, tapered quartz rods; fiberoptics; and even glass lenses. The most interesting of these with respect to clinical investigations are the curved, tapered quartz rod developed by Rockwell and the fiberoptics systems, especially the single, precise quartz fiber of Nath. The advantage of these aids is that the laser beams of high intensity are developed from a flexible, precise, and also sterilizable operating probe. These high-output laser beams also may be transmitted through endoscopes and operating microscopes.

Table 23-1 shows the systems that are ordinarily available to the dermatologist. In the future, the other systems, such as the semiconductor lasers, gallium arsenide, and the chemical lasers, with their high efficiency, may find uses in the field of dermatology.

For use in the treatment phase of dermatology, the three important CW lasers are the argon, the neodymium–YAG, and the CO_2 laser.

Because the CO_2 lasers have a higher output deficiency than do other lasers, they are

245

Table 23-1 *Lasers of Dermatologic Interest*

Laser	Spectral Region	Wavelength (nm)
Ruby	Red	694.3
Neodymium	Infrared	1060.0
Neodymium–YAG	Infrared	1060.0
Argon	Blue–green	499.5–514.5
Krypton	Visible	476.2–647.1
CO_2	Far infrared	10,600.0
Helium–neon	Red	632.8
Ultraviolet	Ultraviolet	265.0–360.0
Tunable dye	Varies	

of current interest. The CO_2 laser may include various systems, such as the high-power CW, the pulsed and Q-switched, the oscillator amplifier, and the stabilized single frequency system. Two recently developed systems are the TEA CO_2 laser (*t*ransverse *e*xcitation *a*tmospheric pressure laser) and the "COFFEE Laser" (*c*ontinuously *o*perating *f*ast *f*low *e*lectrically *e*xcited laser).

The two instruments currently in use in dermatology are the high-output CO_2 operative laser of the American Optical Company and the CO_2 laser of Israel Industries, Ltd. The carbon monoxide laser has simpler optics than does the carbon dioxide laser, as well as a high efficiency rate and infrared output. This, as well as the new holmium laser, will also be used for investigative dermatology in the near future.

The new ultraviolet laser systems, which will also be of considerable use to dermatologists in the future, include the nitrogen laser and the fourth harmonic from the neodymium–YAG at 266 nm. The ultraviolet lasers are cur-

rently under investigation in Germany and by Parrish et al with respect to studies on vitiligo, psoriasis, and other dermatologic disorders.

Another group of laser systems of more significant interest in diagnostic dermatology, especially with respect to the new techniques of cytofluorography, are the tunable dye lasers (Fig. 23-1). These can be tuned over the whole visible spectrum into the near infrared and the ultraviolet. Various dye systems are used to produce these laser systems. Cytofluorography includes scanning of nuclear fluorescence, immunofluorescence, bacteria, and viruses, and also, recently, cellular sorting, ie, sorting polymorphonuclears, monocytes, and lymphocytes into selected groups. When higher outputs are available the tunable dye lasers will probably also be used for the treatment phases of dermatology. The new laser nephelometer is used in immunology for quantitative analysis of various immunoglobulins, IgA, IgG, Ig ManaC 3C.

Chemical lasers have a high efficiency and will be used more frequently in the future. They are presently under detailed investigation for laser-induced thermonuclear fusion.

Studies leading to coherent emission in the x-ray region are now in progress. New lasers are increasingly approaching the x-ray region. Actual x-ray lasers are not available as yet but studies continue in that region of the electromagnetic spectrum. X-ray lasers will reveal the 3-dimensional molecular structure of matter, and may help develop cancer therapy.

After a laser is selected, the question of safety is considered for all applications of the laser system. For an analysis of safety factors,

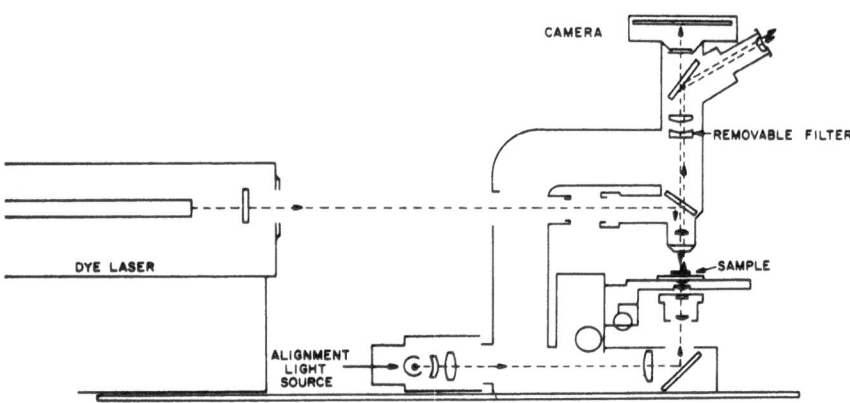

Figure 23-1.   Tunable dye laser set-up for immunofluorescence study. Courtesy of Electro-Optics System Design.

it is necessary to know, in brief, the effects of the laser in living tissue.

Laser Reactions in Tissue

As mentioned previously, lasers, unlike some of the other modalities discussed in this volume, have almost unlimited energy and power densities and differential wavelength absorption in tissue. The darker the skin color, the greater the absorption from the near infrared and visible lasers. Therefore, the color of the target area is important.

For an accurate determination of the skin color, the direct reading spectrophotometer is often used. The instrument used in the Laser Laboratory of the Medical Center of the University of Cincinnati has been the Color EYE of Kollmorgen. The chart used measures the reflectance curves from the skin surface for from 400 to 680 nm [3].

The reaction in tissue due to a laser beam is predominantly a thermal-induced coagulation necrosis, nonspecific in character, resembling, according to Richfield, the dermatopathologist of the Laser Laboratory of the Medical Center of the University of Cincinnati, the necrosis produced by deep electric burns. Steam bubbles are present in tissue also. The thermal effects of laser radiation have not been studied as intensely as have the thermal effects of significant heat burns [6].

In addition to the thermal effects there are a host of nonthermal reactions in tissue. These include the following:

1. Elastic recoil and pressure wave formation
2. Tissue ionization
3. Harmonic frequency generation
4. Multiphoton absorption processes
5. Free radical formation
6. Inverse bremsstrahlung
7. Photochemically induced photooxidation
8. Photohydration, especially of the pyrimidine bases of nucleic acid
9. Raman and Brillouin scattering "subsequent formation of additional frequencies and sound waves of hypersonic frequencies" [10]

These nonthermal effects are produced especially by the pulsed laser systems. The lasers used for the bulk of operative surgical procedures, the continuous wave lasers, mostly generate the thermal effects in tissue. These CW lasers do not produce dispersion of target fragments as do the pulsed lasers. This dispersion has been shown to spread viable cancer fragments in animals but not in man. However, this has not occurred in animals using CW lasers for cancer treatment. More studies of the basic laser reactions in tissues are to be done, especially with the chronic exposure techniques.

Research of more than 15 years duration has shown no carcinogenic effect of the laser systems used in either animal experimental work or human exposure [12]. The human skin exposure also included chronic exposures. The nonspecific fibrosis shows none of the endarteritis, abnormal fibroblasts, or the telangiectasia characteristic of x-ray reactions in tissue. Recent experiments by Ehlers and Florian [1] with ruby laser impacts on the skin of brown mice, with red-filtered xenon light as a control, suggested, but did not prove, precancerous cytologic changes in the skin cell nuclei. Additional experiments regarding this problem must be performed.

Laser Safety

As indicated previously, before working with a laser one must review laser safety for the protection of the patient as well as the operator. The areas of concern, in order of importance, are the eyes, the skin, and the respiratory system. Both area control and personnel control are taken into account.

In area control, one must consider the following safety factors.

1. The prevention of spectral reflectance
2. The prevention of air pollution from making contact with the target
3. The monitoring of electric hazards (high-power output systems are used)
4. The monitoring of cryogenic materials (often used in many laser applications)

For personnel protection, the most important precaution is the use of protective glasses (Fig. 23-2). These allow the operator to see and at the same time offer significant eye protection. It is important to remember that there is not one single type of protective glasses. Each laser system demands a specific eye protection.

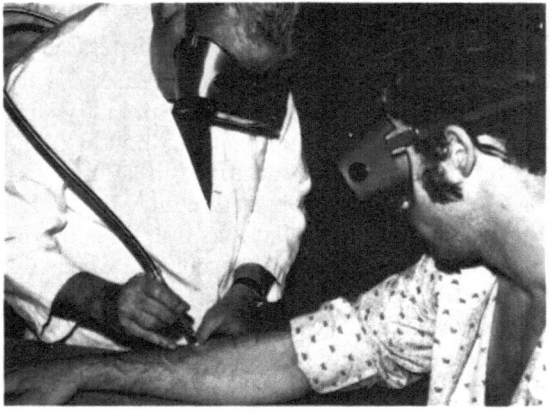

Figure 23-2.   Argon laser with the flexible fiber of Nath for the treatment of tattoos.

Gloves and clothing protect the skin. Often, acute burns of the skin are the result of an accident.

Current research in safety concerns new lasers and chronic exposure experiments. These experiments have been done on the skin of the lower back, a protected area; on actinic pigmentations in keratoses [12]; on benign seborrheic warty growth; on scars; and on the ink pigments incorporated in skin. These experiments provide one of the few sources of data for chronic exposure effects on the living tissue in man. These experiments have been and are being done at 694.3 nm. They have indicated no evidence of any carcinogenic activity. For the control of air pollution, of more concern for material processing in industry and in the military than in dermatology, adequate ventilation systems, exhaust systems, and so forth, are required, especially when working with hazardous materials.

Investigative laser treatments are usually considered to be high-risk exposures and detailed safety programs must be provided. If a laser facility is established a laser safety officer must be designated whose job is to survey and monitor the ongoing laser programs and to revise and update them as new technological developments occur.

For adequate details of laser safety programs, one is referred to the 1977 publication of the American National Standards Institute (ANSI), Z-136 Committee, *Standards for the Safe Use of Lasers.** This publication lists US

*American National Standards Institute Inc., 1430 Broadway, New York, N.Y., 10018.

standards for use of the laser systems now available. It is hoped these will soon be adopted as international standards.

Laser Applications

When one is familiar with laser systems and with associated laser safety programs, one can then consider the applications of the laser. In dermatology, there are essentially three phases: laboratory investigative studies, laser diagnostic techniques, and investigative laser dermatologic surgery.

The laser, which is a light beam of many wavelengths, is precise in its application; therefore, it can be used for microirradiation studies in the dermatologic research laboratory. The laser beam transmitted through the optis of the microscope can provide beam sizes varying from less than a micron, on up according to the optics of the microscope. Thus, it is possible to irradiate portions of living tissue, cells, and individual cellular components, including chromosomes. When vital dyes are used, the wavelength dependency of the tissue is realized. This has been possible with vital dyes, even quinacrine, for laser cellular tissues, and has enabled microsurgery to be done on chromosomes, mitochondria, and other single structures of the cell. For the dermatologist, the microsurgery of tissue cultures melanoma has been especially of interest.

Another phase of microirradiation techniques is laser microemission spectroscopy, employing direct analysis of tissues and dried blood samples for cations. This has been analyzed in unstained frozen skin sections for calcium, arsenic, gold, and lead. The sections are then stained and the impact areas of the microprobe analysis become evident [2].

Another phase of laser microprobe analysis is the study of lead poisoning in children. In this technique, microirradiation impacts are done on hair shafts for microemission spectroscopy. The lead concentrations at various levels along the hair shaft can be determined quantitatively. Unlike atomic absorption spectroscopy, these analyses can be done in tiny areas of the hair without its complete destruction. Actually, laser microprobe analyses can also be done without discomfort or hazard to the child. Attempts have been made to correlate these studies with the analyses of lead levels in children with lead poisoning.

With Vahl [14], there have been detailed examinations of the laser impact areas with ultramicroscopic analyses using scanning electron microscopy (SEM) and transmission electron microscopy (TEM), with x-ray crystallography to develop pictures of those structures in the hair shaft that give rise to the lead. These studies can be adapted to many trace-metal analyses. Thus, laser microirradiation provides the dermatologist with a technique that may be used on living skin without complete destruction of the area under investigation. It has been used in the analysis of tattoo pigments, in cation analyses, and in the spectroscopic study of cancer, argyria, Wilson's disease, and other reactions. Raman and Brillouin spectroscopy also provide techniques for dermatologic analyses. Obviously, laser chemistry, especially in the field of photochemistry, provides many investigative opportunities.

Thus, optical qualities of living skin can be studied in detail with laser systems. As laser technology develops, there will be further dermatologic applications, with opportunities to study the basic mechanisms of nonionizing radiation. It will be possible to compare the basic reactions at cellular level with those due to other forms of nonionizing radiation, ie, microwave, ultrasonics, and ultraviolet. These reactions in tissue will then be compared to those due to ionizing radiation.

At present, there is much interest in the dermatologic applications of phototherapy, due to studies of the effects of photoreactor compounds on psoriasis and herpes simplex. There is current research on skin test models with laser ultraviolet and photosensitizers. This is important for research on current PUVA therapy in dermatology.

Diagnostic Laser Techniques in Dermatology

New developments in holography, which is sometimes called 3-dimensional lensless photography, and microholography, are recently being applied to dermatology.

In brief, a light wave from a laser is reflected from an object to a photographic plate. Simultaneously, another portion of the beam impacts directly on the photographic plate.

This image is subsequently reproduced by laser or other light and a 3-dimensional image is produced. This will make it possible in the future to provide 3-dimensional color photography and a view of the dermatologic lesion as a whole. Until recently, there has been little use of this particular technique in medicine; most of the applications have been in industry for nondestructive testing of stress patterns by so-called interferometry. The medically related development having dermatologic application is acoustic holography.

In acoustic holography, the mechanical vibration form, from the pulsed echo, is used with the surface phenomenon of the disturbances developed by the laser to form a hologram. It is thus possible to "see" below the surface. Current studies using acoustic holography, involving diagnosis of breast cancer; the fetus in utero; dynamic movements of the wrist, hands, and elbow; portrayal of thrombosis; gallbladder pictures; and so forth, suggest that this could have value for soft tissue examination in dermatologic disorders. This would include imagery for tumors, foreign bodies, vascular disturbances, and the tissue changes associated with scleroderma and calcinosis. A new microscope, the Kessler Sonoscope, uses ultrasonics to examine bits of living, unfixed tissue, with the visible image developed by the laser. In dermatology, this can be used to study the influence of external agents on developing skin in the embryo, tissue cultures, and actual living skin test models.

The laser is becoming increasingly important in the fields of information handling and communications. Laser communications have been developed, for example, for the armed services, to be used in the diagnostic field of medicine to expand community medical services. This is similar to medical diagnosis closed-circuit television. Similar techniques have been developed at Mount Sinai Hospital, New York, for pediatric clinics in Harlem. Laser communications have been used in Cleveland for surveillance and in the hospital area for monitoring surgery at a distance. With this technique, patients can be examined in color and, in the near future, in 3-dimensional imagery. Laboratory tests can be served in color. Microscopic sections, in color and at magnification, can also be reviewed, as well as cultures of fungi in microorganisms. These services, provided at a distance from a medical center, can increase community dermatologic service in a practical fashion. Features to be determined include the cost expenditures, after the initial experiments, and patient acceptance of this impersonal type of medical care.

Another communications development involves a 12-inch video disc (MCA) scanned by a helium–neon laser beam and electronically coupled with a color television set. This is certainly revolutionary in information handling and will have a tremendous impact on dermatologic learning. Three-dimensional imagery will also be available.

Investigative Dermatologic Surgery

Laser dermatologic surgery, although in use for more than 15 years, is still termed investigative. Hundreds of patients have been treated, but it is still necessary to consider such treatment as investigative. The need for expensive, sophisticated instrumentation, the multidisciplinary background necessary for laser surgery control, and poor financial support for basic investigative studies are but some of the factors responsible for official disinterest and neglect. This is in spite of the technique's tremendous applications in industry, the military, and communications. Efforts are presently being made to correct this deficiency, with the recent increase in high-output laser surgery in several other medical fields. A high-output CO_2 laser surgical unit is shown in Fig. 23-3. Recent developments have made this laser more flexible and self contained. A CO_2 laser attached to a colposcope is used extensively now in gynecologic surgery. We have been using this for microsurgery.

Laser Dermatologic Surgery

Obviously, in presenting a new technique one is aware of the responsibilities not only as regards patient protection and operator protection, but also concerning the need for critical evaluation. Controls for dermatologic laser surgery must be used. The following surgical instruments were used as controls.

1. Scalpel
2. High-frequency electrosurgical unit
3. Cryogenic scalpel
4. Hot plasma scalpel (at present, only for animal experimentation)
5. Infra-red coagulator of Nath

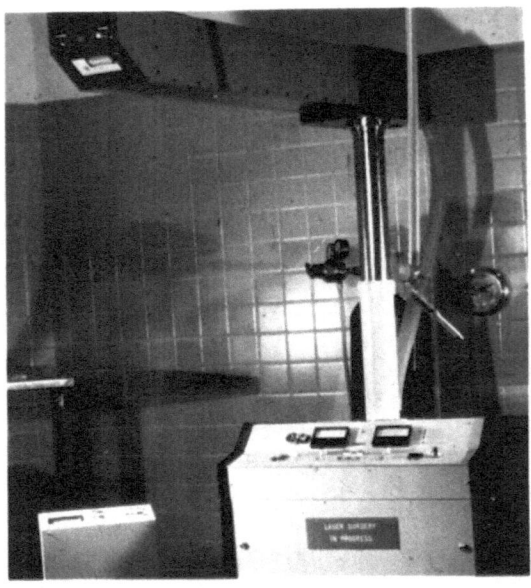

Figure 23-3.   High-output CO_2 laser surgical unit. Courtesy of Israel Laser Industry, Ltd.

In our studies, one hot plasma scalpel for bloodless surgery was found to be hazardous in animal experiments because of mass argon gas embolism formations. Link et al [13] have done many extensive studies with the plasma scalpel. Many basic features have been investigated, such as the vaporization of water contents and the pyrrolization of tissue components. Link et al believe it will be possible to develop a safe hot plasma scalpel in the future. The lengthy dermatologic experience with high-frequency electrosurgery makes the use of this mode rather simple to evaluate, especially for excisional surgery.

The basic advantages of the laser scalpel are (1) fine precision, since a collimated beam is used; (2) bloodless surgery, possible in some areas; and (3) color ie, differential absorption of some lasers in the visible light range; (4) ability to operate on blood vessels without actual contact of the blood vessel. For the hot plasma scalpel, precision is adequate, and perhaps, under some circumstances, bloodless surgery may be possible, but as yet, the color dependency is not available.

The following lesions have been treated by laser dermatologic surgery.

1. Vascular tumors
   a. Port-wine stain
   b. Cavernous

c. Spider angioma
d. Glomus
2. Tattoos, including debris tattoos
3. Warts, especially the current epidemic of massive florid condylomata acuminata
4. Tumors
   a. Melanoma
   b. Multiple basal
   c. Kaposi (small tumors)
   d. Angiosarcomas (small tumors)
5. Miscellaneous
   a. Leukoplakia colored with vital dyes
   b. Subungual hematoma
   c. Basosquamous acanthomas (seborrheic warty growths)
   d. Actinic keratoses

The laser systems used have included the following.

1. The pulsed ruby laser
   a. Normal mode
   b. Q-switched
2. The CW high-output CO_2 laser [11]
3. The argon laser
4. The neodymium-YAG laser [9]

The popular CW helium–neon laser has been used for transillumination in experiments in tissue to determine its value compared to incoherent transillumination techniques.

In tattoos, the presence of color means increased absorption by the laser. The following difficulties may be considered: small target areas, for large tattoos, with the current available pulsed laser instrumentation; and varying depth of pigment deposition in the tattoo.

The laser has been shown to be of value especially for small tattoos of the linear type, where the depth of pigment is not great. The Q-switched ruby laser (Fig. 23-4) has been excellent but until larger beam areas are available, it is not possible to treat effectively the large, broad, tattooed areas. Hypertrophic scarring is more apt to occur with the normal mode, pulsed ruby laser than with the Q-switched laser. Scarring is more apt to occur when "hot spots" are present in the beam, ie, when the beam is not homogeneous.

Laser treatment of tattoos involves the test treatment of 3 or 4 small spots. These are observed for a period of at least 2 months to evaluate healing and efficacy. More extensive treatments can then be done. Other modes

used in the tattoo experiments have included the following.

1. Dermabrasion
2. Salabrasion
3. Chemotherapy, (eg, tannic acid–silver nitrate)
4. Excisional surgery

Current studies include the combination of laser therapy and excisional surgery of resistant or thickened areas. Dermabrasion may be used to smooth down the subsequent hyper-

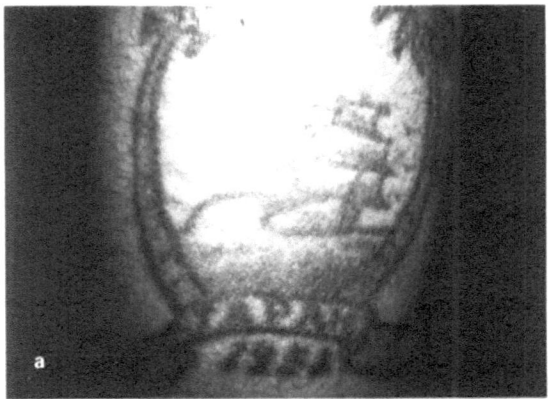

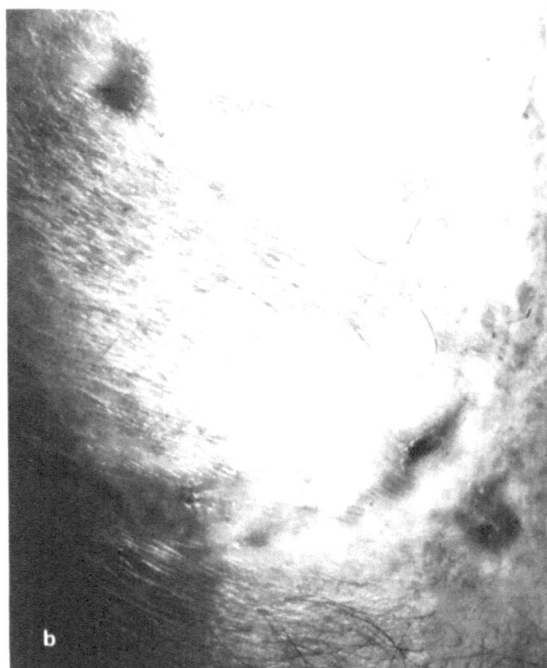

Figure 23-4. Ruby laser treatment of extensive tattoo. *a.* Before treatment. *b.* After multiple treatments.

trophic scarring. Repigmentation has been observed in the treated areas 3 or 4 years after laser treatment. The reactions, in addition to hypertrophic scarring, have included the development of psoriasis, occasional recurrent transient vesicles, and bullae.

An interesting phase of study has been in the treatment of debris tattoos from coal mine and land mine explosions in Viet Nam, and powder burns (Fig. 23-5). If these particles are not too deeply located, the laser has been able to volatilize them. If they are too deep into the deep dermis, pitted scarring may often result. Again, larger target areas are necessary for Q-switched ruby laser systems. The neodymium-YAG laser has also been effective in the treatment of linear tattoos.

It is important that more effective laser instrumentation be provided, especially the Q-switched oscillator–amplifier systems for ruby and neodymium lasers, so that more cosmetically acceptable treatments can be done for larger tattoos. The laser, as indicated, may also be an adjuvant to excisional surgery. The laser dermatome, now under study for the excision of eschar, may also be used for tattoo excision prior to immediate graft replacement. At the Shriners Burns Institute of the Medical Center of the University of Cincinnati, there has been successful use of the laser in excision of eschar with immediate graft replacement through less-

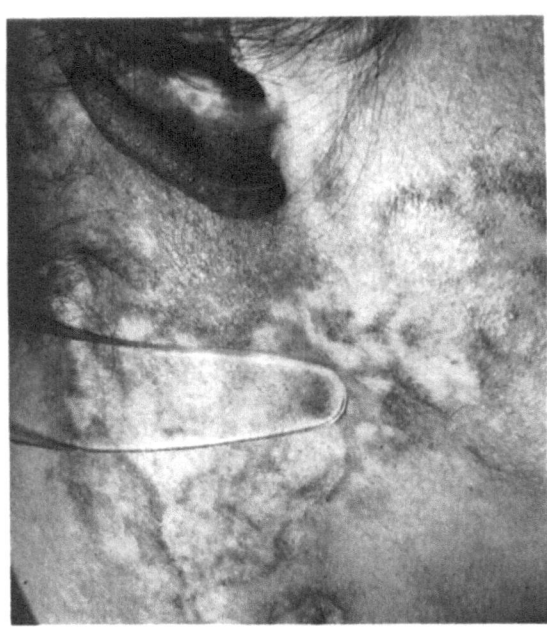

Figure 23-6.   Reticulated appearance of laser treatment of extensive port-wine stain. Diascopy shows depth of residual areas.

ened bleeding and minimal thermal coagulation necrosis.

Vascular Tumors

A few infants with cavernous angiomas on the skull and the genitalia have been treated primarily to show the lack of local tissue radiation hazards with this therapy. Good results were obtained. The most extensive studies have been with intractable port-wine stain (Fig. 23-6). For port-wine stain, the pulsed ruby laser has been used, and recently, in a large number of patients, the argon laser has been employed [8]. Use of the argon laser, according to investigative studies, is more justified because the absorption spectrum of argon relates well to the absorption spectrum of hemoglobin. At present, some five medical centers in this country have established argon laser treatment facilities for the treatment of port wine marks. Most of these are in the division of plastic surgery. The value of the laser in the treatment of port-wine stain has again been limited with current instrumentation, since only small, linear port-wine stains can be so treated. With proper laser protective shields, developed in our laboratory, impacts of the eyelids have also been done successfully.

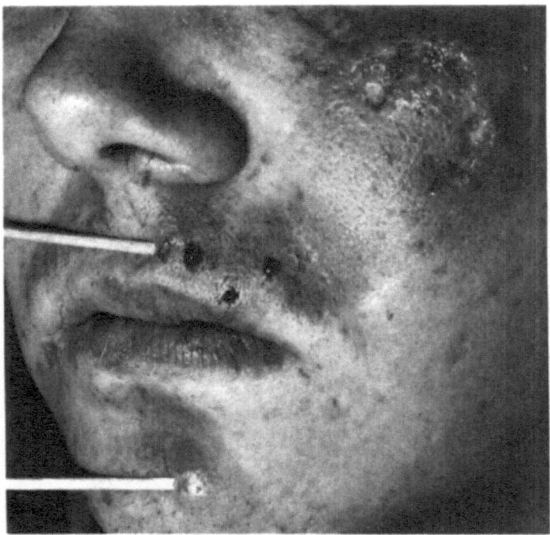

Figure 23-5.   Immediate reaction of laser treatment of debris tattoo from land mine explosion. Small cleared areas resulted.

Mixed port-wine stains and cavernous angiomas, when they are not quite extensive, have also been treated effectively with the laser. Here, too, excisional surgery has occasionally been combined with laser treatments. In the older individual with sagging and bulging of the vascular masses, the laser has been effective even in the large areas. Occasional development of the cavernous spot, or granuloma telangiectaticum, on port-wine stain has also been treated with the laser.

Laser treatment for port-wine stains begins with test treatment of one or two postage-stamp size spots. Local anesthesia is used around the target area. For children, initial laser testing is begun around the age of 6 or 7 since cooperation of the patient is necessary for eye protection. If the laser is effective, multiple treatments are given under general anesthesia, either with halothane or ketamine. New argon lasers are to be used to treat large areas (Fig. 23-7). Complications have included occasional hypertrophic scarring, especially around the lip and chin. Rarely is there revascularization of the lesion. If tissue involvement is intense and deep, the laser may not be effective. Also, the darker the lesion, the more effective the laser absorption. Patients with Sturge-Weber syndrome have been treated. With eye involvement of the port-wine stain, the patient should

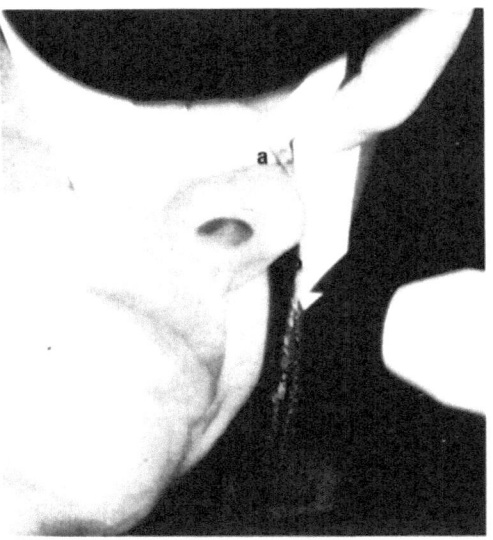

Figure 23-7. Argon laser treatment of port-wine stain of the lip. Diffusing lens used to make treatment spot larger.

be checked for glaucoma. Hemorrhage has not been a result of laser action on tissue.

Multiple lesions of glomus tumors have been treated with the ruby laser under partial focus with good scarring. If the lesions are extensive, laser treatment is not practical at present.

Spider angiomata have also been treated with the laser if the central feeder is not too deep. Transillumination has been used to attempt to study the feeder branches in extensive progressive angiomas of the face, head, and pharynx of infants. It has not been possible to critically evaluate experiments with topical and oral corticosteroids combined with laser radiation. As yet, the laser had not been used for severe progressive angiomas of the head and neck nor the intracranial extensions of Sturge-Weber syndrome. Development of high-output laser systems with bloodless surgery will facilitate these procedures.

It is evident that more effective laser instrumentation is necessary to be able to treat more extensive types of persistent vascular lesions, for which there is often no other therapy.

Multiple Malignancies

The patient with multiple basal cell malignancies obviously offers an opportunity for critical evaluation of local laser treatment. With the excellent results obtained from the combination of curettement, electrosurgery, and electrocoagulation necrosis, it is difficult to compare the results with the laser except as an investigative procedure (Fig. 23-8). The patient with multiple basal cell malignancies, then, is offered laser treatment when the usual modalities cannot be used. At present, many lesions have been treated and some patients followed for over 8 years. The recurrence rate is not as low as it is for curettement and electrosurgery. The recurrence rate of our original series was 12%. This has now been reduced to less than 5%, but it is still inferior to that of other current therapies. Control studies have been done at intervals after laser treatment with Mohs's controlled chemosurgery to monitor the extent of immediate laser-induced thermocoagulation necrosis. Tattooing or coloring nonpigmented basal cell malignancies has also increased the effectiveness of laser radiation. Vital dyes and sterile ink suspensions have been used.

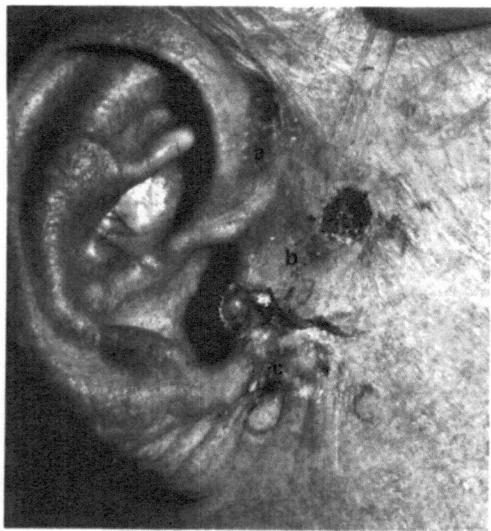

Figure 23-8. Technique of controlled experimentation for laser treatment of multiple malignancies immediately following therapy. All areas healed in a similar manner. *a*. Curettement and electrosurgery. *b*. Laser treatment. *c*. Laser treatment.

Ferrofluids and colloidal ion suspensions have also been injected into nonpigmented basal cell malignancies and then irradiated with the laser to show increased absorption and effectiveness of these compounds. There has been no toxicity. These experiments are part of a study of the combined use of ferrofluids and microwaves to induce tissue hyperthermia and cancericidal effects. High magnetic fields move the ferrofluids into desired depot areas such as lymphatic regional glands and metastases. [7] These new fiber optics will permit transmission of high output laser systems for those metastases already treated with iron and microwaves. Such investigative studies with ferrofluids and other iron compounds in multiple skin malignancies will help to develop more important applications in cancerous conditions.

The most extensive and significant laser cancer research, including both animal and human studies, has been with melanoma. At present, of course, primary melanoma is treated only very rarely with the laser, and then only when conventional treatments cannot be applied. For lentigo maligna, large areas in elderly, debilitated patients have been treated with laser radiation to show its effectiveness. Only a few patients have been observed for

long periods and no recurrences have been found. When conventional treatments are not applicable, as in recurrent melanoma of the lower leg associated with congestive heart failure, the laser has been used as an adjuvant in patients with multiple cutaneous metastases refractory after surgery radiation, chemotherapy, and infusion techniques. Recently, the CO_2 laser has been used to excise melanomas and, immediate graft with replacement where needed.

Attempts have also been made to study immunologic aspects of melanomas with laser therapy using the following procedures: (1) tissue culture of the patient's melanoma cells, laser impacts of the tissue culture, and injection of the extract of the tissue culture; (2) reinoculation into dermis of laser-irradiated melanoma metastases with controlled, electrocoagulated masses, x irradiated masses, and surgically removed masses; (3) BCG vaccination of metastatic laser melanoma; and (4) DNCB sensitization.

Perilesional leukoderma, often reported, developed in one patient under laser treatment with spontaneous disappearance of many lesions but not the visceral metastases. Disseminated cutaneous melanomas still have a poor prognosis, even after extensive laser treatment.

Florid Condylomata Acuminata

One of the features of the current venereal disease epidemic is the increased incidence of florid condylomata acuminata with the the development of giant lesions. This increased incidence is due to the widespread use of oral contraceptives, and increased sexual freedom. The frequency of the florid cases is quite astounding. They are usually too far advanced for topical therapies of any type, especially podophyllin. Oral therapy with methionine, used for some years at our laboratory as a chemotherapeutic agent, has not been effective. Operative procedures are therefore necessary for the patient with extensive condylomata acuminata. Occasionally, the lesions are so extensive that, in the female, vulvectomies have been required, and destructive scarring of the penis has been observed in the male with florid lesions. It is the flat type rather than the pedunculated lesion that offers the greatest difficulty in operative surgery. Current experiments include the use of the high frequency electrosurgical instrument as the control for the laser surgical unit. The technique of Kaplan [2] for laser excision of the pendulous growth has been excellent. Under general anesthesia, the vegetative lesion is held and the base is cut with the high-output CO_2 laser with no bleeding. For broad-based oozing, the high frequency electrosurgery, excision, and sutures must be used. The CO_2 laser, at present, has not been able to correct extensive bleeding. Perhaps, for broad-based, extensive lesions in the moist perineum of the female, a graft replacement, even in the presence of infectious lesions, may be necessary. At any rate, these cases provide extensive material for investigative laser surgery. Plantar warts, after paring down resistant intractable, recurrent tissue, have also been treated with high-output laser systems. It is not evident whether the results are due to psychologic factors or actual physical cures.

We have established at our laboratory an extensive, cooperative study of laser treatment of early preinvasive malignancies with special laser operating microscopes (Fig. 23-8), and of treatment of advanced cancer with high-output

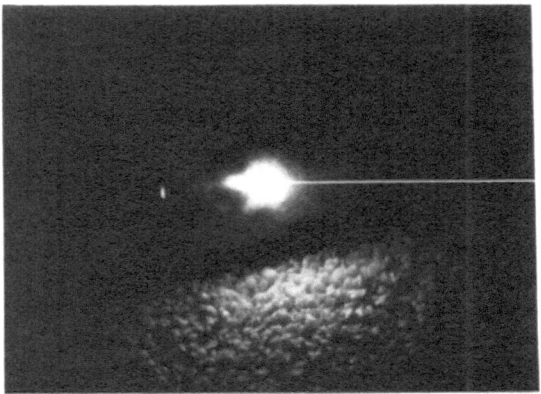

Figure 23-10. Low-output helium–neon laser for treatment of chronic ulcer.

systems. The services included in this study include dermatology, general surgery, maxillofacial surgery, and gynecologic surgery [4,5].

Future Developments

Some miscellaneous future developments include laser epilation, laser acupuncture, and study of the relationship of the laser to Kirlian chemoluminescent photography. This latter field, concerning electric coronal discharge or bioplasma, offers much interesting material for the dermatologist if proper controls and repetitive pictures can be obtained.

Russian investigators are using the laser instead of conventional needles for acupuncture. The reported relief of pruritus may lead to controlled acupuncture treatment studies in dermatology.

Recently, low-output helium–neon lasers have been used for stimulating phagocytosis, for healing chronic ulcers, and for delaying graft rejection (Fig. 23-10). Control studies in the future will help to determine the role of the laser as a stimulating agent.

References

1. Ehlers G, Florian HJ: Kanzerogene Wirkung von Laser strahlen? Fortschr Med 91:832, 1973
2. Goldman L: Applications of the Laser, CRC Press, Cleveland 1973
3. Goldman L, et al: High power neodymium-YAG laser surgery Acta Derm Venereol 53:45, 1973
4. Goldman L: Laser Cancer Research. Springer-Verlag New York 1966

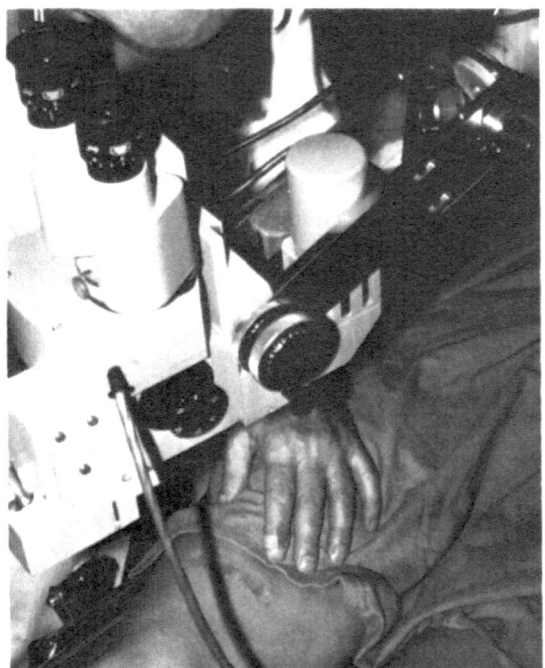

Figure 23-9. The new argon laser microscope for studying preinvasive cancer of the skin, oral cavity, and cervix.

5. Goldman L: Laser surgery for skin cancer. New York State J. Med. 77:1897, 1977

6. Goldman L: Trauma from Visible and Infrared Lasers. In Day SB (ed): Pathobiology of Trauma. New York, Plenum, 1975

7. Goldman L, Dreffer R: Microwaves, magnetic iron particles and lasers as a combined test model for investigation of hyperthermia treatment of cancer. Arch Derm Res 257, 227, 1976

8. Goldman L, Dreffer R, Rockwell RJ Jr, et al: Treatment of Portwine marks by an argon laser. J Dermatol Surg 2:385, 1976

9. Goldman L, Nath G, Schindler G, et al: High-power neodymium-YAG laser surgery. Acta Derm Venereol (Stockh) 53:45, 1973

10. Goldman L, Rockwell RJ Jr: Lasers in Medicine. New York, Gordon and Breach, 1971

11 Goldman L, Rockwell RJ Jr, Naprestek Z et al: Some parameters of high-output CO_2 laser experimental surgery. Nature 228:1344, 1972

12. Goldman L, Rockwell RJ Jr, Richfield F: Long-term laser exposure of a senile freckle. Arch Environ Health 22:401, 1971

13. Link WJ, Incropera FP, Glover JL: Development and Evaluation of the Plasma Scalpel, a Tool for Bloodless Surgery. Techn Rep No HTGDL-9. West Lafayette, Ind, High Temperature Gas Dynamics Laboratory, School of Mechanical Engineering, Purdue University, 1973

14. Vahl, Jhana: Personal communication.

24

The Plasma Torch

Hugh M. Crumay

The Plasma Torch: The Plasma Scalpel

The plasma torch is a poorly understood, little known prodigy among the physical modalities used in medicine. It is unknown to most physicians because it is presently an experimental tool, references in the medical literature are sparse, and it masquerades under several aliases. For example, the plasma torch has been called the plasma arc, the plasma jet, the plasma scalpel, and the arc plasma scalpel. Reasons for the variety of names will be elucidated below. The last two terms emphasize cutting ability; jet scalpel and plasma jet scalpel would be other acceptable terms. In general, considering both industrial and medical applications, we believe the term plasma torch may best describe the true nature of this device. However, when it is used to cut tissue, plasma scalpel is a more appropriate term.

In any event, it is a unique surgical tool of great potential. A surgeon can use the plasma torch to incise and excise with minimal hemorrhage ("bloodless surgery"). This makes it of immediate interest to the surgeon who incises organs beneath the skin, or excises fresh burns. Tissue is cut by an open all-consuming jet plasma "flame," that may be thought of as a very sophisticated, extremely hot welder's torch. Where and how it will be used in dermatology is not presently clear.

Plasma used in this sense is not, of course, related to blood plasma. To the physicist, plasma is a state of matter: a hot, partially ionized gaseous discharge in which ionized atoms are equally divided into light particles (free electrons, negatively charged) and heavy particles (ions with positive charge). In as much as charges are equal, plasma is electrically neutral. Plasma differs from ordinary gas: it is a good conductor of electricity, due to free electrons, and it is affected by a magnetic field. Plasma develops whenever any gas is highly energized in some fashion. Most plasmas contain un-ionized molecules or atoms, since complete ionization can occur only at extremely high temperatures. True plasmas can vaporize any known substance; hence, they cannot be contained for prolonged periods of time. Plasmas occur naturally in the atmospheres of stars and they are also familiar as lightning and the aurora borealis. The glow area of an electric arc is man-made plasma. Link [5] states that "a plasma gas is a high temperature, electrically conductive, partially ionized gaseous mixture which is electrically neutral."

It is now evident that plasma gas may be generated by various methods; all of them depend on conversion of electric energy into thermal energy. The plasma torch (Fig. 24-1) is "an arc-gas device capable of heating gas to extremely high temperatures" [11]. Any gas (eg, argon, helium, hydrogen, nitrogen) or a mix-

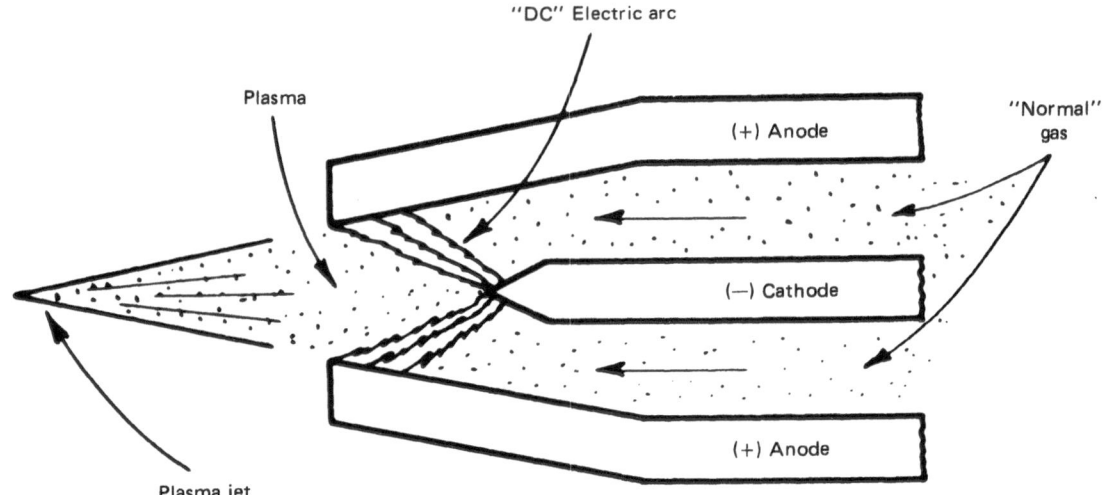

Figure 24-1. Schematic of the operating chamber of a plasma torch—specifically of the water-cooled plasma scalpel shown in Fig. 24-2. This is an example of the nontransferred-arc type of plasma torch. A transferred-arc type, where the uncooled material to be cut becomes the anode, is also used in industry.

ture of gases (eg, air, or argon and helium) is forced into a chamber, commonly cooled by water (or gas), containing both a positive and a negative electrode (anode and cathode). When a direct electric current supply is turned on, an electric arc can form between the two electrodes. As gas passes through the arc it is continuously energized and partially ionized—increasing temperature soars (as electric energy of the arc becomes thermal energy of the gas) and pressure rises as conductivity of the system increases. Grimm and Kusnetz [3] state that "the processes in the arc, where the electric energy is transferred, are extremely complex." Plasma is formed as soon as temperature reaches a critical level. Grimm and Kusnetz [3] conclude that "magnetohydrodynamic forces and the pressure which is built up in the chamber cause the plasma to be ejected through the orifice." Then, as Link [5] states, "as the energy of the plasma is expended, the electrons recombine with the ions . . . resulting in the 'normal' gas with which we began."

Controlled generation of plasma became possible early in this century; yet, reliable plasma torches have been available to industry only since World War II. Plasma temperatures may rise to 60,000 F (more than 33,000 C) and jet velocities of gases passing through the arc may reach 10,000 miles/hr. The beam (jet) of the plasma torch must obviously be narrow if it

is to serve as a scalpel that will cut precisely. Inert argon–helium gas mixtures are capable of producing the necessary slim, miniature jet which operates at a temperature of about 10,-000 C [1]. In 1973 Link et al [7] developed an efficient plasma scalpel with an average operating jet temperature of 3000 C (Fig. 24-2).

This plasma scalpel prototype is the size of a large fountain pen, about 0.5 by 6 inches, and may be comfortably held in the hand (Fig. 24-3). Argon and/or helium are passed through a direct current electric arc near the operating end of the device. The anode serves as the attachment site of the electric arc and also as a nozzle (port) through which the plasma is ejected. The cathode is spring-loaded at the supply end so that it may be advanced momentarily to contact the anode. Then, as it retracts a direct current electric arc is struck if current is flowing.

During operation the anode becomes much hotter than the cathode; hence, water is used to cool the anode, while the flow of "normal" gas under pressure partially cools the cathode. Even so, both electrodes, like the water-seal ring and the nose cone, deteriorate to some extent, consumed by the vary plasma they help create. The cathode is adjustable and may be advanced to compensate for erosion of its tip, thus prolonging its life. Cables connecting the scalpel to the support system are quite

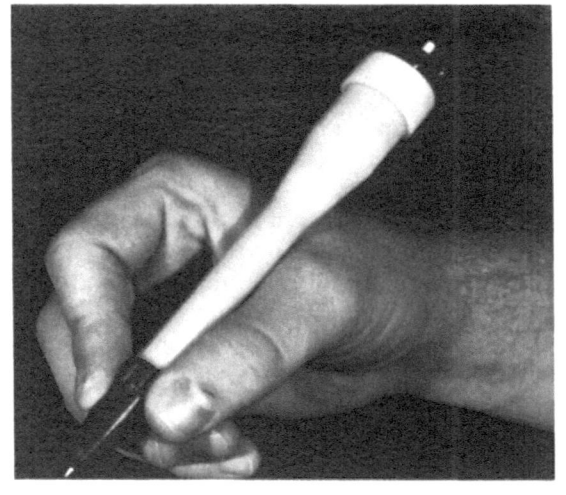

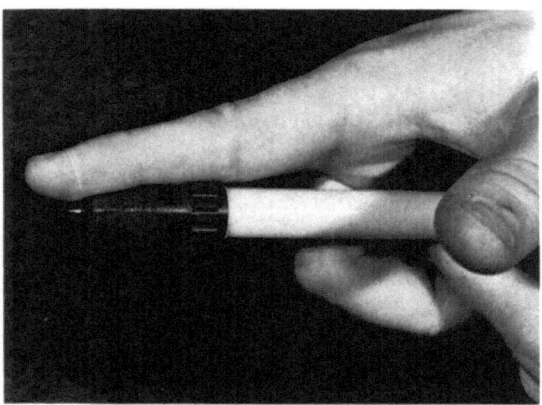

Figure 24-4. The plasma scalpel developed by Link et al [7]. Heat is largely confined to the visible portion of the jet. Courtesy of Link et al [7].

less, depending upon the speed at which the scalpel is moved. Accumulation of blood in the incision does not interfere with cutting, if the plasma scalpel is submerged in the pool of blood and contact with the tissue surface is continued. During surgery, recalcitrant bleeding sites may be sealed by holding the tip of the torch 0.5 inch from the tissue surface and directing the jet of hot plasma gas on the site. Apparently, optimum simultaneous cauterization and incision depend on plasma scalpel cutting speed, gas flow rate, arc current, and a mixture of 50% argon and 50% helium.

Link et al [6] determined that plasma scalpel incisions heal without complications—specifically, that incisions in mouse skin heal much like similar incisions made with the electrosurgical scalpel. Healing times of plasma scalpel incisions and diathermy electrode incisions are much the same. As expected, cuts made by cold steel heal faster—scars were 40 to 60% larger than those made by electrosurgical scalpels, which in turn caused scars double the size of those made by steel scalpels. Intravascular ingestion of operating gas (both dissolved form and embolic) occurred during canine hepatectomies. Gross, ultrasonic, and mass spectrometric evaluation revealed that amounts of gas were comparatively small, and were removed in a single pass through the pulmonary circulation; none reached the left side of the heart and no adverse physiologic effects due to gas ingestion were observed [4].

New, full-thickness burns in pigs may be excised to the deep fascial plane with the plasma scalpel; also, split thickness autographs are successful [9]. Excision time, percentage of takes, healing time, and size of scars for plasma scalpel excisions and grafts, when compared to steel scalpel excisions and grafts, are similar; however, loss of blood was 5 times greater when the steel scalpel was used.

Although use of the described plasma scalpel seems quite safe, it is wise to recall that Powell et al [10], while evaluating the "potential health hazards associated with the use of the medium output plasma torch in biologic research," pointed out that the following dangers may accompany the employment of high-pressure output plasma torches in industry: possible harmful amounts of ultraviolet light emitted at 365, 320 to 280, and 254 nm wavelengths; heat sufficient to cause thermal burns; high overall noise levels; and excessive amounts of toxic ozone and oxides of nitrogen. Grenz-ray output was negligible. A history of keratoconjunctivitis was elicited. Others have detected emission of ultraviolet radiation below 110 nm and have noted that particulate matter resulting from industrial applications could be toxic. These studies indicate the necessity of protecting the eyes, ears, and skin of some industrial plasma torch operators, and stress the importance of providing adequate ventilation. Fortunately, except for the chance of a heat burn, physicians using the plasma scalpel are not exposed to such risks.

The plasma torch promises to become a valuable surgical tool in the future. Size, ease of use, and probable future cost suggest practicability. Techniques of burn excision and successful autograph repair may be utilized to remove large skin tumors. Mainly because of the theoretical possibility of gas embolism, the plasma torch should be the subject of further investigative studies before it is recommended for human surgery.

References

1. Freeman MA, Incropera, FP: Operational Characteristics of a Prototype Arc Plasma Scalpel. Presented at the 23rd ACEMB Meeting, Washington, DC, November 15–19, 1970
2. Goldman L, Solomon H JR, Rockwell RJ Jr et al: Plasma torch reactions in the skin. J Invest Dermatol 48:478, 1967

3. Grimm RC, Kusnetz HL: The plasma torch. Arch Environ Health 4:295, 1962

4. Henderson MR, Link WJ, Glover JL, et al: Gas transport resulting from plasma–scalpel surgery. Med Biol Eng 12:208, 1974

5. Link WJ: Description of a plasma gas. Personal communication, 1974

6. Link WJ, Glover JL, Edwards JL, et al: Wound healing of mouse skin incised with a plasma scalpel. J Surg Res 14:505, 1973

7. Link WJ, Incropera FP, Glover JL: Development and Evaluation of the Plasma Scalpel. A Tool for Bloodless Surgery. Techn Rep No HTGDL-9. High Temperature Gas Dynamics Laboratory, School of Mechanical Engineering, Purdue University, Lafayette, Ind, 1973

8. Link WJ, Incropera FP, Glover JL: The Thermal Response of Tissue Subjected to Plasma Scalpel Heating. 73-WA/Bio-32. Presented at the ASME Winter Annual Meeting, Detroit, 1973

9. Link WJ, Zook EG, Glover JL: Plasma scalpel excision of burns. An experimental study. Plast Reconstr Surg. 55(6):647, 1975

10. Powell CH, Goldman L, Key MM: Investigative studies of plasma torch hazards. Am Ind Hyg Assoc J 29:381, 1968

11. Speicher HW: Plasma jet. Arch Environ Health 2:278, 1961

25

Ultrasound

Hugh M. Crumay

Before the beginning of the 19th century, Spallanzani recognized the existence of sound that is inaudible to human ears, after noting that bats did not fly into unseen obstacles unless their hearing was impaired. The physiologic potential of ultrasound was probably first recognized by Langevin in 1917, when he saw small fish killed by sonic waves. Medically speaking, ultrasound was given its greatest impetus in 1944 when Horvath reported successful ultrasonic treatment of sarcomatous disease and other types of superficial malignant growths [17]. Use of ultrasound grew rapidly in Germany, but it was not widely accepted in the United States until 1952, following the first report of the Council on Physical Medicine and Rehabilitation.

Ultrasound is a form of acoustic or mechanical vibration, identical to that of sound, occurring at frequencies too high to be detected by humans with a keen sense of hearing. Usually man cannot hear sounds with a frequency above 17,000, or at the very most 20,000, hertz. Vibrations between 12 hertz and 17 to 20 kilohertz are called sound waves; above 20 kilohertz they become ultrasound waves. Supersonics commonly refers to speeds greater than the velocity of sound rather than to frequency, although supersound and ultrasound are defined as synonyms.

Ultrasound may be considered a form of diathermy if one defines diathermy as the use of high frequency currents to produce heat, especially deep heat, in the body. Currently the dermatologist has little interest in the production of deep heat, but must be aware that it occurs with ultrasonic applications. Ultrasound causes little temperature rise in superficial tissue, despite the fact that biophysical research suggests it is the most effective deep heating agent.

More energy can be added to the patient per unit time by ultrasound than by moist heat, ultraviolet, infrared, or electromagnetic diathermy. This is because greater depth of penetration causes a primary, more uniform rate of deep tissue temperature rise than can result by other means, when most of the energy is absorbed by superficial tissue with only secondary heat transfer to deep tissue. Griffin [5] observed that penetration and transmission are synonymous, but that penetration and absorption are inversely related. Obviously, deep tissue heating may appeal to most physicians, but not to a dermatologist.

Physics and Biophysics

When diathermy is applied the following chain of events takes place [12]:

1. Heat formation occurs concurrently with energy absorption by the biologic medium. Electric or mechanical energy interacts with

tissue molecules and is eventually transmuted.

2. Heat conduction occurs with transfer of heat from sites of higher temperature to those of lower temperature. The total or net temperature rise in tissue mass is due to heat production.

3. Physiologic change follows temperature rise. Ion transfer is accelerated at higher temperatures and hence metabolic activity increases. If temperature is sufficiently elevated blood vessels dilate, blood flow increases, and, in turn, increased metabolic activity is further supported.

4. Clinical change results from physiologic alterations. We do not fully understand why such physiologic effects benefit certain diseases, but biochemical reactions, as well as heat, may play an important role. Changes are significant only if documented by controlled and statistically reliable studies.

Limitations of space preclude an adequate discussion of the biophysics of ultrasound. A more complete review is provided by Schwan [15]. Except for differences in frequency, the physics of ultrasound and acoustic sound are identical. Therapeutic frequencies of ultrasound, currently applied, usually vary between 0.7 and 1 megahertz.* For surgical purposes, James [7] notes, frequencies between 1 and 9 megahertz may be employed. Medical applications, including diagnostic frequencies, according to Wells [18], may be as high as 15 megahertz. Recently, an ultrasonic "bath" operating at comparatively low frequencies of 50 to 200 kilohertz and low voltage has been introduced [8]. This machine has multiple transducers using a small amount of wattage over a large area, which should make it safer and reduce the need for close supervision. However, Griffin [5] advises that "clinical claims must be evaluated in light of Summer's and Patrick's report that at frequencies less than 300 kilohertz there is no significant temperature rise, regardless of the intensities used."

Frequency is directly related to velocity, but inversely related to wavelengths:

*Therapeutic frequencies of ultrasound and "long wave" surgical diathermy are similar, but only valve tubes (never spark gaps) are used in ultrasound oscillatory circuits.

$$\text{Frequency} = \text{Velocity/Wavelength}$$

Velocity of sound in tissue is little influenced by change in frequency; therefore, it is frequency independent. Because of high water content the velocity of sound in soft tissue is approximately the same as that in water at room temperature; velocity is only slightly less in fat and a little more than doubled in bone. The following figures for velocity are approximate. The velocity of light (3.0×10^8 m/sec) is 900,000 times the velocity of sound in air (3.3×10^2 m/sec). Sound travels faster in media of greater density, so that velocity is 5 times greater in water and tissue (1500 m/sec) and 15 times greater in iron or steel (4500 m/sec). Sound is not propagated in a vacuum.

Tissue absorption, on the other hand, is frequency dependent. The absorption coefficient of tissues is larger than that of water. The reasons are not entirely clear, but tissue absorption is directly related to the molecular absorption properties of protein. Ultrasound is relatively slowly absorbed by fat, rapidly by muscle, and very rapidly by bone. A vibration rate of approximately 1 megahertz is usually selected for therapy because with that frequency the absorption coefficient of muscle results in optimal deep heating. Absorption becomes too small to cause satisfactory tissue heating when frequencies are much below 0.7 to 1 megahertz; as the absorption coefficient gets smaller, depth of penetration approaches or is greater than body (tissue) dimensions [15]. As frequencies become higher than 2 to 4 megahertz, depth-related absorption increases rapidly, and with increased frequency eventually only surface heating results.

If velocity of sound in water and tissue is 1.5×10^5 cm/sec and the frequency of ultrasonic vibrations is 1 megahertz, the wavelength is 0.15 cm. As indicated, a frequency of 1 megahertz is purposely selected to produce optimum deep heating with presently available therapeutic applications. Structures much larger than the wavelength of ultrasound can be much smaller than the wavelength of audible sound. Tissue structures and interfaces transparent to low frequency audible sound waves may reflect or scatter the short waves of ultrasound.

At tissue interfaces longitudinal oscillations may be partially transformed to transverse oscillations (sheer waves), which are more rapidly absorbed. This may result in local heat build-up and pain. The proportion of energy transferred into sheer waves depends on a complicated relationship between the differences in acoustic properties of adjoining tissues, the angle at which sound waves strike the interface, and the frequency of the oscillations [15]. Formation of sheer waves and heat will be greater when the tissue interfaces are of very different acoustic properties (eg, bone and soft tissue).

Tissues too thick or dense to permit transmission of ultrasound may be transparent to long audible sound waves. The amount of energy reflected at tissue interfaces or membranes depends on the mismatch of acoustic impedance, which is a function of the specific acoustic impedance and the membrane thickness. Acoustic impedance is proportional to the product of tissue density and sound velocity in the medium, assuming that sound wave incidence is perpendicular to a plane tissue layer [11]. Transmission of ultrasound in tissue is maximal and reflection minimal if tissue layer thickness equals an even multiple of the quarter-wavelength in the membrane; conversely, if thickness is an uneven multiple maximal reflection and minimal transmission occur.

Griffin [5], as recorded earlier, points out that transmission is synonymous with penetration; absorption and transmission are inversely related. To effect a tissue change, energy added to a patient must be absorbed (Grotthus–Draper law). In turn, the amount of tissue change depends on how much energy is absorbed (Arndt–Schultz principle). Addition of (1) a subthreshold quantity of energy causes no demonstrable change, (2) a threshold or above threshold quantity stimulates normal function, and (3) too great a quantity prevents normal function or destroys the absorbing tissue. Resultant principles of absorption are true for all types of energy added to the patient.

All kinds of energy may be absorbed, transmitted, reflected, or refracted. In the human patient especially, it is difficult to determine how much of each takes place. Clinically, dosage must be determined by physician observation and patient sensation (mild heat); both these responses are highly individualized. This is emphasized in ultrasonic therapy in which patient sensation is a particularly unreliable

guide, because the skin largely transmits, rather than absorbs, ultrasonic energy.

Ultrasonic beams can be sharply focused and aimed. Sound is propagated in the form of longitudinal compressional waves, compared to transverse electromagnetic waves. Since propagation requires a compressible medium, sound is not transmitted through a vacuum. Therapeutic applications produce sound beams almost cylindric in shape. Intensity across the beam is not uniform, varying most nearest the applicator [12].

The principal physical effects of ultrasound are agitation, particle streaming, cavitation, and, especially, production of heat. Primary reactions occurring within an ultrasonic beam at therapeutic intensities are directly related to particle movement (agitation and particle streaming) resulting from wave propagation.

Alternating rarefaction and compression displaces particles in the medium. These particles are subjected to an acceleration 100,000 times that of gravity. Great differences in wave pressure of about 1 to 5 atmospheres occur over the short distance of one-half wavelength. At therapeutic frequencies of 1 megahertz intensities up to 40 W/cm² have been easily obtained without focusing. Lehmann [11] compares therapeutic ultrasonic intensities of 4 W/cm² to a "noise level produced by ten thousand high-output speakers in a room of one cubic centimeter." Such powerful mechanical forces are apt to create secondary reactions in tissue.

Energy is converted into heat by the physical properties of the absorbing medium. In the body, transformation of electric or radiant energy into heat is determined by the electric properties of the absorbing tissue; conversion of ultrasonic energy into heat is controlled by the mechanical properties. Cavities can be produced in fluid and tissue during the rarefaction phase. Since gases are always present in biologic material we are concerned with gaseous cavitation. Gas moves out of the bubble into the surrounding fluid during the compression phase of ultrasonic vibration. During the subsequent rarefaction phase, the bubble expands and the gas moves from the fluid into the cavity, creating larger bubbles. Gas bubbles may expand to tear tissue or vibrate in such a manner that shock waves are formed [12]. Cavitation may therefore destroy

stroy tissue, but proper dosage and technique (massage and pressure) prevent damage.

Too little attention has been paid to the fact that depth of penetration of ultrasonic energy in living tissue is dependent upon frequency as well as absorption and transmission [5]. If the frequency is 90 kilohertz, about 50% of energy will penetrate soft tissue to a depth of 10 cm; if the frequency is 1 megahertz the same amount of energy will penetrate to 5 cm; if the frequency is raised to 4 megahertz a similar amount of energy will penetrate to a depth of only 1 cm. This probably explains why ultrasound of 89 kilohertz frequency benefitted more patients with osteoarthritis than did 1 megahertz ultrasonic energy [6].

The Generator

Ultrasound energy is mechanical vibration produced by transforming electric energy into mechanical energy. A generator much like the usual diathermy machine, in all but one respect, is used to produce a high frequency alternating current. The 3 basic components of the ultrasound generator are the power circuit, to increase voltage; the oscillatory circuit, to increase frequency; and the transducer (treatment or sound head), to convert electric into mechanical (acoustic) vibration. Obviously, the transducer is the significant component; it is essentially a piezoelectric crystal connected to two electrodes (Fig. 25-1).

High frequency alternating energy (voltage) is converted into mechanical vibration by reversal of the piezoelectric effect. An alternating electric charge applied on the surfaces of the transducer crystal deforms the crystal so that there is an alternating increase and decrease in crystal thickness, depending on the

polarity of the applied charge, and this results in usable mechanical vibration. The amplitude of the vibration is maximal at the mechanical resonance frequency of the crystal; consequently, the capacitance and inductance of the oscillatory circuit are selected to produce the same resonant frequency.

Natural pure quartz, ceramic materials (eg, barium titonate), and artificially grown perfect crystals (eg, lithium sulfate) may be used as piezoelectric crystals. Required voltage to produce 3 W/cm^2 may vary from approximately 100 to 2000 V, depending on the crystal. Pure quartz requires the highest voltage because of its high impedance; ceramics require the least voltage [17]. The front of the crystal is cemented to the treatment face of the metal housing of the transducer (sound head) which acts as a ground connection. The metal housing (treatment or sound head, applicator) is shaped to make an air chamber against the back of the crystal (Fig. 25-2). Ultrasonic waves are reflected by air and transmitted by metal to the body.

Ultrasonic energy is measured in watts. The total wattage given off by the total surface of the crystal or the covering metal face is divided by the area of the surface. If the total wattage is 10 and the area 5 cm^2, the sound head gives off 2 W/cm^2. Ultrasound is prescribed in terms of watts per square centimeter. Although generators used for therapy in the United States may deliver up to 4 W/cm^2, clinically the power level rarely exceeds 2 W/cm^2. Applicators with a surface smaller than 5 cm^2 are seldom used therapeutically because the angle of divergence of the beam becomes too large. On the other hand, as the radiating surface of the applicator gets larger the angle of beam divergence gets less. However, a larger

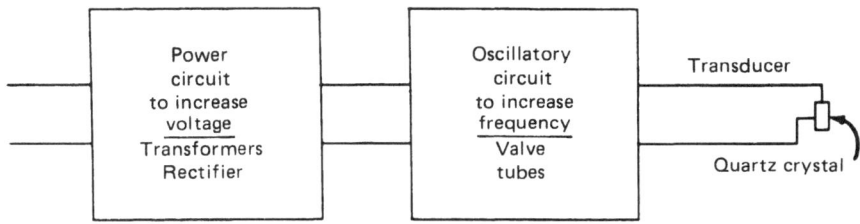

Figure 25-1. Diagram of basic components of an ultrasound generator. Circuitry is similar to that of the electrosurgical diathermy generator, but the electrodes are attached to a quartz crystal to form a transducer.

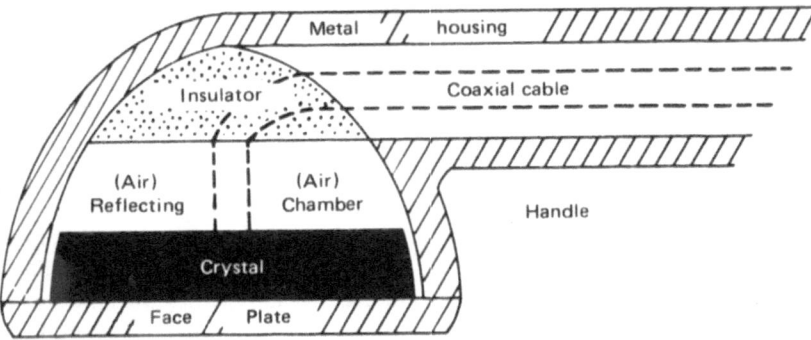

Figure 25-2. The "sound head" of a transducer (schematic).

applicator makes it harder to maintain constant contact with concave and convex body surfaces, and size must be limited.

Physiologic Effects

Literature concerning physiologic effects of ultrasonic energy is confusing because parameters are often incomplete and conclusions are muddled. One must realize that the physiologic effects of ultrasonic energy are just beginning to be understood [5]. The most important effect of therapeutic ultrasound on tissue is deep heating. As expected, the usual physiologic responses following all types of increased heating occur and presently are believed to be responsible for most therapeutically significant reactions. Uniquely, ultrasound also causes heating at tissue interfaces such as those of muscle and bone. We have seen that peripheral arterial blood flow can be increased and tissue metabolism altered. Hyperemia, increased vascularity, edema, and even tissue necrosis have been observed experimentally. Nerve stimulation or sedation, and alteration of conductivity to the point of temporary blocking, may result from different applications. Pain thresholds can be elevated and muscle spasms relieved.

Heating can occur only concurrently with absorption, which apparently takes place at the molecular level. Absorption of ultrasonic energy is directly related to the protein content of tissue; protein may account for 80% of soft tissue absorption. Increased tissue density also promotes absorption. On the other hand, tissues with high water content absorb little ultrasonic energy. Bone, with a dense cortex and a matrix of high protein content, absorbs about 10 times more than does muscle. Absorption in

muscle, in turn, is half that in nerve, double that in fat, and 10 times that in whole blood (Table 25-1).

As anticipated, when ultrasonic energy is added to the body more heat is produced in muscle than in fat. The heat differential produced in bone will vary and be less than expected because thermal conductivity, reflection, and refraction all reduce temperature rise. Furthermore, reflection and refraction probably divert more than 35% of the applied energy to softer adjacent tissues.

Temperature elevation is chiefly responsible for increased permeability of membranes and change of membrane potential. Nonthermal reactions play a lesser but probably a definite role during exposure to ultrasound. In most cases these have been incompletely studied and are not completely understood. Increased membrane permeability and accelerated diffusion of ions are apparently due to "streaming of fluids in the ultrasonic field and a resultant stirring effect" [12]. Reactions in muscle, tendon, and nerve cannot be entirely explained by increased temperature.

Table 25-1 *Absorption Coefficient of Tissues (1 megahertz ultrasonic energy)*

Tissue	Absorption Coefficient (approximate)
Blood plasma	1
Whole blood	3
Fat	15
Skeletal muscle	30
Peripheral nerve	60
Whole bone	300

Adapted from Griffin [5]; data from Griffin [5] and Lehmann [12] (1965).

Gaseous cavitation in tissue can cause destruction of tissue, but is not observed with clinical dosage and can be prevented by transducer pressure. Cavitation from gas bubbles does not occur due to viscosity of suspension fluids, density of suspended cells, continuous movement of the transducer, suitably filtered ultrasonic output, higher frequencies, or comparatively low ultrasonic energy.

Metallic implants such as disks, cups, and nails have much greater impedance than does surrounding soft tissue, and reflection may cause harmful localization of ultrasonic energy. With clinical dosages prescribed, however, there is no danger. High dosages, multiple beam, or focused ultrasound can be used to destroy tissue and tumor cells, but the exact mechanism is not understood and all malignant cells cannot be destroyed. Most experts agree there is no good evidence to prove that pulsed ultrasound is better than continuous sound. Pulsing reduces average output and resultant reactions under usual conditions, but continuous wave output can be controlled to duplicate the effects of pulsed ultrasound.

Application Technique

Slight variations in technique of application can cause appreciable change in penetration and biologically effective dosage. The general physical condition of the patient should be checked before applying ultrasound. The skin must be checked for sensation and integrity before therapy and examined for injury after treatment. The transducer head may have to be tuned to the oscillator circuit after a warm-up period. Preferred machines do not need tuning and some incorporate protective systems to prevent overheating and crystal damage. The output dial is set so that the ultrasonic energy delivered is 1 to 4 W/cm², and usually not more than 2 W/cm². The output meter shows watts delivered to, but not watts received by, the body. Treatment periods usually last 5 to 15 min and are terminated by an automatic timing device.

Transmission of ultrasound from the treatment head to the body requires good contact. Nonconducting air gaps (bubbles) between the sound head and skin surface are intolerable. Good coupling is most often achieved by coating the skin with mineral oil or

some similar material. The sound head is pressed firmly enough to assure good contact. Massage technique is used to keep the transducer moving slowly, either in a rotary fashion, or with short, back and forth strokes in a linear fashion. Such movement reduces the chance of appreciable refraction and prevents undesirable hot spots. Ultrasonic machines incorporating a warning device to signal poor coupling are desirable.

Underwater coupling may be used to treat uneven surfaces, such as those of the distal extremities, and sensitive areas. The body part to be treated and the transducer head are immersed in a bath; the water acts as the coupling medium and direct contact is unnecessary. Dissolved gases such as oxygen and carbon dioxide are often pulled out of solution to form bubbles, which tend to accumulate on the face of the energized treatment head. These bubbles reduce energy transfer and should be repeatedly wiped off (with a finger). Boiling water before treatment or substituting large amounts of oil for water are more or less impractical because of the time factor or the additional expense involved.

Uses of Ultrasound in Dermatology

After extensive personal experience and review of available literature, Veltman [16] recommended ultrasonic therapy for only three conditions: (1) gravitational ulcers, (2) scleroderma circumscripta, and (3) acute pyogenic infections such as boils and carbuncles. He added that "all authors agree about favorable effects in these diseases." Neurotrophic and traumatic ulcers were not considered suitable targets. Because of potential hazards one is warned not to treat postthrombotic conditions and malignant skin tumors. We should recall that ultrasonic therapy was readily accepted and widely used in Europe when comparatively little interest was evident in the United States. Probably few, if any, dermatologists in this country are using ultrasound to treat dermatoses.

Ultrasound may raise skin temperature in Raynaud's phenomenon. A large number of skin diseases, including dermatitis, psoriasis, tinea capitis, neurofibromatosis, and keloids, as well as varicose and decubital ulcers have been treated; but such therapy is not recommended. Many different in vitro viruses have been inactivated by ultrasound. Just how this relates to disease caused by in vivo viruses is unknown. Derickson and his collaborators [2] treated 88 cases of herpes simplex. Approximately 90% of those treated thought they were helped, but statistically placebo therapy was just as effective.

In 1958 Kent [9] reported dramatic destruction of warts with an apparent cure rate of 90% in a small group of 10 patients. He thought that wart necrosis might be due to "either a vascular, molecular, or viral effect." Rowe and Gray [14] successfully treated 22 to 25 patients who had from 1 to 70 plantar warts; residuals that were "small, dry, and so superficial it was no longer a problem" were counted as successes. They do not attempt to estimate the percentage of cure. In a controlled study, Cherup and his associates [1] related no adverse reactions while curing 80% of 55 "feet on 49 patients." Occasionally, warts on one foot persisted despite disappearance on the opposite sole. Five patients, and presumably 5 feet, used as controls showed no improvement.

In 1969 Kent [10] recorded the results of treating 1000 patients (690 females and 310 males) who had diverse types of warts. He does not state how many had plantar warts, but 584 "had foot involvement." Unfortunately, but perhaps understandably, 574 did not complete treatment; 426 with diverse types of warts completed treatment; 346, representing a corrected satisfactory percentage of 81.3%, were clear of warts without recurrence for 2 years. The overall average number of treatments, at an arbitrary optimum interval of 1 week, was 12.6 (14.7 average for females and 10.4 average for males). Maximum number of treatments was 134 to a female and 53 to a male.

On the other hand, Quade and Radzyminski [13] gave 2 treatments each week to 15 patients and only 3, or 20%, were cured. It is interesting that all cures were accomplished in 3 weeks and that 12-week courses did not reduce the number of failures. Kent's work and our experience with other methods of therapy suggest that continued treatment might have resulted in a much higher cure rate, questionably from "tincture of time." Gersten [3] no longer treats plantar warts with ultrasound "because I was not satisfied with the effective-

ness of the technique in my own experience, nor was I impressed by the results achieved by others." Ultrasound is not used to treat warts at the Hospital of the University of Pennsylvania.

Equipment and technique used to treat warts were similar in all studies. Continuous wave ultrasound was employed most often. Pulsed ultrasound was used and preferred by Kent in almost 50% of his cases; he thought higher dosages could be safely given with the pulsed wave. Frequency varied from 800 kilohertz to 1 megahertz. Maximum effective acoustic output varied from 15 to 21 W while the effective radiating area of the transducers was 5 or 6 cm^2, so that average intensities of 0.1 to 3 W/cm^2 could be generated.

A dosage of 0.1 to 2 W/cm^2 was prescribed for 15 min and usually applied with a moving sound head. Treatments were given routinely once each week, sometimes 2 or 3 times weekly, and once 5 times per week for 3 weeks. A rather heavy oil was the most common coupling agent; but some preferred water, especially for extensive involvement and uneven surfaces. Dosage should be influenced by the wave form, the coupling agent, a stationary or moving sound head, the proximity of wart to bone, and perhaps most of all by individual preference. Dosage below 1 W/cm^2 appeared just as effective as that between 1 and 2 W/cm^2. Griffin [4] stated that "if the patient's sensation is normal, and he feels a comfortable warmth in the area being treated without onset of dull aching pain during treatment, the intensity is probably adequate and not too strong."

All agree, apparently, that ultrasound is a safe, painless, and more or less effective method for treating plantar warts. No doubt many physicians will object to the time required for each visit; the only other objections are those common to other safe, nonscarring treatment modalities—weekly visits for protracted periods. Young warts and virgin (untreated) warts seem to respond best. In most cases, pain is relieved early in the course of treatment. It seems that wart location and patient age bear little relation to cure rate. There is less agreement about size. Cherup et al [1] found that "the more the lesions, the better the response to therapy"; this can hardly be said about other treatment modalities.

Conclusions

The physiologic effects of ultrasonic energy are not fully understood. Apparently, most of the beneficial effects result from the formation of heat, but the real importance of nonthermal reactions has yet to be determined. Skin is thin and transparent to ultrasound; hence little heat is produced in the skin by conversion of sonic energy. Proper parameters for treatment of skin lesions probably have not been determined; it seems plausible that they would be different than those considered optimal for "deep" heating. Perhaps ultrasonic frequencies higher than 1 megahertz will prove more valuable. In the light of present knowledge and because of technical difficulties as well as individual variation, Schwan [15] points out that "it is not surprising that success depends to a great extent on intuitive ability to properly apply the chosen form of diathermy." Thus, chance and intuition may account for success and failure. In the meantime, there is good evidence that the interested dermatologist may find ultrasound of value in the treatment of plantar warts. Safety and lack of pain are most desirable qualities if we can prove effectiveness of therapy. Offhand, it seems logical that the skin specialist might be interested in ultrasonic generators operating at greater frequencies of 4 or more megahertz to cause relatively superficial, rather than deep, heating. Until cooperative efforts of the biophysicist, physiologist, engineer, and clinician change the picture, widespread use of ultrasound in dermatology is not anticipated.

References

1. Cherup N, Urban J, Bender LF: The treatment of plantar warts with ultrasound. Arch Phys Med Rehabil. 44:602, 1963
2. Derickson BA, et al: Treatment of herpes simplex with ultrasound. Preliminary report. Arch Phys Med Rehabil 50:454, 1969
3. Gersten JW: What's the answer? Phys Ther 51:83, 1971
4. Griffin JE: What's the answer? Phys Ther 51:82, 1971
5. Griffin JE: Physiologic effects of ultrasonic energy as it is used clinically. Am Phys Ther Assoc 46:18, 1966
6. Griffin JE, et al: Results of frequency differences in ultrasonic therapy. Phys Ther 50:481, 1970
7. James JA: Therapeutic aspects of ultrasound. Br J Radiol 42:72, 1969
8. Kaiser HS: New method of applying ultrasonic therapy. J Am Podiatry Assoc 60:280, 1970
9. Kent H: Plantar wart treatment with ultrasound. Arch Phys Med Rehabil 40:15, 1959
10. Kent H: Warts and ultrasound. Arch Dermatol 100:79, 1969
11. Lehmann JF: Ultrasound therapy. In Licht S (ed): Therapeutic Heat and Cold. Baltimore, Waverly Press, 1965
12. Lehmann JF: Ultrasonic diathermy. In Krusen FH, Kottke FJ, Ellwood PM (eds): Handbook of Physical Medicine and Rehabilitation, 2nd ed., Philadelphia, Saunders, 1965
13. Quade AG, Radzyminski SF: Ultrasound therapy in Verruca plantaris, J Am Podiatry Assoc 56:503, 1966
14. Rowe RJ, Gray JM: Ultrasound therapy of plantar warts. Arch Dermatol 82:1008, 1960
15. Schwan HP: Biophysics of diathermy. In Licht S (ed): Therapeutic Heat and Cold. Baltimore, Waverly Press, 1965
16. Veltman G: Ultrasonic therapy in dermatology. Br J Phys Med 15:21, 1952
17. Watkins AL: A Manual of Electrotherapy, 3rd ed. Philadelphia, Lea & Febiger, 1968
18. Wells PNT: Physical aspects of the application of ultrasonics to diagnosis and treatment. Br J Radiol 42:72, 1969

26

Cryosurgery in Dermatology

Setrag A. Zacarian

Nearly one-half of all integumentary disorders that confront the dermatologist necessitate the use of some form of physical modality for effective management. Liquid nitrogen has been the ideal refrigerant. It is readily available, nonexplosive, and extremely cold, having a boiling point of -196 C. This last characteristic is most essential if one is to treat malignant tumors of the skin. Dry ice (CO_2, -78.5 C) and instruments that employ liquid nitrous oxide (LN_2O, -89.5 C) are effective only for the treatment of benign and precancerous growths, including the management of acne. The anatomic depth of skin cancers precludes coolants with a low boiling point (Table 26-1). The cryogen must be sufficiently cold, as with liquid nitrogen, to overcome the microcirculatory barrier of the integument and allow the ice front to develop and extend into the subcutaneous tissue and beyond.

From the turn of the century to the early 1960s, cotton-tipped applicators were used to administer liquid nitrogen. This limited its use to the treatment of benign growths of the skin [1,12,22,23]. Modern cryosurgery commenced in 1962 with the implementation of sophisticated cryogenic instrumentation, using liquid nitrogen for the amelioration of neurologic disorders [5]. Liquid nitrogen was subsequently employed in the treatment of various malignant tumors [4,9], both as a primary approach and also for palliative measures.

The Pathogenesis of Cryonecrosis

A minimum temperature of -25 C within and below the neoplasm is essential for effective cryonecrosis [6]. The rate of freezing and subsequent thawing are important considerations; the more rapid the freeze and slower the thaw phase, the greater is the degree and magnitude of tissue necrosis. Cryogenic temperatures are effective at two anatomic sites: at the cellular level [15–17] and within the microvessels [13,-14,26,28]. The latter undergo both stasis and thrombosis with inevitable and irreversible tissue necrosis. It has been demonstrated [19] that a distinct, albeit small, cell population of normal or malignant cancer cells will survive subzero temperatures of -196 C. The microcirculatory system, particularly of the integument, cannot maintain its integrity at temperatures much below 0 C. Infarction and ischemic necrosis of surrounding normal and malignant tissue insidiously follow thrombosis of the tiny vessels, which develops at nominal subzero temperatures. Cancerous cells which may otherwise resist extreme cold will not survive the consequences of the cryogenic microcirculatory arrest [28].

Subjecting a given target of skin or neoplasm to either the direct spray of liquid nitrogen or a closed probe or disk initiates an immediate heat exchange at the point of contact. As the heat sink (the coolant) draws heat, the un-

Table 26-1   *Current Refrigerants Used in Cryogenic Surgery*

Agent	Boiling Point	General Use Applications	
Ethyl chloride	+ 12.2 C	Surgery	Local anesthetic
Freon^r 114	+ 3.8 C	Dermatology	Dermabrasion, etc.
Freon^r 12	− 29.8 C	Ophthalmology	Cryoextraction of cataracts; retinal surgery
Freon^r 22	− 41.0 C	Otolaryngology	Tonsillectomy; Meniere's disease
Carbon dioxide (sublimation temperature)	− 78.5 C	Gynecology	Cervical disease; condyloma; carcinoma in situ
Nitrous oxide	− 89.5 C	Gynecology	
Liquid nitrogen	− 195.6 C	Dermatology General Surgery Otolaryngology Plastic surgery Neurosurgery Urology	Benign and malignant; tumors; hemangiomas; tonsillectomy; head and neck surgery; Parkinson's disease; prostatic surgery

From Zacarian [24]. Courtesy of Charles C. Thomas.

derlying skin or neoplasm undergoes a physical transformation, changing from tissue with a 99% water content to a solid compartment of ice. A series of isotherm waves of cold energy extends downward and peripherally as with dissipation of electron energy when using irradiation. The depth and extent of the cryolesion depends in part on the counteracting homeostatic response of the underlying circulation. With liquid nitrogen as the coolant, the underlying circulatory barrier is overcome, allowing the advance of the ice front even beyond the subcutaneous tissue of the integument. This is totally impossible with either dry ice, the freon derivatives, nitrous oxide, or cotton-tipped applicators dipped in liquid nitrogen [3,11,27]. If a series of microthermocouple needles were inserted at various zones within the emerging hemisphere of the cryolesion, from the cutaneous surface to the lowest extent of the ice front to the subcutaneous tissue, one would monitor divergent temperature profiles. The temperature of the frozen tissue immediately below the heat sink (refrigerant source) may range from −120 to −80 C; several millimeters below and peripheral to the original target, one will observe diverse temperature recordings (Fig. 26-1).

Freezing is a function of time. Temperatures will alter within seconds during a freezing period at various zones within the cryolesion. This temperature gradient, or "thermal his-

tory'' [18], is a vital concept. The success or failure of complete eradication of neoplasic tissue by cryosurgery depends upon proper recording of the temperature profile below the neoplasm [24].

Instrumentation

In my own experience a host of benign and precancerous growths can be eliminated effectively with the employment of liquid nitrogen as the cryogen of choice. This same coolant, when employed through a sophisticated yet simple device, will unquestionably eradicate cancers of the skin. There are several cryogenic instruments available to the dermatologist. The CE-8 (Frigitronics, Inc., Shelton, Conn.) is a floor model and strictly for office use. The liquid nitrogen can be sprayed or allowed to circulate through a closed probe. The continuous flow of the coolant is a desirable feature. The hose through which liquid nitrogen passes will at times become rigid and hinder easy movement. Ten portable units are presently available. They are quite efficient, but most do not have the built-in measurement devices so essential in monitoring malignant tumors. Working closely with the engineers at Frigitronics, this author helped develop a new cryosurgical instrument which is portable and yet possesses the versatility of the larger floor models (Fig. 26-2). This unit, referred to as the

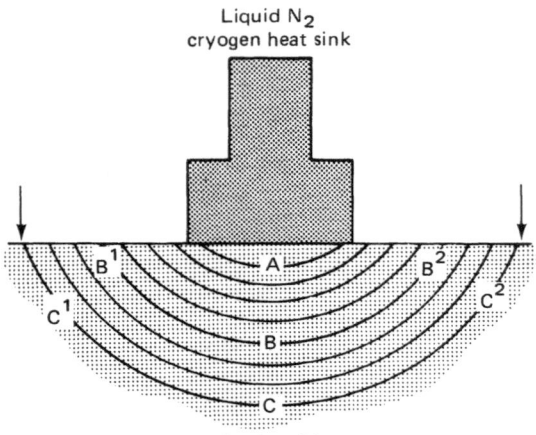

Liquid N$_2$
cryogen heat sink

In vivo skin
thermal gradients within the cryolesion

Temperatures of ice front: A = −120°C; B = −50°C; C = −25°C

Temperatures of ice zones: B$_1$ & B$_2$ = −30°C; C$_1$ & C$_2$ = −5°C

Figure 26-1. Thermal gradients when skin or tumor is subjected to cryogenic temperatures. The lateral spread of freeze from the heat sink (disk or cone) is equivalent to the central depth of the ice front. From Zacarian [25]. Courtesy of Charles C Thomas.

CS-76, has been used by this writer for the past 2 years. A single filling will last from 8 to 12 hours depending upon its use and it requires no electric outlet to generate liquid nitrogen. It is supplied with interchangeable intradermic needles for spray, disks, and cones of various diameters. The unit is portable and self-pressurizing, with safety valves and a pyrometer with inserts for the placement of thermocouple needles.

Treatment of Benign Disorders of the Skin

As outlined in Table 26-2, there are a large number of cutaneous disorders amenable to cryosurgery. Verruca vulgaris and plantaris perhaps constitute the most common problems we see. With the exception of paronychial and mosaic warts, I find the liquid nitrogen spray effective and useful. The spray is directed onto the center of the wart for a few seconds and continued intermittently until the ice front extends peripherally to a hairline distance outside the circumference of the wart onto the normal skin. A single freeze–thaw cycle is satisfactory. Invariably, the patient presents multiple or clustered warts (Fig. 26-3), and one can rapidly freeze them successively within 15 to 30 seconds and cure the patient (Fig. 26-4). Avoidance of undue infiltrations of local anesthesia and electrocautery is thereby attained.

Actinic keratoses are extremely common

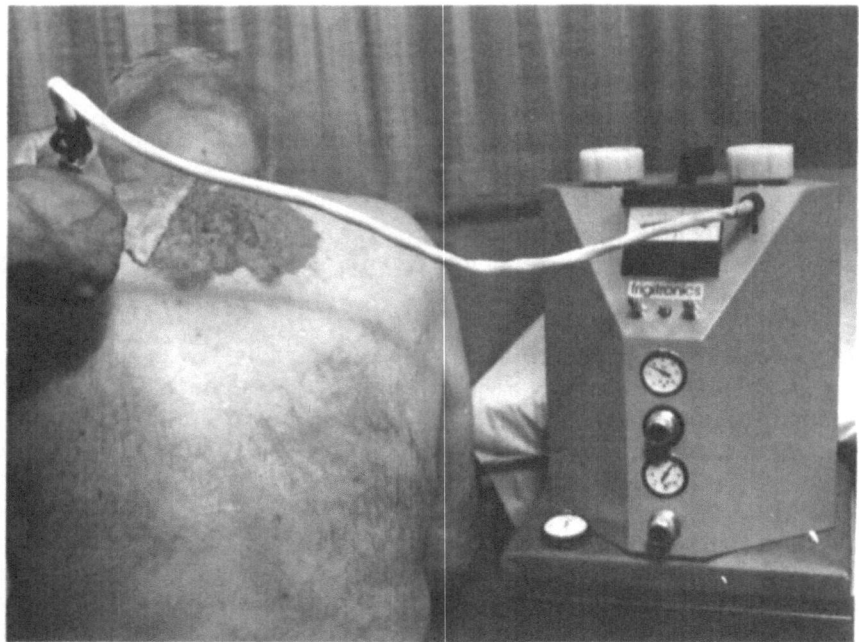

Figure 26-2. Demonstration of cryosurgery of an extensive basal cell carcinoma of the back with direct spray of liquid nitrogen from the CS-76 cryosurgical unit. From Zacarian [25]. Courtesy of Frigitronics, Inc. and Charles C Thomas.

Table 26-2 *Cutaneous Disorders Amenable to Cryosurgery with Liquid Nitrogen*

Benign Disorders	
Acne vulgaris	Lymphangioma
Chondrodermatitis nodularis chronica helicis	Molluscum contagiosa
Cutaneous tags	Porokeratosis of Mibelli
Dermatofibromas	Sebaceous cysts
Discoid lupus erythematosis	Seborrheic keratosis
Granulama pyogenicum	Spider angiomata
Hemangtoma (strawberry mark)	Synovial cysts
Hypertrophic acne scars	Trichoepithelioma
Keloidal acne (keloidal folliculitis)	Verruca acuminata
Ketoids (Small)	Verruca vulgaris and plantaris
Keratoacanthoma	Verrucoid linear and nevus
Larva migrans	
Precancerous Disorders	
Cutaneous horn	Keratoses
	Actinic (senile) and arsenical keratoses
Leukoplakia	Xeroderma pigmentosa

From Zacarian [24]. Courtesy of Charles C. Thomas.

and often multiple. They are readily eliminated with an application of 5-fluouracil (5-FU). I find, however, that many of my patients object to the prolonged use and the lengthy 6- to 8-week period of treatment management. The other distinct disadvantage is that 5-FU cannot be used during the summer because of phototoxicity. With a few seconds of liquid nitrogen spray on each lesion, one can treat from 1 to 20 within minutes. The vesiculation and ensuing scab is followed with complete healing within 10 to 12 days. Seborrheic keratoses, cutaneous tags, and papillomata are treated similarly. In the past year or so, I have noticed an increasing number of patients with verruca acuminata, both on the genitals and in perianal areas. For the larger lesions the application of podophyllin appears to be ineffectual. The direct spray of liquid nitrogen is simple and if lesions appear at the anal orifice, one can apply vaseline gauze to prevent undue diverted spray.

The management of acne with cryosur-

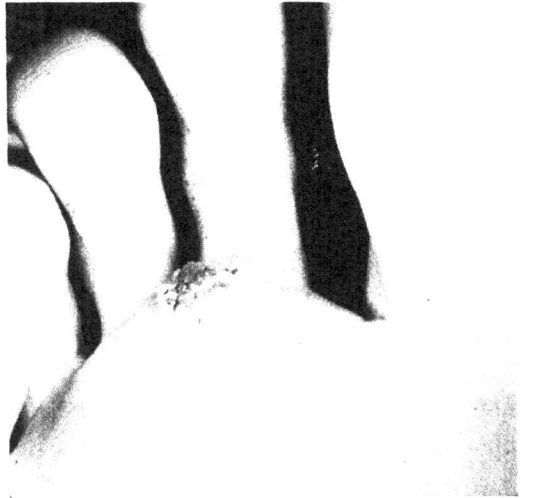 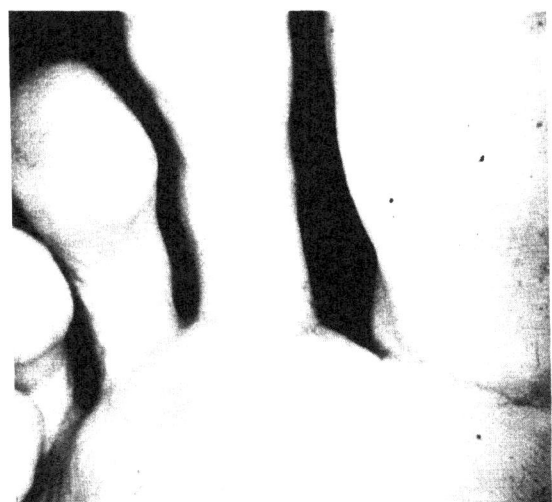

Figure 26-3.   Cluster of warts prior to cryosurgery. This cluster was subjected to 20 sec of single freeze with liquid nitrogen spray. From Zacarian SA: Cryosurgery of Skin Cancer and Cryosurgical Techniques in Dermatology, 1969. Courtesy of Charles C Thomas.

Figure 26-4.   Four weeks following cryosurgery, the plantar warts are eliminated. From Zacarian SA: Cryosurgery of Skin Cancer and Cryosurgical Techniques in Dermatology, 1969. Courtesy of Charles C Thomas.

gery is relatively new. The initial work of Graham [10] appears to be most promising. She applies a small device to her cryosurgical unit spray head which allows an even, wide spread of liquid nitrogen vapor over a large surface of skin. My own experience with acne has been limited to the elimination of keloidal acne scars and hypertrophic acne scars. Small sebaceous cysts respond quite well to 5 to 10 sec of liquid nitrogen spray. We need more experience to fully evaluate the cryosurgical approach to acne scars by means of simple freezing.

Small keloids are quite amenable to cryosurgery. In my experience, keloids up to 2.5 cm in diameter respond favorably to freezing. I tend to use a disk or cone to confine the freeze rather than an open spray. I thus achieve a greater depth without undue peripheral spread of the ice front (Figs. 26-5 and 26-6).

Treatment of Malignant Tumors of the Skin

The cryosurgical approach to the management of skin cancers has been well established [4,6,-9,20,24–26]. The technique is not difficult to master. Once the diagnosis has been established with microscopic examination, the skin is outlined with a marker 4 to 5 mm outside the visible margin of the cancer. A small area outside the tumor margin is anesthetized with Xylocaine. The microthermocouple needle is in-

serted, directing the needle at approximately a 25° angle until its tip lies subcutaneously and midcenter below the neoplasm (Fig. 26-7). At times, the needle proximal to the hub will be exposed. A small ribbon of Scotch tape is placed over the hub to keep the needle intact.

Microthermocouple needles are very delicate. The sensitive area is at the tip, wherein the copper and constantan are delicately fused together under a dissecting microscope. Following freezing and its removal, the needle can be cleaned; and after replacing the protective shield, the entire needle with the attached wiring can be safely autoclaved.

For the average skin cancer, I attach a 19- or 20-gauge plastic needle to the CS-76 unit and commence freezing. The liquid nitrogen spray is directed onto the center of the lesion, 1 or 2 sec on and 1 sec off, to allow the gradual extension of the ice front both peripherally and below the tumor. Spraying is continued until the entire neoplasm is frozen and the edges extend to the previously outlined margin from the lesion (Fig. 26-8). Intermittent freezing is continued until the pyrometer records −25 to −30 C. Spraying is then terminated, complete thawing is allowed, and freezing is begun again. The second freeze time will be approximately one-half the initial freeze to reach the desired temperature.

Following the second thaw, the microthermocouple needle is removed and the tumor

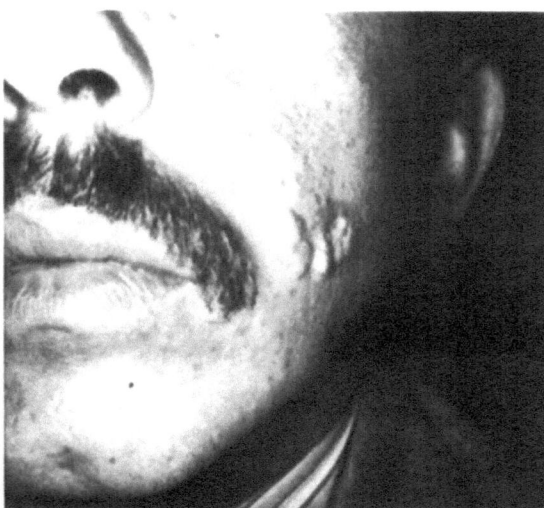

Figure 26-5. Keloid of left cheek, 2 cm in size, of 3 years' duration.

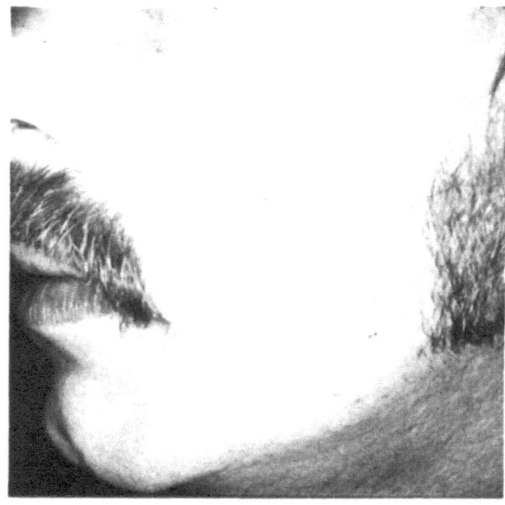

Figure 26-6. Following a single freezing for 60 sec, the keloid is totally eliminated 4 weeks later.

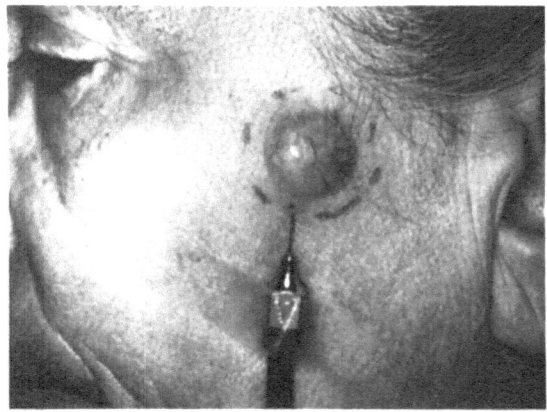

Figure 26-7. Basal cell carcinoma of the left cheek. A 4-man outline is made beyond the visible margin of tumor and the microthermocouple needle is placed subcutaneously below the tumor to monitor the ice front. From Zacarian [24]. Courtesy of Charles C Thomas.

is dressed with a bandage. The average skin cancer may take between 1 and 2 min for complete freezing. The monitored temperature will invariably dictate the termination of cryosurgery. If the entire tumor is to be infiltrated with Xylocaine with epinephrine, the freezing time will be shortened; local anesthetics tend to cause appreciable vasoconstriction of the microvessels and allow a more rapid extension of the ice front below the skin surface.

The patient is informed that he may experience some discomfort both during the freezing period and, particularly, the thaw phase. Tumors frozen on the forehead, temple, and scalp will produce a transient headache during the cryosurgical procedure. Within hours, there follows local edema at the treated site with development of hemorrhagic bullae and serosanguineous exudation. Daily change of dressings is required for several days. Once an eschar has formed, there is no further need for dressings. The treated site can be washed and cleaned. I have never had occasion to employ antibiotics. Cancers of the skin situated on the scalp, forehead, or temples, or near the upper bridge of the nose, when subjected to freezing, will always produce periorbital edema for a day or so. The patient should always be warned of this sequel and perhaps seen the following day after cryosurgery to allay possible concern. Within 4 weeks the eschar is shed and healing is almost complete. Large multicentric carcino-

mas of the chest, back, or lower extremities take twice as long if not longer to heal.

The overall end-results following cryosurgery of skin cancers are quite satisfactory. The wound healing is superior to that of other existing modalities. I have never observed the formation of a keloid, even with patients with this diathesis. Hypertrophic scars are extremely rare except in the midchest and the vermillion border of the lips. Should this develop, intralesional injection of triamcinolone very often corrects this defect. The occasional leukoderma and hyperpigmentation will correct itself over a year or so.

A more accurate measurement of freeze depth is by means of a template or acrylic jig. This small triangular plastic template will allow accurate measurement from 3 to 5 mm below the cutaneous surface when the thermocouple needle is passed through it (Fig. 26-9). The tumor is frozen until the pyrometer records the exact temperature at −25 or −30 C at the specified depth (Fig. 26-10). The cancer is allowed to thaw completely and is refrozen. Some 5 weeks following cryosurgery, the neoplasm is clinically eradicated (Fig. 26-11).

The nose is one of the most common sites for the development of cancer of the face. The patient shown in Fig. 26-12 had an extensive basal cell carcinoma. This was subjected to a double freeze–thaw cryosurgical procedure

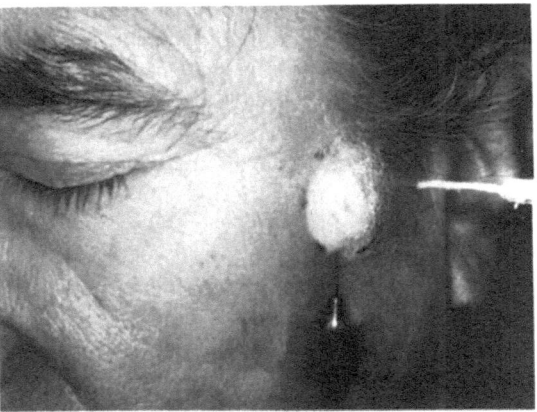

Figure 26-8. The carcinoma in Fig. 26-7 is subjected to an intermittent spray of liquid nitrogen until the desired temperature of −25 to −30 C is achieved below the neoplasm and the marginal spread of freezing has extended beyond the tumor margin as delineated. From Zacarian [24]. Courtesy of Charles C Thomas.

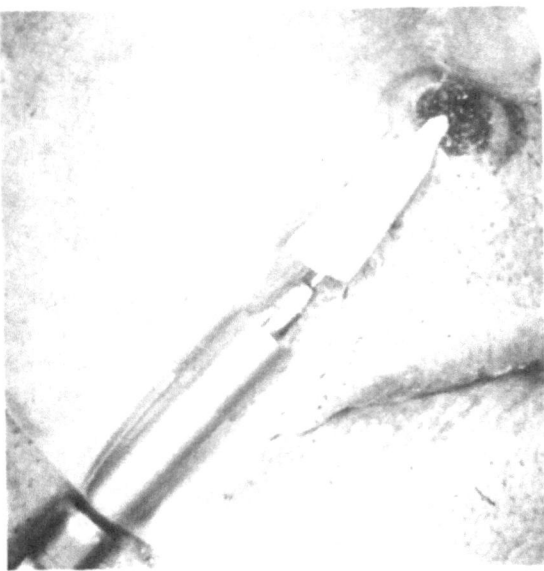

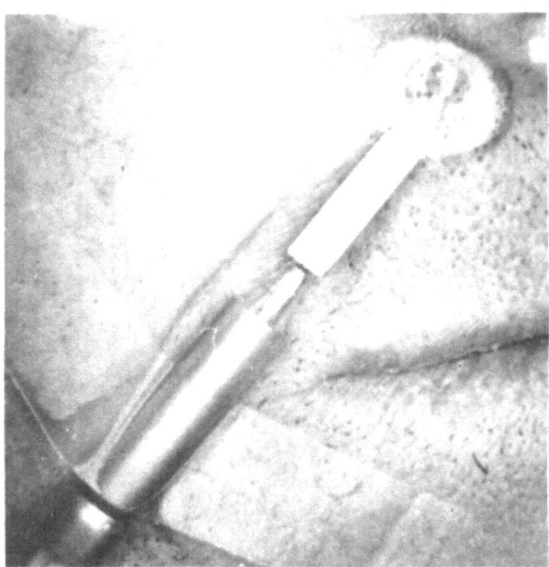

Figure 26-9. Placement of the microthermocouple needle through the 4-mm tract of the template, prior to cryosurgery of a basal cell carcinoma of the right nasolabial fold. (The template is manufactured by Frigitronics, Inc, Shelton, Conn.)

Figure 26-10. After 2 min of initial freeze of the cancer, the ice front has extended to a safe margin beyond the tumor edge and the registered temperature at 4-mm depth below the surface is −30 C. From Zacarian [25]. Courtesy of Charles C Thomas.

with liquid nitrogen spray. Four weeks following cryosurgery, the neoplasm was completely eradicated (Fig. 26-13). No recurrence was noted in 5.5 years. In 13 years of cryosurgery of skin cancers, I have found at least one-third to involve the nose and ears. The underlying cartilage tolerates freezing extremely well. I have never encountered any degree of cryonecrosis of cartilage wherein adequate repair did not follow. There have been occasions where I have frozen through the entire ear with final healing and absence of chondronecrosis or perforation. The nose and ear are critical areas, where irradiation therapy for malignancy is contraindicated and cryosurgery ideally serves as the physical modality of choice.

Early epidermoid carcinomas of the lip with no clincal evidence of metastasis to regional glands respond favorably and effectively to cryosurgery (Fig. 26-14–26-16).

Approximately 5 to 7% of skin cancers develop upon the eyelids, particularly the lower lids. Neoplasms in this location offer a challenge to all cancer therapists. To date, I have treated 100 patients with cancer of the lids with 8 recurrences [25]. There has been considerable interest by ophthalmologists in the treatment of eyelid cancer with cryosurgery, partic-

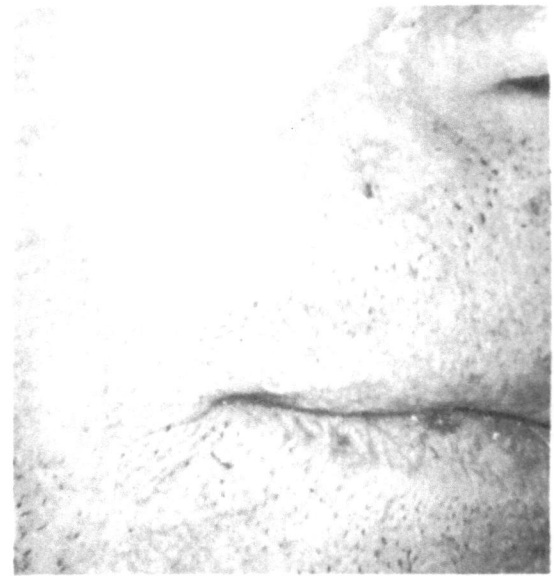

Figure 26-11. Five weeks following cryosurgery, the cancer is clinically eradicated with some hyperpigmentation at the site which will soon disappear. From Zacarian [25]. Courtesy of Charles C Thomas.

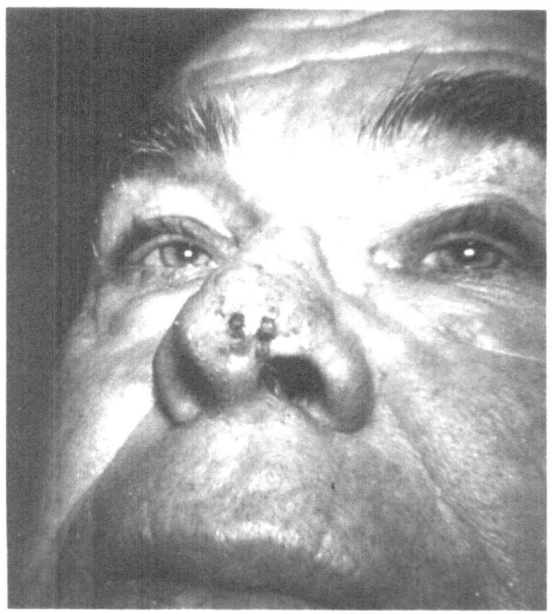

Figure 26-12. Basal cell carcinoma of the lobule of the nose prior to treatment.

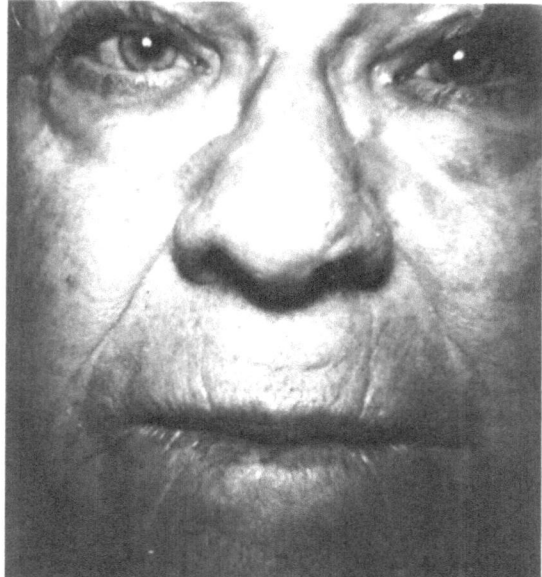

Figure 26-13. Five weeks following cryosurgery, there is no evidence of the carcinoma or recurrence for 5.5 years. From Zacarian [24]. Courtesy of Charles C Thomas.

ularly by Beard [2] and Fraunfelder [7,8]. The recurrence rate tends to be higher in this location regardless of the therapeutic modality, short of Mohs's chemosurgery. Cryosurgery is no exception. I have found no permanent damage to the lacrimal duct in those lesions where freezing was applied to the inner canthus. The tarsal plate, as with cartilage, appears to tolerate cryosurgery quite well [25]. Once the tumor has invaded the bulbar conjunctiva, cryosurgery is contraindicated and a more definitive

plastic and reconstructive surgery must be considered. The patient in Fig. 26-17a (p. 279) presents an ulcerated basal cell carcinoma of the medial canthus including the left paranasal area as well as the upper lid. Placement of the Jegher plastic retractor affords protection from liquid nitrogen spray to the globe. The tumor is frozen (Figs. 26-17b and c on p. 279). Four weeks following cryosurgery, there is no clinical evidence of the epithelioma (Fig. 26-17d on p. 279).

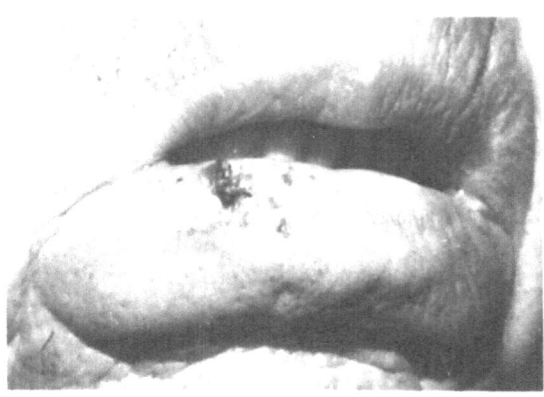

Figure 26-14. Epidermoid carcinomas of the lower lip prior to treatment. From Zacarian [25]. Courtesy of Charles C Thomas.

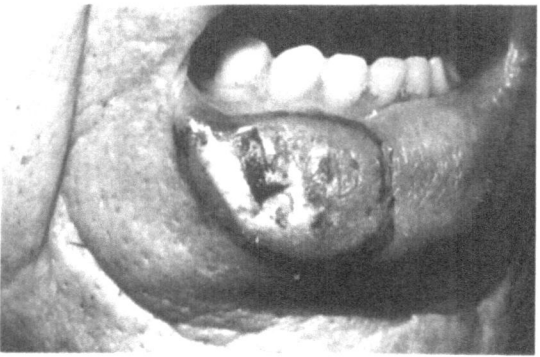

Figure 26-15. During the initial thaw following the primary freeze. This tumor was frozen for 90 sec and followed with a second freeze. From Zacarian [25]. Courtesy of Charles C Thomas.

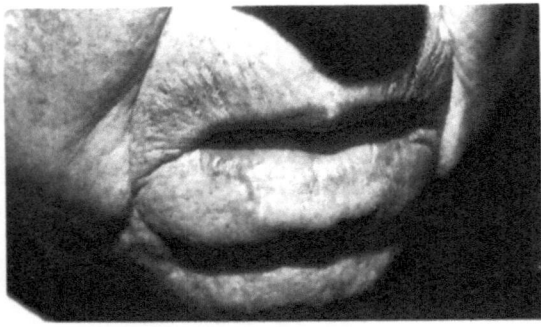

Figure 26-16. Five weeks following cryosurgery, total elimination of the carcinoma with no residual and no recurrence for over 2 years. From Zacarian [25]. Courtesy of Charles C Thomas.

Reflections Following Thirteen Years of Cryosurgery

1. For benign and precancerous disorders of the skin, liquid nitrogen spray is an ideal modality.

2. Cryosurgery for most primary skin cancers is both effective and curative.

3. Cryosurgery can be employed for recurrent cancer from previous surgery or irradiation with no fear of unsatisfactory wound healing.

4. A double freeze–thaw cycle is a necessity for all cancers. [19] Monitoring the desired temperature below the tumor will enhance the cure rate, with particular use of the template at 4- or 5-mm depth for accurate in-depth measurement of freezing.

5. Carcinomas of the scalp carry a high recurrence rate with all modalities, including freezing. Tumors in these locations can best be managed with wide and deep surgical excision.

6. Large, bulky tumors cannot be adequately treated with freezing unless most of the mass is initially dissected away with a bipolar cutting current, followed by freezing at the base of the cancer.

7. Cryosurgery as a palliative measure has an *important* place in cancer management.

8. Cryosurgery is preeminently effective for skin cancers overlying cartilage, as with the nose and ears. Cancers situated at the ala nasi must be frozen deep and wide, since recurrences in this area are more common than in any other location of the nose.

9. Large multicentric carcinomas of the skin of the chest and back can be frozen without monitoring, as these lesions are superficial. Wide margins of normal skin outside the visible tumor should be frozen. If a tumor is very large, ie, 10 or 15 cm, one can freeze one-half initially and freeze the other half 2 months later.

10. Multiple lesions can be subjected to cryosurgery at a single office visit.

11. Morphealike basal cell carcinomas or the sclerosing type are not amenable to cryosurgery.

12. Cryosurgery is a useful and effective modality for cancers of the eyelids and particularly of the medial canthus.

Statistical Data

In the past 12 years, this author has cryosurgically treated 1801 patients with a combined total of 2713 malignant tumors of the skin [25]. The histologic classification of these tumors is as follows: 2441, basal cell carcinoma; 148, epidermoid carcinomas; 73, basosquamous cell carcinoma; 40, Bowen's disease (carcinoma in situ); 3, Kaposi hemorrhagic sarcoma; and 8, lentigo maligna. During this entire period of careful follow-up there have been 56 recurrences, representing a failure rate of 3.4%. Two-thirds of these recurrences were noted in patients treated with the application of liquid nitrogen–chilled copper disks between 1964 and 1966, a technique long abandoned. The direct spray of liquid nitrogen as outlined in this chapter for the management of skin cancer has been most rewarding and effective. Complications from this modality include edema and blister formation: Hypertrophic scars, respond to intralesional triamcinolone. Hyperpigmentation and hypopigmentation will improve or disappear in due time. Neuritis and neuropathy following cryosurgery are also reversible with time. For extensive cryosurgery for acne, one should be cautious that the patient does not have underlying collagen disease and, in particular, cryoglobulinemia or cryofibrinogenemia.

Cryosurgery offers the clinician an excellent modality for the management of both benign and malignant tumors of the skin with superior wound healing and absence of keloid scars (see Figures 26-18a and b on p. 279.)

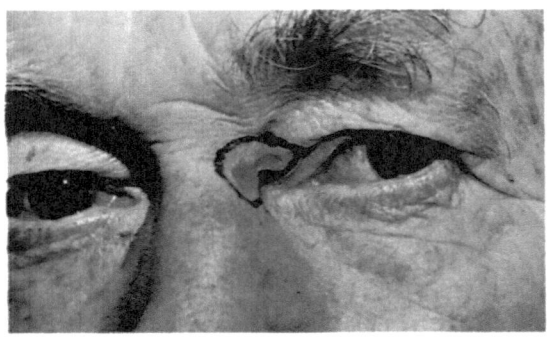
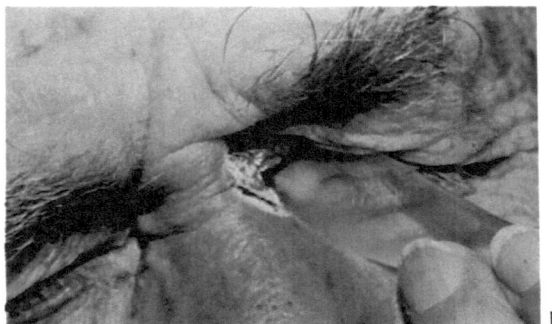
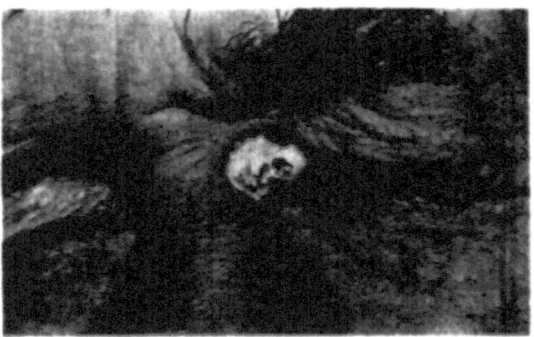
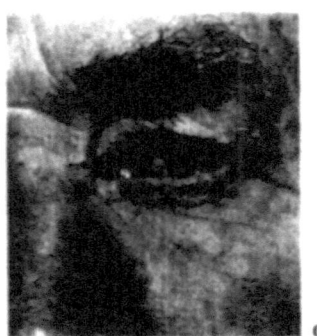

Figure 26-17. *a*. Basal cell carcinoma of left medial canthus of the lower lid extending to upper lid and left paranasal area. *b*. After a drop of 1% Pontocaine is instilled in the eye, a Jegher plastic retractor is placed in the eye to avoid liquid nitrogen spray to the globe. (Plastic retractor obtained from Storz Instruments, St. Louis, Mo.) The tumor is vigorously treated with 90 sec of intermittent spray of liquid nitrogen. *c*. The cryosurgical site after a single freeze. Note the freezing has been extended to outside the visible margin of the tumor. Following a complete thaw, a second freeze was initiated. I have recently subjected eyelid tumors to a triple freeze–thaw cycle. *d*. Six weeks following cryosurgery, there is complete elimination of the carcinoma without obstruction of the lacrimal apparatus or notching of the lid. From Zacarian [25]. Courtesy of Charles C Thomas.

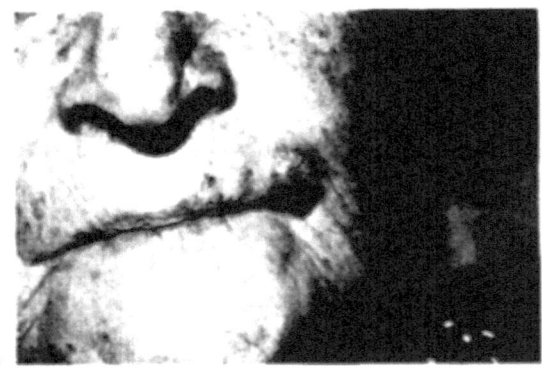
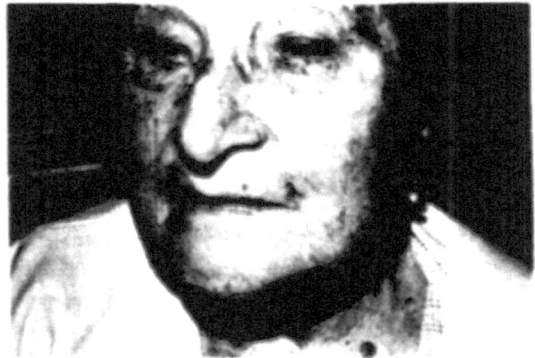

Figure 26-18. Biopsy proven basal cell cell carcinoma of the upper lip. *a*. Prior to cryosurgery. *b*. Same patient, 5 weeks post cryosurgery of BCC. A slight erythema of the site which six months follow-up has disappeared.

References

1. Allington HV: Liquid nitrogen in the treatment of skin disorders. Calif Med 72:153, 1960
2. Beard C, Sullivan JH: Cryosurgery of eyelid disorders including malignant tumors. In Zacarian SA (ed): Cryosurgical Advances in Dermatology and Tumors of the Head and Neck, Springfield, Ill, Thomas, 1977
3. Brodthagen H: Local freezing of the skin by carbon dioxide snow. Acta Derm Venereol (Stockh) 41 (Suppl 44):9, 1961
4. Cahan WG: Cryosurgery of malignant and benign tumors. Fed Proc 24:S241, 1965
5. Cooper IS: Cryogenic surgery of basal ganglia. JAMA 181:600, 1962
6. Cooper IS, Grossman F, Gorek E: Cryogenic congelation and necrosis of cancer. J Am Geriatr Soc 10:2899, 1962
7. Fraunfelder FT, et al: The future of cryosurgery for periocular and ocular lesions. J Dermatol Surg, 3:422 1977
8. Fraunfelder FT, Wallace TR, Farris HE, et al: The role of cryosurgery in external ocular and periocular disease. Trans Am Acad Ophthalmol Otolaryngol in press 1978
9. Gage AA, Emmings F: Treatment of human tumors by freezing. Cryobiology 2:24, 1965
10. Graham GF: Cryotherapy against acne vulgaris yields "good to excellent results." Dermatol Practice 5(3):2, 1972
11. Grimmett RH: Liquid nitrogen therapy. Histological observations. Arch Dermatol 83:563, 1961
12. Hall AF: Advantages and limitations of liquid nitrogen therapy of skin lesions. Arch Dermatol 83:562, 1961
13. Kreyberg L: Stasis and necrosis. Scand J Clin Lab Invest 15(Suppl 71):1, 1963
14. Kreyberg L: Local freezing. Proc R Soc Lond [Biol] 147:546, 1957
15. Mazur P: Causes of injury in frozen and thawed cells. Fed Proc 24:S175, 1965
16. Meryman HT: The interpretation of freezing rates in biological materials. Cryobiology 2:165, 1966
17. Meryman HT: Mechanics of freezing in living cells and tissues. Science 124:124, 1956
18. Rinfret AP: Thermal history. Cryobiology 2(4):171, 1966
19. Stone D, Zacarian SA, DiPeri C: Comparative studies of mammalian normal and cancer cells subjected to cryogenic temperatures in vitro. J Cryosurg 2(1):43, 1969
20. Torre D: Cryosurgery of premalignant and malignant skin lesions. Cutis 8:123, 1961
21. Torre D: Cryosurgery in dermatology. In von Leden H, Cahan G (eds): Cryogenics in Surgery. Flushing, Medical Examination Publishing, 1971, pp 500–529
22. White AC: Possibilities of liquid air to the physician. JAMA 36:426, 1901
23. Whitehouse HH: Liquid air in dermatology, its indications and limitations. JAMA 49:371, 1907
24. Zacarian SA: Cryosurgery of Tumors of the Skin and Oral Cavity. Springfield, Ill, Thomas, 1973, Chap 1
25. Zacarian SA: Cryosurgical Advances in Dermatology and Tumors of the Head and Neck. Springfield, Ill, Thomas, 1977
26. Zacarian SA: Histopathology of skin cancer following cryosurgery. Int Surg 54:255, 1970
27. Zacarian SA, Adham MI: Cryogenic temperature studies of human skin temperature recordings at 2 mm human skin depth following application with liquid nitrogen. J Invest Dermatol 48:7, 1967
28. Zacarian SA, Stone D, Clater M: Effects of cryogenic temperatures on the microcirculation in the golden hamster cheek pouch. Cryobiology 7:27, 1970

Index